THE ENCYCLOPEDIA OF

POISONS AND ANTIDOTES

Third Edition

THE ENCYCLOPEDIA OF

POISONS AND ANTIDOTES

Third Edition

Carol Turkington
and
Deborah Mitchell

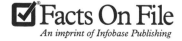
Facts On File
An imprint of Infobase Publishing

The Encyclopedia of Poisons and Antidotes, Third Edition

Facts On File
An imprint of Infobase Publishing
132 West 31st Street
New York NY 10001

Library of Congress Cataloging-in-Publication Data

Turkington, Carol.
The encyclopedia of poisons and antidotes / Carol Turkington with Deborah Mitchell ; foreword by Shirley K. Osterhout. — 3rd ed.
p. ; cm. — (Facts on File library of health and living)
Rev. ed. of: The poisons and antidotes sourcebook. 2nd ed. c1999.
Includes bibliographical references and index.
ISBN-13: 978-0-8160-6401-4 (hardcover : alk. paper)
ISBN-10: 0-8160-6401-6 (hardcover : alk. paper)
1. Toxicological emergencies—Handbooks, manuals, etc. 2. Poisoning—Handbooks, manuals, etc.
I. Mitchell, Deborah R. II. Turkington, Carol. Poisons and antidotes sourcebook. III. Title. IV. Series:
Facts on File library of health and living.
[DNLM: 1. Poisons—Encyclopedias—English. 2. Antidotes—Encyclopedias—English. QV 13 T939e 2010]
RA1224.5.T873 2010
615.9'08—dc22   2008050407

CONTENTS

ACKNOWLEDGMENTS

The author would like to thank the librarians at the National Library of Medicine and the medical libraries of Hershey Medical Center, the University of Pennsylvania Medical Center and Reading Medical Center, the staffers at the National Institutes of Health and the countless people from national organizations, services, and government agencies around the country concerned with toxicology and poisons. A special thank you to Heather Albright and Catie Fisher for valuable Internet research assistance.

INTRODUCTION

"Everything is poison, there is poison in everything. Only the dose makes a thing not a poison." This quote, attributed to Paracelsus, the Swiss physician and alchemist born in 1493 who has been called the father of toxicology, still rings true. It seems barely a day passes that we are not made aware of a new toxic substance that threatens our children or are informed by the media about the dangers of toxins found in our food, air, and water. Poisons and toxic substances are commonplace in everyday modern life.

Yet poisons and other toxic substances have been a subject of fascination since ancient times. Archaeologists have found evidence that primitive humans used poisons with their hunting weapons to hasten the death of their prey. Humankind's great interest in poisons eventually extended to ways they could be used against their own kind, and this use bred a great deal of fear, especially among people in positions of power who were afraid that poisons would be used against them. One such individual was Mithridates VI, a king of Pontus in ancient northern Turkey about 114 B.C. He was so paranoid about being poisoned that he dedicated much of his life to finding antidotes to known toxic substances of his time. He left behind a wealth of notes about poisons and antidotes, including the 54 ingredients of an antidote he had concocted to ward off any attempts by his enemies to poison him.

Leap ahead several millennia to the 21st century where people are exposed to literally tens of thousands of poisonous and toxic substances, with new ones being introduced all the time. Being poisoned today is often accidental and happens frequently in children, in whom poisoning is the fourth most common cause of death. Most accidental poisonings can be prevented simply by keeping harmful substances out of the reach of children. Other cases of poisoning can be avoided with a healthful dose of knowledge and common sense, such as knowing which household chemicals should not be mixed, keeping certain plants away from pets, always wearing protective clothing when using pesticides or certain paint materials, and being aware of toxins in the home and other environments that can cause insidious effects. Although antidotes are more available today than in the past and scientists are always working to develop new ones, prevention will always be better than treatment.

This revised edition reflects many changes in the world of toxicology. Foremost is new research in the field that includes not only information on new toxic substances that can impact health but important, updated data on former entries. Among the many new entries are:

- bisphenol: A potentially deadly toxin that is found not only in canned foods but in the ubiquitous water bottles and baby toys, including those children chew and suck on

- flunitrazepam: Under the trade name of Rohypnol, it is commonly used as a date rape drug

- mold: It has always been around, but in recent years it has become a huge health (and legal) concern when it is found in homes, schools, and other buildings. Black mold is associated with toxicity, but what about other common molds? We take a closer look.

- polonium-210: A known poison that recently (2006) made headlines when it was used to cause the demise of Russian dissident Alexander Litvinenko. Apparently this rare radioactive element is more accessible than previously thought.

Many changes in toxicology have occurred over the past 10 years, so each of the original entries in this book has been reviewed and updated, as needed, with relevant information. This updated edition also has been partially reformatted to make it easier for readers to locate essential information. Thus the first 38 pages of the first edition, which covered critical topics such as "What To Do in a Poisoning Emergency," "How to Prevent Poisoning in Your Home," "How to Prevent Food Poisoning," and "Poisons by Symptom," have been incorporated into the A-to-Z format that makes up the rest of the book (except for the appendixes).

As before, this book is designed as a guide and reference to a wide range of poisons and antidotes. *It is not a substitute for prompt medical attention from a poison control center or an experienced physician trained in toxicology.* All cases of suspected poisoning should be reported immediately to a poison control center.

Specific entries include poisonous and toxic substances and their antidotes. All commonly encountered poisonous and toxic substances, plants, and creatures have been included, together with a fair representation of more unusual varieties found throughout the world.

To make information more accessible, entries relating to poisonous and toxic substances have been subdivided by category into "poisonous part" (where applicable), "symptoms," and "treatment." Entries are listed by common names, with Latin names in parentheses; additional common names or nicknames are also provided for all poisonous and toxic entries. All entries are extensively cross-referenced.

Information in this book comes from the most up-to-date sources available and includes some of the most recent research in the field of toxicology, but readers should keep in mind that changes are occurring all the time. Although this book can serve as a comprehensive, concise, and convenient source of critical information, its format and space limitations do not allow it to address all the needs of its readers. Thus the appendixes, which have been updated extensively for this edition, provide the latest relevant information on home testing kits, hotlines, newsletters, organizations, poison control centers, sources of educational materials, and more—all for parents, teachers, health professionals, and all other curious readers who want to keep their finger on the pulse of change in the extremely complex field of toxicology.

ENTRIES A TO Z

AAPCC Toxic Exposure Surveillance System (TESS) A method of collecting poison data from the American Association of Poison Control Centers (AAPCC). This system, formerly known as the National Data Collection System, has grown steadily since its inception in 1983. TESS is the only comprehensive poisoning surveillance database in the United States and serves as a valuable resource for product safety managers, medical directors, and regulatory affairs directors.

TESS contains detailed toxicological information on all human poison exposures reported to U.S. poison centers. The database is updated daily, with approximately 6,500 new cases added each day, or more than 2.3 million per year. Approximately 44 percent of cases are followed up to determine the course and outcome of the exposure.

acetaminophen This widely used painkiller is also known as paracetamol or by its chemical name, N-acetyl-p-aminophenol (APAP). Acetaminophen is sold under the trade names Tylenol, Tempra, or Panadol and generally is not poisonous unless ingested in large amounts—usually accidentally by children, as a means to commit suicide, or inadvertently when combined with various cough and cold medications, many of which also contain acetaminophen. Some of those medications include hydrocodone with acetaminophen (Lortab, Vicodin), tramadol with acetaminophen (Ultracet), propoxyphene (Darvocet), oxycodone (Percocet), pamabrom, pyrilamine (Midol, Pamprin), and Tylenol with codeine.

Although researchers are still unsure about the key to APAP's painkilling action, it is known that the drug can damage the kidney and liver when taken in excessive amounts. Research suggests that combined with even small amounts of alcohol, APAP can cause liver toxicity.

Symptoms
If a toxic dose has been taken, symptoms will appear within 24 to 36 hours and include nausea, vomiting, abdominal pain, lethargy, and jaundice at 48 hours or later. The minimum toxic dose in adults in a single ingestion is 7.5–10 grams; in children younger than 12 years it is 150 milligrams/kilograms. Chronic toxicity among alcoholics has been reported after daily ingestion of high doses (5–6 grams).

Treatment
Empty the stomach as soon as possible by lavage or with syrup of ipecac. Specific treatment is determined by a blood level of the drug after four hours. The specific antidote is N-acetylcysteine (NAC), which, for maximum liver protection, should be given within eight to 10 hours of ingesting acetaminophen. NAC is given in 17 doses in a hospital. Provide general supportive care for kidney or liver failure; liver transplant may be necessary.

acetylcysteine Antidote for acetaminophen overdose and possibly for carbon tetrachloride and chloroform poisoning. Acetylcysteine often causes nausea and vomiting when given by mouth. In rare cases, generalized urticaria has been observed in patients receiving oral acetylcysteine. If this occurs or other allergic symptoms appear, acetylcysteine treatment should be stopped. If the drug is vomited, it should be given again. Rapid intravenous administration can cause a drop in blood pressure, and at least one death has been reported when a child received a rapid intravenous dose.

See also ACETAMINOPHEN.

acids   Acids are chemical substances that have a sour taste, are soluble in water, and turn litmus paper red. They produce pain and corrosion to all tissues with which they come in contact. Problems in swallowing, nausea, intense thirst, shock, breathing problems, and death can result from ingesting acids.

Acid poisonings should be treated like any other poisoning emergency: Give the person fluids to drink and call the poison control center for specific instructions. DO NOT INDUCE VOMITING.

Acids are identified by their pH value, which ranges from 0 to 14; acidic substances are listed from strongest (0) to weakest (6). Neutral pH is 7; 8 through 14 are alkaline (base).

Many of the foods we eat and drink are slightly acid or base, as are our body's fluids. One of the most common acids is vitamin C (ascorbic acid). Others include

- sulfuric acid: found in automobile batteries, metal cleaners, and polishes
- hydrochloric acid: metal cleaners and polishes
- nitric acid: cleaning solutions
- oxalic acid: cleaning solutions, furniture and floor polishes, waxes, and bleach
- phosphoric acid: metal cleaners and polishes
- carbolic acid or phenol: antiseptics, disinfectants, preservatives

See also DIMETHYL SULFATE; PHENOL.

aconite   See MONKSHOOD.

aconitine   The chief active ingredient in the dried, powdered root of monkshood (aconite). Aconitine is an unstable alkaloid used in some liniments.

Symptoms
This central nervous system stimulant causes a burning sensation of the mouth, tongue, lips, and throat nearly immediately after ingestion. Other symptoms include nausea, vomiting, diarrhea, restlessness, vertigo, slow breathing, low body temperature, and convulsions. As little as two to five milligrams (approximately one teaspoonful of the root) may cause death from paralysis of the cardiac muscle or respiratory system.

Treatment
Symptomatic. There are separate reports that amiodarone and magnesium sulphate may be effective in suppressing ventricular tachyarrhythmia (fast rhythm in the heart's lower chambers) caused by aconitine toxicity.

See also MONKSHOOD.

acrylamide [Other names: acrylamide monomer, acrylic amide, propenamide.]   This flaky crystal is a rather strong toxin used to make polyacrylamide, a nontoxic substance used to clear and treat drinking water, to strengthen paper and for other industrial uses. It melts at fairly low heat and dissolves easily in water; it can be swallowed, inhaled, or absorbed through the skin.

Symptoms
This neurotoxin affects the skin, eyes, and nervous system and can cause severe (sometimes permanent) brain damage. Symptoms, which may not appear immediately, include peeling, reddened skin on the hands and feet, a numbness in the feet and legs, and sweaty palms and feet. When poisoned with acrylamide, the patient may appear to be drunk, with an awkward, stumbling gait and muted reflexes.

Treatment
If there is no vomiting, administer a slurry of activated charcoal followed by gastric lavage with saline cathartics. Daily doses of vitamins B_1 and B_{12} over 45 days may protect the central nervous system. Pilocarpine may cause a temporary improvement in motor activity in some patients, and aspirin or phenylbutazone may be given to ease muscle pain.

Actifed   See DECONGESTANTS.

adder   Any of several poisonous snakes of the viper family (Viperidae), plus the death adder, a viperlike member of the cobra family. (The name may also be used for the harmless hognose snake.) Adders in the viper family include the common adder, the puff adder, and the night adder. No adders are found in the United States.

Although they are related to cobras, adders look more like vipers—thick bodies, short tails, and broad heads. They range from 18 to 35 inches long, with gray or brown skins and dark crosswise bands.

Symptoms

The symptoms caused by the bite of an adder depend in large part on which species makes the bite. Some people experience nothing more than pain and minor swelling at the bite site; others are plagued with chills, fever, falling blood pressure, convulsions, and bleeding from the gums, eyes, and nose. To see symptoms that are specific for different species of adders, see the entries below.

Treatment

Some adder bite victims do not require treatment; others will die of cardiorespiratory failure unless they receive the antivenin. With proper treatment, drowsiness and nausea are the worst adverse effects, followed by severe bruising and swelling at the bite site. For the most effective treatment for adder bites, see the individual entries below.

See also ADDER, COMMON; ADDER, PUFF; ADDER, NIGHT.

adder, common *(Vipera berus)* This adder is a member of the viper family (also called the European viper) and is the snake that has most commonly made its way into literature. It is found throughout Europe and Asia, ranging north of the Arctic Circle in Norway, where it survives by hibernating through a very long winter. As is typical of the more northerly adders, the common adder is darker than some of its southern cousins; it is usually gray with a black zigzag band on the back, with black spots on the side, and its maximum length is about 30 inches. Its bite is rarely fatal.

This snake is the only venomous snake in the British Isles, where it is regarded with loathing and fear, although responsible for very few fatalities.

Each spring, mating takes place, and ritual fights occur between two males, who twist the front part of their bodies in a vertical column, each trying to push the other over. It is this typical mating behavior that inspired the two entwined snakes on the staff of Hermes the Messenger. This symbol is often confused with the staff of Aesculapius, the Roman god of medicine, which also features a serpent (the Aesculapian snake, a nonpoisonous variety).

Symptoms

An immediate sharp pain is followed usually within minutes by tingling and local swelling that spreads. Within hours patients experience tenderness, inflammation, spreading pain, enlarged lymph nodes, and bruising. The entire limb may become swollen and bruised within 24 hours, and in children it can affect the whole body. Some people react to a bite with severe anaphylactic symptoms within five minutes or up to several hours. Hypotension is a very critical sign; symptoms may include nausea, vomiting, diarrhea, urinary and fecal incontinence, tachycardia, sweating, lightheadedness, shock, hives, bronchospasm, and edema of the face, lips, throat, tongue, and gums. Bleeding from the nose and gums into the lungs, stomach, genitourinary tracts, and other areas may occur. Other serious complications include coma, seizures, acute renal failure, and acute pancreatitis.

Treatment

Only a minority of people receive enough venom to cause serious complications. Antivenin is available and should be given in a hospital setting in case the patient has a negative response to the antidote.

adder, death *(Acanthophis antarcticus)* This highly poisonous snake resembles and behaves like a viper, although it belongs to the cobra family and lives in an area where no vipers are found. It can be found in Australia and New Guinea, has a thick body and a broad, flat, triangular head and is colored gray or brown with dark crossbands. A bite from the death adder is fatal about half of the time without treatment. Its close relative is the desert death adder *(Acanthophis pyrrhus),* which also has a 50 percent mortality rate.

Symptoms

A bite from a death adder causes paralysis which can be minor initially but results in death from complete respiratory failure within six hours if not treated. Symptoms typically appear within 15 to 60 minutes and include nausea, vomiting, faintness, drowsiness, staggering, slurred speech, hemorrhage, and death in about half of untreated cases.

Treatment

Antivenin is available, but the specific antiserum must be given and patients should be tested for sensitivity prior to treatment. The antidote is CSL death adder antivenin, but it should be given only if there is clear evidence that the person was poisoned and has been tested for sensitivity. If an antivenin is unavailable, anticholinesterases may be administered.

See also COBRA; SNAKES, POISONOUS.

adder, European   See ADDER, COMMON.

adder, night *(Causus)*   A member of the viper family and native to Africa, the night adder is a small, thin snake found south of the Sahara. Gray with dark blotches, these snakes grow up to a meter long and have small fangs and weak venom that causes pain and swelling. There are no recorded human fatalities.

Nocturnally active, this snake spends the day in its termite mound or hiding under rocks; it is generally slow moving but becomes alert and aggressive when attacked, inflating its body, flattening its neck, and huffing and hissing.

Symptoms

The bite of a night adder is extremely painful and causes inflammation and occasionally local necrosis.

Treatment

Antivenin is available and effective against the venom, although it generally is not required since the venom has relatively low toxicity. However, it is always best to treat any bite from a venomous snake.

See also ANTIVENIN; SNAKES, POISONOUS.

adder, puff *(Bitis)*   There are several poisonous species of puff adder. All members of the viper family, they are found in semiarid savanna and areas of rural human habitation in Africa and Arabia. This is a sluggish snake that tends to lie still rather than flee when approached, but it can strike with amazing speed when aroused and is responsible for numerous snakebites every year. It gets its name from the warning it gives by inflating its body and hissing loudly before striking. This extremely poisonous snake grows from three to five feet long and is gray to brown with thin yellow chevrons on its back.

Symptoms

Seriousness of symptoms depends on the amount of venom, if any, injected by the snake. A bite typically causes extreme pain and tenderness and some necrosis. Serious bites cause the limbs to become immovably flexed due to hemorrhaging, which typically resolves. Other symptoms may include watery blood oozing from the wound, nausea, vomiting, blood blisters, hypotension, weakness, dizziness, and painful swelling of the lymph nodes. If not treated properly, necrosis can spread and eventually cause gangrene and loss of limbs or digits. Although a puff adder bite is serious, less than 10 percent of untreated individuals die of a bite.

Treatment

Antivenin is available. Death can be avoided if adequate antivenin is administered.

See also ADDER; ADDER, COMMON; ANTIVENIN; SNAKES, POISONOUS.

Advil **(ibuprofen)** See ANTI-INFLAMMATORY DRUGS.

aflatoxins A cancer-causing by-product of the *Aspergillus flavus* mold found in peanuts, corn, wheat, rice, cottonseeds, barley, soybeans, Brazil nuts, and pistachios. The molds that produce aflatoxin grow in warm, humid climates in the southeastern United States; the mold can also be produced in the field when rain falls on crops, such as corn and wheat, that are left in the field to dry. Aflatoxin-producing mold can even grow on plants damaged by insects, drought, poor nutrition, or unseasonable temperatures.

Aflatoxin has been called the most potent natural carcinogen known to humans; rat studies suggest males are more susceptible to cancer following aflatoxin exposure. Poor diet also seems to predispose animals to cancer in the wake of aflatoxin ingestion.

Still, scientists know very little about why or how the aflatoxins are produced by the mold, and because it is sometimes difficult to see, all susceptible crops are subject to routine testing in the United States. Unfortunately, it is not possible to detect the mold with 100 percent accuracy.

Although the way agricultural products are stored can affect the mold's growth, the length of time of such storage is also important; the longer agricultural products are stored in bins, the greater the chance that environmental conditions favorable to aflatoxin production will be created. Stored nuts or seeds might accidentally get wet, or the storage bin might not facilitate drying quickly enough to stop the mold from growing.

Aflatoxins are more common in poor-quality cereals and nuts; while most of these low-grade products do not enter the human food market, they are sold as animal feed, which can go on to contaminate animal products (such as meat and milk). For this reason, cottonseed meal (a product often contaminated with high levels of aflatoxin) is banned for use as an animal feed. Cottonseed oil, however, rarely contains aflatoxin, since the toxin sticks to the hulls of the seed.

Milk is commonly contaminated with aflatoxin, and powdered nonfat milk can contain eight times more than the original liquid product, since the aflatoxin adheres to the milk's proteins. In addition, measurable levels of aflatoxin can be found in some baby foods that use dry milk to boost the protein content of the product.

Pasteurization, sterilization and spray-dry processing techniques can substantially reduce aflatoxin contamination of dried milk. Meat products are less often contaminated because little aflatoxin is carried over into the meat, except for pig liver and kidneys. Chicken can also become contaminated with aflatoxin when the bird appears to be only mildly sick.

In humans, aflatoxin is believed to cause liver cancer, according to some east African studies that seem to show a correlation between the two. Epidemiological evidence also suggests men are more susceptible than women, and many scientists believe a poor diet and liver disease also increase susceptibility to liver cancer as a result of aflatoxin exposure. Data from the African studies were strong enough to prompt the Food and Drug Administration and the Environmental Protection Agency to develop strict regulations to control levels in food and animal food sold in the United States.

Aflatoxin can also cause aflatoxicosis, a condition that affects both humans and animals who have ingested aflatoxin-contamined food or feed. Aflatoxicosis is characterized by abdominal pain, vomiting, pulmonary edema, convulsions, coma, liver damage, and death. This condition usually only occurs in developing countries, and there have not been any cases of aflatoxicosis reported in humans in the United States.

Consumers are urged not to eat moldy food, especially grains or peanuts, and are urged to be cautious about eating unroasted peanuts sold in bulk.

African milk plant *(Euphorbia)* There are several species of this poisonous African plant family, including *E. candelabrum, E. grantii, E. neglecta, E. giomgiecpstata, E. systyloides,* and *E. tirucalli,* as well as the non-toxic poinsettia. The plants, which are reportedly used by African women to eliminate troublesome husbands, are found throughout the continent. While some of the plants are used for medicinal purposes, they are also used as arrow poisons (especially the varieties *E. candelabrum* and *E. neglecta*). While others (notably *E. systyloides*) are used to treat hookworms, too much of the plant can cause delirium, convulsions, and death within six hours.

Poisonous part

The latex of some species is poisonous, with the toxic part being complex terpenes.

Symptoms

Irritation of the skin on contact, which may be quite corrosive depending on the species. Ingestion may cause gastritis.

Treatment

For patients experiencing vomiting and stomach upset, provide fluids to offset dehydration.

See also POINSETTIA.

Agent Orange   See DIOXINS.

akee (Blighia sapida)   [Other names: ackee, aki, arbre, fricasse, vegetal] Named for Captain Bligh, captain of the *Bounty,* this tree produces a fruit that, if eaten unripe and unopened, can cause serious intoxication and death. The tree grows to 30 or 40 feet tall with long pairs of leaflets and small, greenish white flowers. A conspicuous red fruit pod splits at maturity, with shiny black seeds inside. Native to western Africa, akee can be found in the West Indies, Florida, and Hawaii.

Poisonous part

Although the fruit is perfectly edible when eaten ripe and fully opened, the unripe and the rancid, spoiled fruit are equally poisonous. Both the fruit capsule and its seeds are poisonous, as is the water in which the fruit is cooked.

Symptoms

Poisoning reaches epic proportions during the winter months on the island of Jamaica, where it is called "vomiting sickness," and it is often fatal. Victims typically experience one of two forms of symptoms: vomiting with a remission of eight or 10 hours followed by more vomiting, convulsions, and coma—or convulsion and coma present immediately. It may take from six hours to a day after ingestion for symptoms to appear, although death can occur within 24 hours after eating. About 85 percent of victims experience convulsions. In cases

of fatal ingestion, hemorrhages can often be found in the brain.

Treatment

Gastric lavage, fluids, treatment of symptoms and intravenous glucose to offset severe hypoglycemia (low blood sugar).

Alar (daminozide) This pesticide has been the focus of massive public attention since the 1980s in the wake of data suggesting it causes cancer and tumors and that it commonly remains as a residue on fruits (particularly apples). Assurances by growers and the Food and Drug Administration that residue levels are very low were suspect, since the toxic substance cannot be detected by the FDA's routine testing procedures for pesticide residues, although specific Alar detection methods are available.

Acceding to public pressure, the manufacturer voluntarily withdrew Alar from the market in 1990. Although Alar is no longer being sold in the United States, no restrictions were placed on the sale and use of remaining stocks.

A 1987 study by the Natural Resources Defense Council claimed that 38 percent of the U.S. apple crop was treated with Alar (especially varieties such as Red and Golden Delicious, McIntosh, Jonathan, and Stayman). Residues have not only been detected on fresh produce; the residue also appears to concentrate in various processed foods, including apple juice, peanut butter, cherry pie filling, and Concord grape juice. In 1989, the release of a new report by the NRDC pointed out that young children are at greater risk from residue than adults because they metabolize food differently.

Although often considered a pesticide, Alar is actually a plant growth regulator. It was introduced in 1967 for use on apples, peaches, pears, prunes, cherries, nectarines, and peanuts. It has also been used on cantaloupes, brussels sprouts, tomatoes, and grapes. The chemical stops fruit ripening, prevents fruit from dropping prematurely and allows the fruit to develop a deeper, more uniform color.

Several studies show that Alar causes cancer, although the data are not complete; a 1987 study by the National Academy of Sciences estimates the risk of benign or malignant tumor formation associated with exposure to Alar to be greater than the one in 1 million risk considered acceptable by the Environmental Protection Agency. There is not enough information to determine whether it causes mutations, birth defects, or other problems, although evidence suggests it is not a mutagen or a teratogen. It is of low toxicity when ingested or applied to the skin.

aldicarb   One of the most toxic pesticides in use today, aldicarb has been registered for use since 1970. A carbamate insecticide, it is effective against a variety of insects, mites, and roundworms. Because it is an acutely poisonous pesticide, it is not registered for home or garden use, although it is registered for use by certified applicators for a variety of crops (such as sweet potatoes, peanuts, potatoes, oranges, sugar beets, pecans, some seed crops, soybeans, and sugarcane).

Several mass poisoning incidents have been reported involving the illegal use of aldicarb on unapproved vegetables and fruits; although it is not approved for use on watermelons, for example, several hundred consumers were poisoned in 1985 after eating watermelon tainted with aldicarb residue. In the long term, exposure to aldicarb has been linked with colon cancer. The Agricultural Health Study results published in 2007 in the *International Journal of Cancer* found a 4.1-fold increased risk of colon cancer associated with exposure to aldicarb among pesticide applicators.

Aldicarb leaches from the soil and has been found in groundwater in New York, Florida, Wisconsin, Connecticut, Maine, Virginia, Maryland, and New Jersey. The problem is especially acute in sandy, acidic soils and warm, moist climates, which help move the poison into groundwater. A 2005 study conducted in the Pacific Northwest, California, Texas, Southeast, and Mississippi Delta region analyzed samples from 1,673 drinking water wells that were within 300 meters of fields treated at least once between 2002 and 2006 with aldicarb. High-performance liquid chromatography found all residues were below the U.S. Environmental Protection Agency Health Advisory Limit of 10 micrograms per liter.

The manufacturer has specifically prohibited the use of aldicarb in areas where drinking water has been contaminated. Because it is a systemic insecticide, residues of aldicarb probably cannot be eliminated by washing produce, although heat in cooking may reduce the levels. It is also prohibited for use near habitats of endangered bird species, because aldicarb is highly toxic to birds, honeybees, freshwater fish, and invertebrates.

Symptoms
It only takes a very small dose for fatal effects in humans. While it is quickly absorbed in the gastrointestinal tract, most is excreted within two days after exposure. Tests with rabbits suggest it is also readily absorbed through the skin. Symptoms include dizziness, muscle weakness, stomach cramping, diarrhea, excessive sweating, nausea, vomiting, blurry vision, and convulsions. Although studies on long-term exposure are inconclusive, there are hints that it may affect the immune system. There is also a potential link to reproductive problems.

Treatment
Atropine is an antidote for aldicarb poisoning, as it is in all carbamate toxicities.
See also CARBAMATE.

Aldomet (methyldopa)   This is one of a group of antihypertensive drugs used to lower blood pressure. It is available as a white tablet or liquid. Aldomet's effects are strengthened if it is taken with other antihypertensives; if taken with alcohol, the sedation is deepened and blood pressure falls dangerously low. The effects of a range of other drugs are also increased if taken with Aldomet, including anticlotting drugs, lithium, or tolbutamide. Behavior problems may appear if combined with Haldol, and blood pressure will soar if combined with monoamine oxidase (MAO) inhibitors or tricyclic antidepressants.

Symptoms
Within 20 minutes to an hour after ingestion, patients taking an overdose experience drowsiness, headache, dizziness, weakness, tiredness,

skin rash, joint/muscle pain, impotence, fever, and nightmares.

Treatment

Atropine or caffeine are used to counteract the effects of excessive Aldomet. Activated charcoal and cathartic also may be used. Gastric emptying is not necessary if activated charcoal is given promptly. In unresponsive patients, dopamine or noradrenaline may be administered.

aldrin [Other names: Aldrine, compound 118, octalene]   A component of chlorinated hydrocarbon, aldrin is the most toxic substance used as an insecticide dust to control grubs and wireworms and as a spray against caterpillars. Used since the late 1940s, aldrin is a white, odorless crystalline solid that is most poisonous when eaten or inhaled, although chronic skin contact can be fatal. A relative of DDT, it stimulates the central nervous system and is toxic to warm-blooded animals. Along with other chlorinated hydrocarbons, aldrin has been banned by the Environmental Protection Agency since 1974 because of the injurious effects on those exposed to it, but European brands are still used for termite control. Experimental evidence suggests a potential carcinogenic effect.

Symptoms

Symptoms begin within one to four hours of exposure and include headaches, dizziness, nausea, vomiting, malaise, convulsions, coma, respiratory failure, and death about six hours later. If convulsions begin more than an hour after ingestion, recovery is likely.

Treatment

The body must be decontaminated, and in cases of severe poisoning, an amyl nitrate capsule is given under the nose for 15 seconds of every minute until sodium nitrite and oxygen treatments are started.

See also CHLORINATED HYDROCARBON PESTICIDES; DDT; INSECTICIDES.

alkaline corrosives   The chemical opposites of acids, alkalies can be extremely corrosive. The most dangerous poisons include sodium hydroxide, or lye (found in aquarium products, drain cleaners and small batteries); potassium hydroxide (some small batteries and cuticle remover); sodium phosphate (abrasive cleaners); and sodium carbonate (dye removers and dishwasher soap). Milder alkalies (ammonia or bleaches) generally do not irreparably burn the esophagus, and the burns usually heal without scarring. Mixing alkaline corrosives with ammonia, toilet bowl cleaners or household cleaners can release hazardous gases and is extremely dangerous.

Inquisitive toddlers in particular are vulnerable to injury from alkaline corrosives, which are often kept under the sink or in old soda bottles in many households. Each year, more than 120,000 American children under age six ingest such corrosive chemicals—mostly household products such as detergents and drain openers.

These extremely corrosive substances can eat right through skin. When ingested, they quickly burn through internal tissues, injuring the esophagus; damage can be irreparable for those who survive.

Because of the dangers of ingestion of lye in particular, federal legislation has required safety caps on containers of more than 2 percent concentrations of lye. Since then, there has been a decrease in the occurrence of these types of poisoning.

Symptoms

Alkalies cause an immediate reaction upon contact, burning whatever tissues they touch and turning the tissue to a fatty liquid. Upon ingestion, there is severe pain followed by the inability to handle secretions, respiratory problems, collapse, and sometimes death.

Treatment

Vomiting is never induced in cases of alkali ingestion, because it brings up the poison and causes more injury. Administration of an antidote in the case of alkaline corrosive poisoning is controversial, since by the time the person reaches the emergency room, it is too late for an antidote. Instead, immediate treatment at home should only be at the direction of a medical professional or poison control center. Once the alkali enters the stomach, it will usually be neutralized by gastric acids. All persons who ingest alkalies need to be seen as soon as possible in a medical facility. The major problem is constricted esophagus.

While the corticosteroid prednisone has remained the treatment of choice for the past 30 years, several studies have questioned its use. Recent studies at the Children's National Medical Center in Washington, D.C., revealed that those treated with prednisone healed as well as those who were not.

In an editorial published in the *New England Journal of Medicine* (September 6, 1991), Frederick H. Lovejoy of Children's Hospital in Boston writes: "Corrosive injury to the esophagus in children is a completely preventable disease." New studies questioning the role of prednisone "remove any false security derived from believing that an effective medical treatment exists."

If contamination is on the skin or in the eyes, wash the area with lukewarm water for 30 minutes.

In the ingestion of alkaline disk batteries, there have been reports of gastrointestinal bleeding and perforation of the esophagus; X-rays are important in these cases. If the battery gets as far as the stomach and the person reports no symptoms, no further action is required.

See also AMMONIA; BLEACH; LYE.

alkaloids A class of bitter, unpleasant-tasting nitrogen-containing compounds including more than 5,000 types, ranging from very simple to extremely complex. They are found in as many as 10 percent of plant species and in a variety of animals; the compounds can be isolated for use as a drug or poison. Chemically similar to alkalies (bases), alkaloids can have strong effects—both positive and negative—on the human nervous system, and some affect internal organs as well.

Some of the most deadly alkaloids include nicotine, taxine, gelsemine and atropine. While most alkaloids do occur in closely related plants, a few alkaloids are also produced by ladybugs, millipedes, ants, toads, and some types of poisonous frogs. Researchers at the University of Chicago have recently uncovered evidence that suggests that at least one variety of bird may also produce alkaloids; a yellow and black bird in New Guinea contains the chemical batrachotoxin, the same chemical found in some types of poisonous frogs. The fingers of anyone who handled the bird immediately became numb as a result of contact with the alkaloid. While there had been no previous evidence of birds containing a chemical defense system, no one had ever looked for such evidence, scientists report.

Symptoms

When ingested, most alkaloids produce a very strong physiological reaction, usually acting on the nervous system in ways that are still little understood.

Treatment

Potassium permanganate.

See also ATROPINE; GELSEMINE; NICOTINE; TAXINE.

amanita mushrooms Of the *Amanita* genus of about 100 mushrooms of the family Amanitaceae, between 25 and 35 are found in the United States. Some of the amanitas are extremely poisonous and include the false morel, fly agaric, panther mushroom and—most deadly of all—the destroying angel or death cap *(Amanita phalloides).* Mycologists disagree about the classification of many of the closely related amanita mushrooms, however, and other sources may differ in these classifications.

Most of the cases of mushroom poisoning in the United States can be traced to the amanitas, particularly *A. muscaria* and *A. phalloides,* which are also sometimes referred to as toadstools (from the German word for "death"). They have been known to be poisonous since ancient times.

Particularly dangerous are the snow-white to pale green or tan amanitas. The amanitas typically have white spores, a ring on the stem slightly below the cap, a veil that is torn as the cap expands and a cup from which the stalk arises.

Poisonous part

There are two types of toxic compounds in the amanitas, which cause two separate syndromes in those who consume them. In *A. phalloides,* the substance amanitine is responsible for the major symptoms;

phalloidine produces degenerative changes in the kidney, liver, and heart muscles. Cooking the deadly *Amanita* does not destroy their toxicity, and it is estimated that just one *A. phalloides* cap can kill an adult. Amanitas that feature amatoxins and phallotoxins include *A. phalloides, A. verna, A. virosa, A. bisporigera, A. ocreata, A. suballiacae,* and *A. tenuifolia.* Amanitas that contain the toxins muscimol and ibotenic acid include *A. muscaria, A. pantherina, A. gemmata, A, cokeri,* and *A. cothurnata.*

Symptoms

In *A. muscaria,* rapid poisoning occurs from a few minutes to two hours after ingestion, depending on the amount of toxin present; symptoms include salivation, sweating, cramps, diarrhea, vomiting, circulatory failure, mental disturbances, coma, and convulsions. Death is rare from *A. muscaria* poisoning. A more deadly poisoning occurs from *A. phalloides,* whose symptoms never appear before six hours after ingestion. When they do appear, they include the sudden onset of colicky abdominal pain, vomiting, and severe diarrhea that may contain blood and mucus. This type of diarrhea is so severe that it is very similar to the symptoms of cholera. Even without treatment, the victim may appear to begin recovering but two to four days after ingestion will experience liver, heart, and kidney damage, circulatory failure, convulsions, coma, and death.

Treatment

Many antidotes to *Amanita* poisoning have been reported, but most of this information has been anecdotal. Some victims of severe *Amanita* poisoning have been treated successfully with a combination of thioctic acid, glucose, and penicillin, or by filtering the blood through charcoal. Gastric lavage is indicated, if the patient has not vomited already, followed by activated charcoal and saline cathartics.

See also AMATOXINS; DESTROYING ANGEL; FLY AGARIC; MUSHROOM POISONING; MUSHROOM TOXINS; PANTHER MUSHROOM.

amatoxins A group of very toxic peptides found in a few species of poisonous mushrooms, including *Amanita phalloides, A. virosa, A. ocreata, A. verna, Galerina autumnalis, G. marginata* and a few types of *Lepiota.* Amatoxins are among the strongest toxins in the world; the lethal dose is just 0.1 milligram per kilogram, but one amanita mushroom cap may contain between 10 and 15 milligrams of toxin.

The Meixner test may detect the presence of amatoxins in mushrooms; their presence is indicated by a blue color that appears after one drop of concentrated hydrochloric acid is added to dried juice from the mushroom cap dripped onto unrefined paper. However, this test should not be used to determine whether it is safe to eat a mushroom.

See also AMANITA MUSHROOMS; MUSHROOM POISONING; MUSHROOM TOXINS.

americium In 1944, four American scientists produced a radioactive rare earth metal called americium by bombarding plutonium-239 with high-energy neutrons. The plutonium-240 changed into plutonium-241, which then decayed into americium-241, which consists mainly of man-made radioactive isotopes.

Americium can be produced in large quantities, but the element has few practical uses. Because it is radioactive it must be handled with caution. Generally, it is used in smoke detectors and medical diagnostic devices, to help make flat glass, and as a portable source of gamma rays in radiography. However, it is extremely expensive to produce in usable quantities.

Humans are typically exposed to high concentrations of americium through food, breathing, or skin contact associated with the release of the metal during nuclear production and accidents, or by working in or living near nuclear power plants. Low levels of americium may be present in water and soil because of atmospheric nuclear weapons testing prior to the nuclear test ban of 1963, as the element can remain in the atmosphere for decades and travel around the globe, settling to earth over time. Because the isotopes decay very slowly in the environment, they have the potential to damage animals that are exposed to high levels. Americium that enters the soil may end up in plants, but typically only in very small, nontoxic amounts.

Symptoms

Once americium is in the body, it can become concentrated in the bones, where it will remain for a long time and slowly decay, releasing radioactive rays and particles. The rays can alter genetic materials and cause bone cancers. Damage to organs is very unlikely, however, because americium does not remain in organs for long.

Treatment

Oral dose of a simple aqueous solution of zinc-diethylenetriaminepenta-acetic acid (DTPA) is effective in treatment of poisoning with pure americium.

ammonia This colorless, strong-smelling poison gas is formed by blowing steam through incandescent coke. Extremely toxic when inhaled in concentrated vapors, ammonia is irritating to both eyes and mucous membranes. It is one of the top five most common inorganic chemicals produced in the United States, where it is used in refrigerants, and to manufacture detergents, permanent wave lotions and hair bleaches, and cleaning agents. It is also used in the manufacture of explosives and synthetic fabrics, herbicides, fertilizers, and pesticides.

Ammonia has been shown to produce skin cancer in humans in doses of 1,000 milligrams per kilogram of body weight. It also irritates the lungs and can cause swelling of lung tissue. It may even cause explosions if mixed with silver or mercury.

Ammonium hydroxide (ammonia water) is a weak alkali formed when ammonia dissolves in water. This clear, colorless liquid contains between 10 and 35 percent ammonia and is used as an alkali in metallic hair dyes, hair straighteners, and protective skin creams; it is also used in detergents, stain removers, and ceramics.

Symptoms

Ammonia fumes can irritate the eyes and upper respiratory tract, causing vomiting, conjunctivitis and inflammation of the lips, mouth, and throat. Toxic cases of inhalations cause airway obstruction, pulmonary irritation with swelling, cyanosis, bronchitis, and pneumonia. Ammonia can damage cells directly, and skin contact can lead to dermatitis; ingestion can burn the esophagus.

Treatment

The ammonia is diluted or neutralized with water or milk, but the victim should not vomit, as the substance could burn the mouth or throat, especially in concentrations greater than 5 percent. For eye contamination, wash the eyes with running water for 15 to 20 minutes. If ammonia is inhaled, move the victim to fresh air and give artificial respiration.

amnesic shellfish poisoning (ASP) This type of shellfish poisoning was first identified in Canada in a 1987 outbreak that killed three and sickened more than 100 people, leading to significant memory loss and confusion. ASP is associated primarily with mussels. The poisoning is especially serious with older patients and may appear to resemble Alzheimer's disease. All known fatalities have occurred in elderly patients.

Symptoms

Initial symptoms appear within 24 hours, and neurological symptoms follow within 48 hours. ASP can be life threatening, causing stomach problems (vomiting, diarrhea, and abdominal pain). In severe cases, neurological problems (confusion, memory loss, disorientation, seizure, and coma) also appear.

Prevention

Eat only shellfish from reportable sources and approved beds.

amphetamines [Other names: beans, bennies, black beauties, black mollies, copilots, crank, crossroads, crystal, dexies, doublecross, hearts, meth, minibennies, pep pills, roses, speed, thrusters, truck drivers, uppers, wake-ups, whites. Trade names: Aktedron, Benzedrine, Elastonon, Orthedrine, Phenamine, Phenedrine.] This white powder (or colorless liquid) is a highly addictive stimulant, once widely prescribed as a diet pill—but this use has now been banned by the Food and Drug Administration.

Amphetamines were also used to treat Parkinson's disease and similar symptoms, depression, alcohol withdrawal, premenstrual tension, and hyperactivity. Today, they are strictly controlled and seldom administered because of serious withdrawal problems and dangerous side effects.

Usually taken in pill form, amphetamines can also be injected when in solution.

(A form of amphetamine commonly known as "speed" or "meth"—methamphetamine—is usually injected intravenously, although speed also comes in oral doses.)

Symptoms

Amphetamines can stimulate both the sympathetic and central nervous systems, and are toxic in levels only slightly above usual doses, although a degree of tolerance can develop over time. Symptoms appear within 30 minutes to an hour, and when these drugs are taken in too large a dose, the symptoms can include sleeplessness, restlessness, tremors, palpitations, nausea, vomiting, diarrhea, anorexia, delirium, hallucinations, euphoria, nervousness, confusion, irritability, short temper, depression, cyanosis, sweating, convulsions, coma, and cerebral hemorrhages. Brain damage or death may result from ventricular arrhythmia or stroke. When amphetamines are taken in only a mild overdose, symptoms include fatigue, mental depression, and high blood pressure. Those who chronically abuse amphetamines may develop heart problems and behavioral abnormalities (such as picking at the skin) and appear paranoid and anorexic. In fact, appetite suppression in long-term addicts can continue for up to two months after amphetamine use has stopped.

Treatment

Isolate the victim in a quiet, darkened room to avoid overstimulation and possible heart failure. Gastric lavage may be helpful if the person is awake, but emesis is not induced because of the risk of abrupt onset of seizures. Administer activated charcoal and a cathartic. Other symptoms are treated, and Valium may be given to slow the heartbeat.

amyl nitrite   An antispasmodic, this is an antidote of cyanide and ergot that is also used medically to dilate the coronary vessels and lower blood pressure. It has been used as a vasodilator in angina therapy for a long time and has also been used as an industrial chemical and perfume scent. The increasing abuse of amyl nitrite "poppers" led to their restriction and the increased popularity of butyl and isobutyl nitrites (related volatile compounds sold over the counter as room odorizers under such names as "Locker Room"). These are inhaled to produce highs and intensify sexual orgasms and are sometimes sprayed in discos to stimulate dancing.

Symptoms

Inhaling the volatile nitrites dilates blood vessels, causing low blood pressure lasting about 90 seconds. Other symptoms include pulsating headache, rapid flushing of the face, dizziness, confusion, vertigo, restlessness, weakness, blue skin, nausea, and vomiting. In addition, butyl nitrite sniffing has caused mild methemoglobinemia in otherwise healthy patients. Chronic abuse of amyl nitrite can cause anemia.

Treatment

Administration of methylene blue may be effective in treating methemoglobinemia. Other treatment is symptomatic.

Anaprox   See NONSTEROIDAL ANTI-INFLAMMATORY DRUGS.

anectine (succinylcholine)   This extremely fast-acting drug is also known as curare and is one of a group of neuromuscular blocking agents that affects skeletal muscles. It is used to promote muscle relaxation during surgical anesthesia and is sometimes given to control convulsions. It is generally used in the operating room during lung procedures, as it stops normal breathing and allows the patient to be placed on a respirator. Many physicians also use it before surgery as a muscle relaxant because it cuts down on the amount of anesthesia needed. It is also an antidote for strychnine poisoning and an anticonvulsant treatment for tetanus (lockjaw). An effective dose can be fatal if breathing is not maintained artificially. This bitter, white powder dissolves easily in water and can be administered either in the muscle or in the veins.

Symptoms

Almost immediately upon injection, anectine produces respiratory paralysis by blocking the neuromuscular transmissions. Symptoms will continue for one to 10 minutes after the injection is discontinued. Cardiac arrest has occurred during the administration of anectine after a head injury.

Treatment

There is no antidote—anectine works too quickly.

See also CURARE; NEUROMUSCULAR BLOCKING AGENTS.

anemone, sea One of the most abundant of the coelenterates, these immobile flowerlike creatures range in size from a few millimeters to about one and a half feet with long tentacles. Anemones are tube-shaped animals usually fixed to a firm surface, with a mouth slit on top and a range of tentacles around the mouth.

There are thousands of varieties of anemones, which differ from one another in every way. They do share one trait in common, however: the ability to sting and paralyze a victim with specialized cells lining their tentacles, which—while not usually fatal in itself—can cause drowning. Some varieties are poisonous to eat as well as capable of delivering a venomous sting.

While not all sea anemones are poisonous, the Matamalu samasama from Samoa *(Radianthus paumotensis, Rhodactis howesii)* is poisonous when eaten raw or cooked and causes respiratory failure. The *Actinia equina* floats along the eastern Atlantic, in the Mediterranean Sea, the Black Sea, and the Sea of Azov; the hell's fire sea anemone *(Actinodendron plumosum)* is found in tropical waters of the Pacific Ocean and the Great Barrier Reef off Australia; and the rosy anemone *(Sagarita elegans)* inhabits the waters off Iceland to the Mediterranean Sea and the coast of Africa.

Symptoms

Effects of the sea anemone sting are usually local, causing itching, burning, swelling, and reddening followed by sloughing of the skin. The tissues may then slough off followed by a long period of purulent discharge, and multiple abscesses may occur. More generalized symptoms include fever, chills, abdominal pain, nausea, vomiting, diarrhea, headache, thirst, and prostration.

Treatment

Soak the stung area in water as hot as possible without scalding the person for up to one hour, using hot soaks while on the way to the doctor. Observe for signs of shock. The ulcers resulting from a sea anemone sting are usually slow to heal and can be resistant to treatment. Baking soda in a paste with water should be applied to the sting to relieve pain. Calamine lotion will also help ease the burning sensation, and painkillers may help with the stinging pain. (Other local remedies for pain used around the world include meat tenderizer, sugar, ammonia, and lemon juice.)

anesthetics, gaseous/volatile These drugs include ether, chloroform, ethylene, and cyclopropane. They are also found as gases, including ethylene, cyclopropane, and nitrous oxide.

All these anesthetics produce general anesthesia; at cold temperatures, they are volatile liquids before they become gases and can be inhaled or ingested.

Symptoms

Overdose stops respiration and interferes with the action of the autoimmune system, causing unconsciousness, respiratory failure, cyanosis, and heart irregularities.

Treatment

Remove gas, maintain respiration, and keep warm. In the event of fever, lower temperature with wet towels.

See also CHLOROFORM; CYCLOPROPANE; ETHER.

anesthetics, local These drugs are used to numb one particular area of the body either by injection or by topical skin application (and include epidural, spinal, and regional nerve blocks). No two act the same, and their effect on patients varies from one person to another depending on the person's physical makeup. These drugs are all related to cocaine and are synthetic versions of the coca bush alkaloids. Local anesthetics include procaine, lidocaine, marcaine, monocaine, nesacaine, nupercaine, duranest, xylocaine, carocaine, oracaine, unacaine, citanest, and novocaine. Of these, procaine is considered the most dangerous and has caused numerous fatalities; shock can occur with only very small doses, and it enhances the action of muscle relaxants.

All of the local anesthetics are colorless (either liquid or gel) and are injected.

Symptoms

Local anesthetics work by blocking the nerve signals, providing a local loss of sensation. When the drugs are given in overdose, these actions may cause central nervous system and cardiovascular toxicity. Toxic levels can result from a single excessive injection, from a series of smaller injections or by accumulation of drug level by repeated doses. Symptoms of systemic poisoning affect primarily the central nervous system and include giddiness, feelings of oppression, severe collapse, coma, convulsions, dizziness, cyanosis, low blood pressure, tremors, coma, irregular and weak breathing, bronchial spasm, and heart failure. Repeated skin applications of local anesthetic can cause hypersensitivity, including itching, redness, swelling, and blistering.

Treatment

First, the injected drug must be removed from the body and absorption from the injection site lessened by using a tourniquet or ice pack. Treat symptoms, maintain airway and give artificial respiration with oxygen to control convulsions and central nervous system depression.

See also LIDOCAINE; PROCAINE.

aniline (amino benzol) A colorless, oily fluid that turns brown when exposed to air, used in inks for stamp pads, printing, and cloth marking, in addition to dyes, paint removers, and paint. Aniline can be ingested or absorbed as a gas, powder, or liquid.

Occasionally, aniline dye poisonings do occur among infants and young children; newborns have been poisoned by touching—and inhaling fumes from—diapers freshly stamped with aniline dye. It is also possible to become poisoned from absorbing shoe polish that contains aniline dyes. Fortunately, there are few poisonings from this substance today.

Symptoms

Aniline interferes with the transportation of oxygen throughout the central nervous system, and within two hours after exposure, moderate exposure may cause cyanosis of the lips, ears, and cheeks. In more severe cases, symptoms of cyanosis are much more marked, together with headaches, shallow breathing, vertigo, chills, nausea, and vomiting. Infants are apathetic and may exhibit convulsions, coma, and death. Direct contact of aniline dye with the skin will cause dermatitis. Chronic poisoning in the wake of inhalation or skin absorption causes mild cyanosis, anorexia, weight loss, weakness, headache, vertigo, irritability, and anemia.

Treatment

Remove victim to fresh air. If the skin has been contaminated, wash thoroughly with vinegar followed by soap and water. If aniline has been ingested, administer gastric lavage followed by liquid petrolatum and a saline cathartic. Oxygen, doxapram, and blood transfusions may also be necessary. In very severe cases, hemodialysis should be used.

Animal Poison Control Center A 24-hour emergency center staffed by veterinary health professionals trained to handle pet poisonings. Pet owners who can't reach a vet or other local experts can call this center by dialing (888) 426-4435. A $60 consultation charge may be applied to your credit card.

The nonprofit organization, affiliated with the college of veterinary medicine of the University of Illinois, is an operating division of the American Society for the Prevention of Cruelty to Animals. It was begun in 1978 and began charging for its services in 1990. All employees are veterinarians with clinical experience, with additional six months' training in toxicology; two are board certified with the American Board of Veterinary Toxicologists. In addition, the animal poison control center supports a backup laboratory to provide additional toxicological assistance.

The center fields calls equally from private pet owners and veterinarians and maintains an extensive log of poisoning cases from more than 4,000 different toxic agents. The kinds of animal poisoning cases vary according to the time of year: pesticides and flea and tick poisonings in the summer; chocolate and poinsettia poisonings during the Easter and Christmas holidays. Most calls are due to poisoning from insecticides used in and around the house or on the farm. The center handles problems with livestock as well as household pets, from dogs and cats to canaries and potbelly pigs.

Poisonings with human medications make up as many as 20 percent of the calls to the animal poison center, especially heart pills and birth control pills left on nightstands. Toxic plants are a third major category.

anisakiasis   A disease of the intestines caused by a parasitic worm *Anisakis simplex,* which infests small crustaceans eaten by many kinds of fish, dolphins, and whales. Humans become infected by eating improperly prepared fish.

Fewer than 10 cases are diagnosed in the United States every year; however, experts suspect many cases go undiagnosed. Japan has the greatest number of cases because of the large amounts of raw fish the Japanese eat, but it also occurs in Scandinavia and Latin America. Anisikiasis is easily misdiagnosed as acute appendicitis, Crohn's disease, gastric ulcer, or gastrointestinal cancer.

The larvae are found in raw, undercooked, or insufficiently frozen fish and shellfish, and its incidence is expected to increase with the increasing popularity of sushi and sashimi bars. Cod, haddock, fluke, flounder, and monkfish have also been known to host the parasite.

Symptoms

Symptoms usually begin within six hours after consuming raw or undercooked seafood. If the larvae is not coughed up or passed into the bowels, it can penetrate the stomach and cause severe pain, nausea, and vomiting. In severe cases, the pain is akin to acute appendicitis.

Diagnosis

In North America, the infestation is usually diagnosed when the patient begins to feel a tingling or tickling sensation in the throat and coughs up a worm. Alternatively, a physician may need to examine the inside of the person's stomach and the small intestines.

Treatment

Surgically removing the worm(s) may be necessary. Most patients recover without treatment.

Prevention

The worm is killed by cooking or freezing the fish. Marinating raw fish in lemon or vinegar does not kill all the harmful bacteria or parasites that the fish might contain. Sushi lovers should eat only at reputable restaurants and ask whether the fish was previously frozen (freezing reduces the risk of illness by killing larvae of parasites that might have been present in the raw fish). The larval stage of the worms are killed by cooking at 140°F for at least 10 minutes.

Antabuse (disulfiram)   This drug is used to treat alcoholics, who experience an extremely unpleasant side effect if they drink alcohol while taking it. Long-term use of Antabuse can damage the peripheral nerves.

Symptoms

An acute overdose may cause vomiting, clumsiness, lethargy, seizures, and coma. Several deaths have been reported as a result of liver failure. Ingestion of alcohol (including some types of cough syrup or other alcohol-containing products) while taking Antabuse can cause flushing, throbbing headache, anxiety, vertigo, vomiting, and convulsion; the severity of the reaction is tied to the amount of Antabuse and alcohol ingested. It generally takes at least one day on the drug before the interaction will set off this reaction, but the reaction will also occur up to several days after the last dose of Antabuse has been taken.

Treatment

There is no specific antidote. For overdose of Antabuse: Induce vomiting or perform gastric lavage; administer activated charcoal and a cathartic. For interaction of Antabuse and alcohol: once symptoms appear, there is not much that can be done; if the victim drank a large amount of alcohol, gastric lavage and activated charcoal should help.

Anthrax   See BACILLUS ANTHRACIS.

antianxiety drugs   A group of drugs used to relieve symptoms of anxiety; benzodiazepines and beta adrenergic blockers are fast acting and used to be the main drugs prescribed for anxiety, although most are addictive. Among them are Xanax (alprazolam), Librium (chlordiazepoxide), Tranxene (chlorazepate), Valium (diazepam), Dalmane (flurazepam), Ativan (lorazepam), Serax (oxazepam), Centrax (prazepam), and Halcion (triazolam). However, benzodiazepines have been largely replaced by selective serotonin reuptake inhibitors (SSRIs). Among the preferred SSRIs for generalized anxiety disorder are Paxil (paroxetine), Lexapro (escitalopram), and Effexor (venlafaxine). Prozac (fluoxetine) and Zoloft (sertraline) are also prescribed.

Symptoms

Overdose of benzodiazepines and beta adrenergic blockers can bring on drowsiness, weakness, double vision, clumsiness, lethargy, convulsions, coma, cyanosis, and breathing problems. Chronic abuse can cause skin rash, gastric upset, headaches, and blurred vision. Overdose of SSRIs may cause serotonin syndrome, which is characterized by restlessness, hallucinations, shivering, nausea, diarrhea, headache, tremor, agitation, and diaphoresis. Most reports of fatalities with antianxiety drugs involve multiple drug ingestions.

Treatment

For benzodiazepines and beta adrenergic blockers, induce vomiting or perform gastric lavage followed by the administration of activated charcoal and a saline cathartic. Follow with supportive measures, including monitoring of blood pressure and fluid levels. For SSRIs, gastric lavage is generally not indicated unless it can be performed within one hour of the overdose and provided the airway is secure. Airway compromise is highly possible because of deterioration of mental status and neuromuscular dysfunction. Use of activated charcoal should be administered with careful attention to the possibility of such compromise.

See also BENZODIAZEPINES; BETA ADRENERGIC BLOCKERS; DALMANE; SELECTIVE SEROTONIN REUPTAKE INHIBITORS.

antiarrhythmic drugs   Prescribed to control unwanted or abnormal heart rhythms. The American Heart Association lists four main categories of drugs used to treat arrhythmias:

1. beta-adrenergic blockers (e.g., atenolol [Tenormin], carvedilol [Coreq], propranolol [Inderal])
2. calcium channel blockers (e.g., diltiazem [Cardizem], verapamil [Calan])
3. sodium channel blockers (e.g., quinidine, procainamide [Pronestyl], disopyramide [Norpace])
4. potassium channel blockers (e.g., amiodarone [Cordarone], bepridil [Vascor])
5. miscellaneous (e.g., digoxin [Lanoxin], adenosine [Adenocard]). All of these drugs may be toxic and even fatal in doses only slightly above the recommended dose, and for some people they are toxic even within the therapeutic range.

Symptoms

Toxicity with antiarrhythmic drugs primarily affects the cardiovascular and central nervous systems. Symptoms include heartbeat irregularities, dry mouth, dilated pupils, delirium, seizures, coma, and respiratory arrest. Quinidine often causes nausea, vomiting, diarrhea, and, with chronic doses, cinchonism (ringing in the ears, vertigo, deafness, and visual disturbances). Procainamide may cause upset stomach and a lupus-like syndrome with chronic use.

Treatment

Heart problems are treated with hypertonic sodium bicarbonate and possibly insertion of a pacemaker; treat symptoms and monitor vital signs. Do not induce vomiting because of the risk of rapid onset of seizures; perform gastric lavage followed by activated charcoal and a cathartic.

See also BETA ADRENERGIC BLOCKERS; DIGITALIS; QUINIDINE.

anticoagulants Drugs used to keep the blood from clotting too quickly and reduce mortality associated with blood clots. They include (1) warfarin, dicumarol, phenprocoumon, and phenindione, which work by interfering with the production in the liver of various clotting factors that depend on vitamin K; and (2) argatroban, bivalirudin, and lepirudin, newer drugs that inhibit thrombin (clot factors). Warfarin sodium (Coumadin) is the least toxic, and most widely used, anticoagulant. A wide range of factors can influence a person's response to anticoagulants, including changes in diet, environment, and medication.

Symptoms

Sudden rush of blood hemorrhaging of the larynx, trachea or lungs, bloody stools, hermorrhages in other organs, bruising and bleeding into joint spaces, skin rash, vomiting, fever, and kidney damage. Repeated use leads to acute poisoning. Fatalities from kidney and liver damage have been reported after repeated doses, and death may not occur until several weeks after the drug has been discontinued.

Treatment

Complete bed rest; medication is administered to prevent internal bleeding.

See also WARFARIN.

antidepressants A class of drugs used to treat depression and anxiety. There are several different kinds of antidepressants that are grouped according to which chemicals in the brain they affect. Selective serotonin reuptake inhibitors (SSRIs) tend to have fewer side effects than other antidepressants. The SSRIs include citalopram (Celexa), escitalopram (Lexapro), fluoxetine (Prozac), paroxetine (Paxil), and sertraline (Zoloft). These are typically the first choice for treatment of depression. Combination drugs are also high on the list of treatment options and include serotonin and norepinephrine reuptake inhibitors (duloxetine [Cymbalta] and venlafaxine [Effexor]), one norepinephrine and dopamine reuptake inhibitor (bupropion [Wellbutrin]), and a combination of reuptake inhibitor and receptor blocker (mirtazpine [Remeron] and trazodone [Desyrel]). The second line of treatment is tricyclic antidepressants (now more accurately called cyclics, or CAs), which include amitriptyline (Elavil), desipramine (Norpramin), imipramine (Tofranil), maprotiline (Ludiomil), and nortriptyline (Aventyl). The least commonly used antidepressants are the monamine oxidase inhibitors (MAOIs), which include isocarboxazid (Marplan), phenelzine (Nardil), and tranylcypromine (Parnate).

Symptoms

An SSRI overdose infrequently results in the development of serotonin syndrome (characterized by restlessness, hallucinations, shivering, nausea, diarrhea, headache, tremor, agitation, and diaphoresis), but other patients who remain asymptomatic for several hours after overdosing usually do not need medical treatment. Research shows that individuals who take up to 30 times the daily dose of an SSRI typically have few or no side effects. Overdose of cyclic antidepressants, however, can be very serious, and is associated with central nervous system symptoms, including hallucinations, confusion, and lethargy that progresses to seizures or coma. Their most serious effect is on cardiac conductivity, resulting in multiple heart arrhythmias, which may result in death. Acute overdose of MAO inhibitors causes slow heartbeat, confusion, hallucinations, agitation, and convulsions. High blood pressure may quickly reverse to low blood pressure, which is an indication of a very serious prognosis. Beer, wine, and cheese eaten with MAO inhibitors can cause very serious symptoms, including intracranial bleeding, circulatory failure, and death.

Treatment

The victim should be under medical supervision, since induced vomiting could cause seizures or arrhythmias. At a hospital, gastric lavage is followed by administration of activated charcoal and a cathartic. For cases of severe overdose of CA, physostigmine salicylate may be used as an antidote. Hospitalization is strongly recommended. Patients receiving good supportive care will recover within four days.

See also MONOAMINE OXIDASE (MAO) INHIBITORS.

antifreeze   Most types of antifreeze contain ethylene glycol or methanol, both of which are poisonous to drink. About 50 deaths occur each year in the United States from antifreeze poisoning, most of which are among alcoholics who turn to antifreeze as an alternative to alcohol; some people attempt to commit suicide by this method. Antifreeze poisoning is also a problem for household pets, who are attracted by the sweet taste. According to Dr. Steve Hansen of the National Animal Poison Control Center, it only takes one teaspoon of undiluted antifreeze/coolant to kill a seven-pound cat.

Poisonous part

Antifreeze containing ethylene glycol is extremely toxic because of its breakdown products and resulting acidosis.

Symptoms

In small amounts, antifreeze poisoning resembles intoxication from alcohol; large doses cause vomiting, seizures, and coma within a few hours, followed by acute kidney failure within 24 to 36 hours. The lethal dose of ethylene glycol is considered to be 100 milliliters for an adult, although recovery has been noted after ingestions ranging up to 970 milliliters. Antifreeze containing methanol can also cause blindness.

Treatment

The victim should be taken to a medical care facility immediately. Fomepizole is used to treat antifreeze poisoning. If the eyes are contaminated, immediately rinse with warm running water for 15 to 20 minutes.

For antifreeze poisoning in pets, owners should first feed the pet soft food (milk or canned pet food) and then induce vomiting using syrup of ipecac. Fomepizole also may be used for pets. *If the pet is found within one hour of poisoning,* alcohol (such as whiskey) may be given as an antidote after vomiting—one or two ounces for smaller dogs and up to three or four ounces for larger breeds. If more than five hours have elapsed since poisoning, emergency home treatment will be fruitless. *Animal ingestion of antifreeze is a serious emergency that requires immediate, intensive veterinary care. Vomiting and alcohol should be administered at home only when veterinary care is not immediately available.* For advice in an animal poisoning emergency, call the National Animal Poison Control Center at (888) 426-4435 ($60 per call). The center's phones are staffed by trained veterinarians 24 hours a day, seven days a week.

See also FOMEPIZOLE; METHYL ALCOHOL; ANIMAL POISON CONTROL CENTER.

antihistamines   A group of drugs that block the effects of histamine, a chemical released during an allergic reaction. While harmless in normal amounts, they can be fatal when taken in massive overdose (as in a suicide attempt or accidental ingestion by young children). Antihistamines are being used more and more, not only to treat allergies and respiratory infections but also for motion sickness and as sedatives. Many are available over the counter.

Examples of over-the-counter (OTC) antihistamines include brompheniramine (Dimetapp, Nasahist), chlorpheniramine (Chlor-Trimeton), clemastine (Allerhist, Tavist), and diphenhydramine (Benadryl), all of which belong to the first generation of antihistamines. Common second-generation antihistamines include loratadine (Claritin, OTC) plus prescriptions cetirizine (Zyrtec), desloratadine (Clarinex), and fexofenadine (Allegra). Second-generation antihistamines are much less likely to cause drowsiness and dry mouth than are first-generation drugs.

Symptoms

Antihistamines are a central nervous system depressant, causing drowsiness, dizziness, and clumsiness; symptoms also resemble atropine poisoning, including dry mouth, fixed dilated pupils, fever, and flushed and reddened face. Children are particularly susceptible to the stimulating effects of antihistamines and can show excitement, hallucinations, toxic psychosis, delirium, tremors, and convulsions followed by respiratory or cardiac arrest.

Treatment

Induce vomiting followed by the administration of cathartics and activated charcoal. Perform gastric lavage for cases in which vomiting is not indicated, such as with poisoning with phenothiazine-type antihistamines, which are less responsive to ipecac-induced vomiting.

antihypertensive drugs Medications prescribed to lower high blood pressure, they are also classified as belonging to one of several drug families according to the way they work. The subdivisions include drugs that increase the rate at which the body eliminates urine and salt (diuretics); beta adrenergic blockers, drugs that block many of the effects of epinephrine (adrenaline) in the body; drugs that block the entry of calcium into the walls of the small arteries (calcium channel blockers); drugs that block formation of a natural body chemical and dilate small arteries (angiotensin-converting enzyme [ACE] inhibitors); and drugs that directly inhibit the effects of ACE II rather than block its production (ACE II inhibitors). ACE II inhibitors have actions similar to those of ACE inhibitors, but they appear to have a more favorable side effect and safety profile.

Examples of antihypertensives according to drug class include: calcium-channel blockers nifedipine (Adalat) and verapamil (Calan); beta-blockers atenolol (Tenormin) and propranolol (Inderal); diuretic hydrochlorothiazide (Hydrodiuril); ACE inhibitors captopril (Capoten) and enalapril (Vasotec); and ACE II inhibitors losartan (Cozaar) and valsartan (Diovan).

Symptoms

In general, overdose causes a generalized depression of the sympathetic nervous system, including lethargy, pinpoint pupils, slow heartbeat, low blood pressure, low fever, apnea, and coma. Onset of symptoms is usually within 30 to 60 minutes; full recovery occurs within 24 hours.

Treatment

Treatment for antihypertensive overdose includes induced vomiting or gastric lavage followed by the administration of activated charcoal and a cathartic.

See also ALDOMET; BETA ADRENERGIC BLOCKERS; CATAPRES; DIURETICS; EPINEPHRINE; MINIPRESS; QUINIDINE.

anti-inflammatory drugs These medications are used to reduce inflammation and include a wide variety of corticosteroids and nonsteroidal anti-inflammatory drugs (NSAIDS), such as aspirin and ibuprofen. Inflammation is one of the body's defense mechanisms in response to infection and certain chronic diseases such as rheumatoid arthritis. But as inflammation increases blood flow, it causes swelling, redness, pain, and heat. Anti-inflammatory drugs are designed to combat this inflammation.

Normally, anti-inflammatory drugs are not very toxic, but persons with gastrointestinal tract disease, peptic ulcers, or poor heart function or those on anticoagulants should avoid them.

Anti-inflammatory drugs include celecoxib (Celebrex), diflunisal (Dolobid), ibuprofen (Motrin, Rufen, Advil, Haltrain, Medipren, Nuprin, Trendar), fenoprofen (Nalfon), meclofenamate (Meclomen) and naproxen (Anaprox, Naprosyn). None of these should be taken with other nonsteroid analgesics, or with warfarin or other oral anticoagulants, because bleeding time may be prolonged while on anti-inflammatory pain relievers. Antacids, however, may sometimes reduce the effects of an anti-inflammatory drug.

Symptoms

If a person is allergic to aspirin or other analgesic drugs, using another anti-inflammatory medicine could be fatal. Anti-inflammatory drugs become toxic when given to those with kidney problems, since the kidneys cannot cleanse the blood.

Overdose causes kidney failure and severe liver reactions, including fatal jaundice.

Normally, anti-inflammatory overdose produces mild stomach upset, with nausea and vomiting plus abdominal pain and internal bleeding. Occasionally, other symptoms might include sleepiness, lethargy, nystagmus (involuntary oscillation of the eyeball), tinnitus (ringing in the ears), and disorientation. However, with some of the more toxic drugs and significant overdose of ibuprofen (in excess of 3,200 milligrams per day), symptoms can include seizures, coma, metabolic acidosis, kidney and liver failure, and cardiorespiratory arrest.

Treatment

There is no antidote. Maintain symptomatic treatment together with antacids for mild stomach problems; perform gastric lavage, followed by administration of activated charcoal and a cathartic.

antimony This silvery white soft metal is a popular hardening agent used in the production of soft metal alloys and rubber, as a coloring agent and in flameproofing compounds. It is also contained in a wide variety of products, including batteries, foil, safety matches, ant paste, ceramics, textiles, glass, enamels, typesetting metals, and alloys. It is also used medicinally as an emetic and to combat worms. It is present in the dust and fumes produced during mining and refining, and from the discharge of firearms. Stibine (antimony hydride) is a colorless gas produced as a by-product when ore containing antimony is treated with acid.

A strong tissue irritant, antimony is lethal in doses of between 100 and 200 mg. Fatal poisonings from antimony are usually from drug overdoses, not from industrial exposure to vapors or dust. This is an extremely rare toxin.

Poisonous part

The toxic mechanism of both antimony and stibine is unknown, but its chemical action is similar to that of arsenic and arsine. It is believed that antimony compounds probably inactivate key enzymes in the body; stibine, like arsine gas, may destroy red blood cells.

Symptoms

While death is rare following the ingestion of antimony if the patient survives the initial gastroenteritis, symptoms are unpleasant and include nausea, vomiting, and bloody diarrhea, with hepatitis and kidney problems. Chronic antimony poisoning is quite similar to chronic arsenic toxicity, causing itchy skin, conjunctivitis, laryngitis, headache, anorexia, weight loss, and anemia. The inhalation of stibine causes headaches, weakness, nausea, vomiting, jaundice, anemia, and kidney failure.

Treatment

There is no specific antidote. As in arsenic poisoning, treatment for ingestion involves gastric lavage followed by the administration of activated charcoal (although there is no evidence that this is effective). Do not use cathartics. Dimercaprol (to hasten the excretion of metals such as arsenic, gold, and mercury as well) may be administered, as well as narcotics for pain. Hospitalization is recommended. In stibine poisoning, a blood transfusion may be necessary after massive destruction of red blood cells.

See also ARSENIC; ARSINE GAS.

antipsychotic/psychometric drugs These drugs are used to treat psychosis, schizophrenia, bipolar disorder with psychotic manifestations, and agitated depression and are a common choice for suicide. They may also be used before surgery to ease fears, to treat tetanus, and to relieve behavior disorders in children.

With the introduction of a new type of antipsychotic drugs beginning in the 1990s, there are now two groups of antipsychotics. The conventional group include chlorpromazine (Thorazine), fluphenazine (Permitil), mesoridazine (Serentil), perphenazine (Trilafon), prochlorperazine, promethazine, thioridazine (Mellaril), trifluoperazine (Stelazine), thiothixene (Navane), haloperidol (Haldol), loxapine (Loxitane), and molindone (Lidone). The second or atypical group consists of aripiprazole (Abilify), clozapine (Clozaril), olanzapine (Zyprexa), risperidone (Risperdal), and ziprosidone (Geodon).

Symptoms

These drugs seldom cause death because it takes a high dosage to reach toxic levels. There is also tolerance to the sedating effects, and patients on chronic therapy may tolerate much larger doses than normal. Therefore, the toxic dose after acute ingestion is quite variable. Severe intoxication may cause coma, seizures, and respiratory arrest. There may also be jaw muscle spasm, rigidity, and tremor. Further, patients on long-term antipsychotic medication may develop a neuroleptic malignant syndrome (rigidity, high fever, sweating, lactic acidosis).

Treatment

There is no specific antidote. Some experts recommend bromocriptine in the treatment of neuroleptic malignant syndrome, although other treatments for high fever are successful. Induce vomiting or perform gastric lavage if victim is seen within 30 to 60 minutes or if the overdose is substantial (gastric lavage is preferred).

The mainstay treatment for comatose patients is activated charcoal, intravenous fluids, and ECG monitoring; for patients with cardiotoxicity, it is plasma alkalinization with sodium bicarbonate and hyperventilation; for neurotoxicity, it is intubation, plasma alkalinization, and hyperventilation.

See also THORAZINE.

antiseptics and disinfectants Both products are designed to kill microorganisms; antiseptics are applied to living tissue and disinfectants to inanimate objects. Despite the fact that they have never been proven to kill germs, they are widely used in both home and medical applications. Among the most common are hydrogen peroxide, alcohol, and iodine. All of these agents are generally used in diluted solutions and cause very little toxicity. Still, skin contact and vapors can be irritating to skin and the respiratory system. These products are more hazardous when used in aerosol form, since the mist can be inhaled through the nose and mouth.

See also HYDROGEN PEROXIDE; IODINE; ISOPROPYL ALCOHOL.

antivenin A specific treatment for snake, scorpion, spider, or other venomous animal bites. It is produced by inoculating animals (usually horses) with venom from a poisonous animal, which stimulates the production of antibodies in the horse to neutralize the poisons in the venom. A preparation with the antibodies (or antivenins) can then be produced from samples of the horse's blood. When given to a snakebite victim, the antibodies bind to and neutralize circulating venom proteins.

Commercial antivenins are available for bites from all types of pit vipers (rattlesnakes, cottonmouth, and copperhead snakes) and the coral snake. Antivenins for treating the bites of scorpions, spiders, fish, and jellyfish—or snakes that originate outside the United States—can be obtained at zoos and from veterinarians. Black widow spider antivenin is available in some hospitals within the United States; antivenin for the stings of poisonous fish and jellyfish are generally not available in this country.

Experts do warn that the two commercially marketed antivenins for snakebite available in this country cause painful and sometimes serious reactions in the vast majority of treated snakebite victims. While neither poses a life-threatening risk, both trigger a generalized and sometimes severe immunological reaction called "serum sickness" in about 75 percent of individuals.

The most difficult aspect of producing antivenin lics in thc purification—that is, extracting protein from the horse's blood that has the antibodies but not the other, useless proteins. These "useless" proteins from the horse are what trigger the serious reactions when injected into humans, since the human immune system recognizes them as foreign. In response to these foreign substances, a few people go into anaphylactic shock, a life-threatening immune response characterized by flushing and itching, nausea, breathing problems, and lowered blood pressure.

It is possible to test a snakebite victim's sensitivity to horse protein, but the skin test itself can trigger anaphylactic shock, and a positive response would then require a physician to choose between a potential severe reaction to antivenin and death or amputation from the snakebite. And in about 3 percent of cases, victims with negative skin tests go on to have severe reactions to the antivenin anyway.

Recent research suggests that high-tech purification techniques using sheep's blood or chicken eggs instead of horse serum may result in a better antivenin. Chicken-based antibodies cannot trigger the highly inflammatory allergic reaction in humans that horse proteins can (unless there is a history of severe egg allergy); sheep antibodies also seem to cause fewer allergic reactions in humans.

See also ANTIVENIN, BLACK WIDOW SPIDER; ANTIVENIN, CORAL SNAKE; ANTIVENIN, RATTLESNAKE; SNAKES, POISONOUS.

antivenin, black widow spider   The antidote for the bite of the black widow spider, this antivenin is produced by injecting horses with venom and collecting some of the blood, which then contains antibodies to the poison. The antivenin should be given to victims of black widow spider bite in the presence of uncontrolled severe high blood pressure or if the victim is pregnant. Black widow spider bites in pregnant women may cause an abdominal spasm so severe that it sets off a miscarriage or early onset of labor.

As with other types of antivenin produced from horse serum, immediate allergic reaction is possible and a skin test for hypersensitivity should be performed.

See also ANTIVENIN; BLACK WIDOW SPIDER.

antivenin, coral snake   The antidote to the bite of the poisonous eastern coral snake *(Micrurus fulvius)* or the Texas coral snake *(M. fulvius tenere)*. It is not effective against the bite of the Arizona or Sonora coral snake *(M. euryxanthus)*.

The antivenin is produced by injecting horses with venom and then collecting some of the blood, which contains antibodies to the poison. As with other types of antivenin produced from horse serum, immediate allergic reaction is possible, and a skin test for hypersensitivity should be performed.

See also ANTIVENIN; CORAL SNAKE, ARIZONA; CORAL SNAKE, EASTERN.

antivenin, rattlesnake   The antidote for rattlesnake bite is produced by injecting horses with the pooled venoms of the eastern diamondback rattlesnake, the western diamondback, the cascabel, or tropical, rattlesnake and the fer-de-lance. The blood serum from the horse then contains a combination of several antibodies against venom constituents.

When given intravenously to the victim of rattlesnake bite, the antivenin binds to the venom throughout the body. However, it is possible to have an allergic reaction to the antivenin, causing anaphylactic shock even in those who tested negative for horse serum allergy.

See also ANTIVENIN; RATTLESNAKES.

Antizol   Antizol (fomepizole) is the first drug indicated as an antidote for antifreeze (ethylene glycol or methanol) poisoning. Commonly known as 4-MP (4-methylpyrazole), it works by blocking the formation of toxic ethylene glycol metabolites. If unchecked, these metabolites could lead to kidney damage.

Side effects

Reactions to the drug may include headache (14 percent), nausea (11 percent) and dizziness, increased drowsiness and bad taste (6 percent) each. Minor allergic reactions have been reported.

apomorphine   This powerful emetic is an alkaloid salt derived from morphine. It has been used to induce vomiting in cases of oral poisoning, but at the moment, it is rarely used in either adult or childhood poisoning cases because it also strongly depresses breathing. Naloxone is used to treat the respiratory depression that occurs following apomorphine use. Apomorphine is popular, however, in veterinary medicine.

See also NALOXONE.

apple of Sodom *(Solanum sodomeum)*   This common Hawaiian weed is also known as Dead Sea apple. It is a member of a very large genus of 1,700 species, most of which have not been evaluated toxicologically.

Poisonous part

Human poisoning is usually attributed to immature fruit, which contains the toxin solanine glycoalkaloid.

Symptoms

While there is little danger of fatal poisoning in adults, children may ingest a fatal amount of this plant. Symptoms appear several hours after ingestion and include gastric irritation, scratchy throat, fever, and diarrhea. (Solanine poisoning is often confused with bacterial gastroenteritis.)

Treatment

The same general supportive care that would be given in gastroenteritis cases; fluid replacement may be required.

apricot pit See PRUNUS.

aquarium products According to numerous reports at poison control centers around the country, a wide range of fairly nontoxic products sold for the upkeep of home aquariums may end up in the hands of young children, who may inadvertently ingest them. In addition, adults may find them in medicine cabinets and use them mistakenly for eye, ear, or nose drops.

These products include antichlorinc compounds (sodium thiosulfate), pH indicators, vitamins, copper sulfate, aquarium salts, and a range of antimicrobials used to combat algae and fungi. Most are not very toxic, with the exception of some pH kits that contain sodium hydroxide (lye).

See also ALKALINE CORROSIVES.

arrow poison frogs (Dendrobatidae and *Phyllobates*) This tree frog (also called "dart poison frogs") of the Colombian rain forest is one of a group of brightly colored amphibians of South and Central America.

Once captured by the native people, it is carried back to camp, impaled on a sharpened stick and slowly roasted over an open fire; as it dies, the frog secretes a highly toxic mucus from the pores of its skin. This poison will later be applied to the tips of the Indians' blowgun darts and arrows. One specimen in this group is so toxic that one frog contains enough poison to kill about 100 people; handling this frog with bare hands could be fatal.

A supposed source of hunting magic in the rain forest, another type of this frog provides ointment used in prehunt ceremonies in which hunters burn themselves and then rub a stick coated with this frog's chemical on their wounds. According to legend, they awake with much keener senses the next morning. South American natives also rub frogs on wounds and cuts because the frog's skin contains potent antibiotic peptides.

Secretions from still another type of toxic frog will change the color of parrots; rubbing a bit of frog secretion over the spot of a plucked feather will cause a new feather to grow back in a different color.

Some poison frogs grow no bigger than a fingernail, whereas others vary so much in color that even frog experts mistake cousins as separate species. They all are rain forest inhabitants and live on land away from water, as long as there is enough water to lay their eggs. Most of these frogs have only slight water requirements, and some can be found living in the tiny water sac of bromeliad plants high above the forest floor. Most, however, prefer to live among the leaves that litter the rain forest floor, not in trees.

All the arrow poison frogs are very small and beautifully colored and can be handled carefully without danger—as long as they don't get excited. While there are many hundreds of different species, only a few are actually used to treat arrows; it takes up to 50 of them to coat the tips of a quiver. The most common of the poisonous arrow-tippers are

Flat-spined Atelopus (Atelopus planispina), a gold and green Ecuadoran mountain frog with white spots and black markings.
Zetek's frog (Atelopus zeteki), a Panamanian golden frog; males have black blotches.
Yellow-spotted arrow poison frog (Dendrobates flavopictus), a black central Brazilian frog from the uplands, with bright yellow spots and lines.

Boulenger's arrow poison frog (Atelopus boulengeri), a black mountain frog from Peru and Ecuador with creamy spots.

Three-striped arrow poison frog (Dendrobates trivittatus), a South American black and yellow striped frog.

Two-toned arrow poison frog (Phyllobates bicolor), a vivid red frog with black markings from northern South America.

Gold arrow poison frog (Dendrobates auratus), a small gold and green frog from Nicaragua through Panama to Colombia.

Poisonous part

Of the family Dendrobatidae, four genera have skins with alkaloid compounds capable of killing a human if the toxin enters the blood (as from an arrow wound), and more than 50 poisonous species have been documented so far. Herpetologists suspect that the frog alkaloids are a by-product of metabolism.

Symptoms

While the toxin of the arrow poison frogs can be deadly if it enters the bloodstream (and one species, *Phyllobates horribilus,* can be fatal if chewed), skin contact with the frogs causes an irritating skin reaction, with swelling, reddening, and blistering.

Treatment

In cases of skin contact, wash secretions immediately with soap and water. If a person touches the skin and rubs an eye, the eye should be immediately rinsed with water or a saline solution. Significant skin reactions may require a doctor's care and treatment of dermatitis-type reaction; steroids may be helpful.

arsenic [Other names: arsenic trihydride, arsenic trioxide, arsenous oxide, metallic arsenic, white or gray arsenic] The 20th most common element that occurs naturally in pure form, arsenic is present in all human tissue and is a fairly accessible poison. It is used in the manufacture of ceramics, enamels, paint, wallpaper, weed killer, insecticide, rat poisons, and pesticides. In its natural state, arsenic is a gray metal. While arsenic has been used intentionally to murder, poisoning also occurs as a result of industrial accidents or accidental ingestion.

In addition, arsenic (present throughout the earth's crust) contaminates the groundwater around the world. In the United States, the Environmental Protection Agency (EPA) tightened the federal standards for arsenic by lowering the 50 parts per billion (ppb) drinking water standard to 10 ppb. The new drinking water standard was adopted in January 2001, and the EPA gave public water utilities across the country five years (until January 2006) to reduce the level of arsenic in their tap water supplies. The standards apply to the approximately 74,000 community and noncommunity water systems in the United States.

Symptoms

Most toxicologists believe arsenic combines with enzymes to interfere with cellular function, causing severe gastric distress, esophageal pain, vomiting, and diarrhea with blood. The skin is cold and clammy, and blood pressure plummets followed by convulsions and coma.

Arsenic poisoning can be chronic, occurring over a long period of time, and in such cases causes weakness, tiredness, scaly skin, and changes in skin pigmentation, followed by swelling of the lining of the mouth and finally a degeneration of nerves, causing tingling and numbness and moments of paralysis; death comes eventually from heart failure, bone marrow failure, or infection.

Poisoning may also result from a single large dose (acute poisoning), in which case death can come within a day, and sometimes after only a few hours. In acute cases, the arsenic affects the intestinal lining, quickly producing painful symptoms—nausea, vomiting, diarrhea, sweating, and burning of the throat, followed by collapse and death. Individual susceptibility to arsenic poisoning varies, and some individuals can develop a tolerance to doses of arsenic that would kill others.

Because arsenic is an element and cannot be broken down any further, traces remaining in a person's hair, fingernails, and urine can be identified upon urinalysis or autopsy.

Treatment

In acute arsenic poisoning, the patient should be transported to a medical facility. Gastric lavage and fluid replacement are vital, together with the administration of dimercaprol for two or three days followed by penicillamine until the arsenic level in the urine drops. The victim should also be treated for dehydration, shock, pulmonary edema, and liver damage and may be put on a kidney dialysis machine after the dimercaprol. Chronic poisoning is also treated with dimercaprol.

arsine gas This arsenic compound is an extremely poisonous, colorless inflammable gas (AsH_3) composed of arsenic and hydrogen, which occurs when metals containing arsenic are exposed to acids. The gas, also called arsenic hydride, is used as a military poison gas, but most cases of arsine poisoning occur in the metallurgic industries during the refining process and during galvanizing, soldering, and lead plating.

According to the American Conference of Environmental Industrial Hygienists, 0.05 part per million is the maximum safe concentration for prolonged arsine exposure.

Arsine gas has a disagreeable odor, similar to that of onions or carbide.

Symptoms

Inhalation causes vomiting, cramps, and nausea; decrease or cessation of urine output, which is often stained red four to six hours after exposure, followed by the appearance of jaundice. Effects of exposure to arsine gas include damaged kidneys and destruction of red blood cells; chronic exposure leads to gradual loss of strength, diarrhea or constipation, scaling of the skin that can become malignant, paralysis, confusion, and anemia.

Treatment

Physicians advocate early exchange transfusions and the administration of dimercaprol, which is usually not effective. Those with less than fatal doses of gas will recover; those who receive a fatal dose cannot be saved despite treatment. The only true solution to arsine gas poisoning is prevention.

See also ARSENIC.

artane See TRIHEXYPHENIDYL.

asbestos A mineral fiber found in rocks and manufactured into heat- and friction-resistant materials. Asbestos is one of the most widely recognized sources of environmentally produced disease. It was used in a wide variety of ceiling materials, insulation, roofing, shingles and siding, hair blowers, some vinyl floor tiles and vinyl sheet flooring, stoves and furnaces, appliance insulation, walls, and pipes.

Unfortunately, the toxic nature of asbestos (it causes lung and stomach cancer) was not realized until the demand for its use resulted in its incorporation in most buildings and vessels constructed for an entire generation. And even though it has been accepted that asbestos can cause disease in those exposed to it, there is considerable controversy about the dose required to produce disease.

Occupations most at risk for asbestos exposure include insulators, shipyard workers, construction workers, and pipe fitters.

Exposure to asbestos leads to an accumulation of the mineral in the lung, which then migrates to other regions in the body. It can cause asbestosis, a disease characterized by progressive restriction of lung capacity caused by a pulmonary fibrous reaction to the inhalation of asbestos fibers. Other diseases associated with asbestos exposure include lung cancer and mesothelioma (a rare tumor originating in the cells lining the chest and abdominal cavity).

Asbestoslike fibers are commonly found in drinking water sources throughout the United States originating from rock areas in watersheds, from refuse dumps, and in asbestos-containing water pipes. There is no evidence, however, that ingesting these fibers causes disease in humans.

If asbestos is found and must be disturbed, handle it carefully wearing a filtered mask. If at all possible, experts recommend that a trained contractor remove it.

ascorbic acid (vitamin C) This is a powerful reducing agent used in treating methemoglobinemia in conjunction with methylene blue following poisoning with benzene, lead or arsenic poisoning, nicotine intoxication, bacterial toxins, and anaphylaxis.

See also ARSENIC; BENZENE; LEAD POISONING; NICOTINE.

asp   See COBRA, EGYPTIAN.

aspartame   Sold under the trade names Nutra-Sweet Spoonful, Equal-Measure, and Equal, aspartame is an artificial sweetener discovered by accident in 1965. It is a synthetic combination of two amino acids (phenylalanine and aspartic acid).

Although it was kept off the market for many years because one animal study suggested a high incidence of brain tumors, other studies failed to duplicate these results. Eventually it proved to taste better than many alternatives on the market, and it was subsequently approved for use as a food additive after being subjected to one of the most rigorous scientific safety testings.

After more than 100 studies, however, there is still controversy over its safety. Critics say that many of the studies used by the Food and Drug Administration (FDA) to approve the use of aspartame are tainted by excessive food industry support. But FDA reviews show no adverse health effects among laboratory animals tested.

Yet complaints about aspartame accounted for between 78 and 85 percent of all complaints made to the Food and Drug Administration (FDA) from the 1970s until 1992, when the FDA stopped categorizing the complaints as a grievance against aspartame. Instead they put the complaints into general categories such as "death" or "seizure" without mentioning aspartame, even when the death or seizure was reported as a reaction to aspartame. The most common complaint was that it caused severe headaches among sensitive users. In addition, aspartame can cause severe problems for people who have phenylketonuria (PKU). Products using aspartame must carry a label to warn people with PKU disease that the product contains phenylalanine.

According to the results of a review published in *Critical Review of Toxicology* in 2007, the studies evaluated provide no evidence to support an association between aspartame and any type of cancer. The investigators concluded that the evidence from their review indicated that aspartame is safe at current consumption levels. However, another study, also published in 2007, reported the results of a carcinogenicity bioassay, which confirmed and reinforced the first experimental demonstration of aspartame's multipotential carcinogenicity at a dose close to the one deemed safe and acceptable for humans. The study also suggested that when exposure to aspartame begins at the fetal stage, the cancer-causing effects increase. Based on these findings, the National Institute of Environmental Health Sciences recommended that the FDA reevaluate its position on aspartame as being safe under all conditions.

Critics are also concerned about aspartame because it contains phenylalanine and aspartic acid, which in large doses excessively stimulate the brain, similar to the effect of monosodium glutamate (MSG). This overstimulation can damage the brain, perhaps leading to neurological diseases. Studies done on animals also suggest that children, especially infants, could be particularly vulnerable to brain damage caused by aspartate-induced overstimulation of brain cells. For this reason, some scientists recommend that pregnant women avoid using aspartame since studies suggest that—at least in animals—infants are particularly vulnerable to brain damage caused by aspartate's excess stimulation to the brain.

Because of a child's small body weight, aspartame doses per pound of body weight can easily be two to three times higher than that of an adult drinking, for example, the same amount of artificially sweetened soft drink.

While the long-term safety of aspartame has yet to be determined, large acute ingestions require only supportive therapy, if any.

Aspergillus flavus   A species of mold that produces the very toxic substance aflatoxin.

See also AFLATOXINS.

aspirin (acetylsalicylic acid)   This common pain-killer and antipyretic (fever reducer) is a slightly bitter white powder usually sold in tablet form and, in correct dosages, is not poisonous. However, in large doses (such as a child would take in swallowing a bottle of pills) it can cause acid-base imbalance, convulsions, coma and, occasionally, respiratory failure.

Salicylic acid was first isolated from willow bark in 1838, but it was another 60 years before aspirin found its way into clinical practice. Since then, aspirin and other salicylates have been the most widely used medicines in the country. Because of this extensive use, it is not surprising that a large number of overdoses—both acute and chronic—have been recorded.

In the United States, more than 200 different products contain acetylsalicylic acid (aspirin), sodium salicylate, and salicylate acid itself. Salicylates are also found in a number of products designed for topical application, where they can lead to poisoning through absorption through the skin.

There are a number of ways in which salicylate poisoning can occur. Because the metabolic pathways in young children are soon saturated by repeated excessive doses of salicylates during illnesses accompanied by fever, it is fairly easy to give too much aspirin to young children. For this reason and because of the association between aspirin given during certain illness and Reye's syndrome, pediatricians usually prefer the use of acetaminophen with young children. Frequent application of teething gels containing salicylates can also cause toxicity. In addition, deliberate suicide attempts by overdosing on aspirin are common in persons between ages 15 and 35 and sometimes occur in those as young as 8 or 10.

However, according to the poison experts, the incidence of salicylate poisoning is decreasing. Toxicity is decreasing, experts believe, primarily because less aspirin is being used by children and adults and because of child-resistant containers. Unfortunately, there has been a parallel trend of an increase in poisoning with acetaminophen, probably because of increased use of this medicine.

Symptoms
Symptoms of overdose typically appear three to six hours after ingestion and usually involve the central nervous, lung, gastrointestinal, and renal systems. Aspirin in large doses can cause abdominal pain, tinnitus (ringing in the ears), acid-base imbalance, fever, dehydration, and restlessness, while severe toxicity can result in lethargy, convulsions, coma, and respiratory failure.

Treatment
Activated charcoal should be given as soon as possible, and if bowel sounds are present, charcoal may be repeated every four hours until charcoal appears in the stool. Electrolyte abnormalities should be corrected, then alkaline diuresis (increasing production of urine) can be used to increase urine pH. In people who have ingested a large amount of salicylate, hemodialysis may be a very efficient way to eliminate it from circulation.

atropine An alkaloid frequently found in different species of nightshade that can cause problems in swallowing or speaking, rapid heartbeat, dilation of pupils, and very high fever and delirium. Atropine is extracted from deadly nightshade (belladonna) for medicinal purposes—as a premedication before general anesthesia to lessen lung secretions, or as an emergency treatment for an abnormally slow heartbeat. Most homes, in fact, have medications containing atropine, since they are widely used for eye, skin, rectal, and gastrointestinal problems.

The fatal dose of atropine is unknown; while there is wide variance in tolerance from one person to another, estimates suggest that more than 20 milligrams is fatal to children and more than 100 milligrams fatal to adults. Jimsonweed-especially the seeds—is the plant most commonly ingested, usually to obtain a "high."

In terms of benefits, atropine serves as an antidote for poisoning by organophosphate insecticides by treating SLUDGE (salivation, lacrimation, urination, diaphoresis, gastrointestinal motility, emesis), the symptoms typical of organophosphate toxicity. Atropine is also an antidote for nerve gases, including Tabun, Sarin, Soman, and VX. Some nerve gases destroy acetylcholinesterase, which prolongs the action of acetylcholine. Atropine reduces the effect of acetylcholine.

Symptoms

Symptoms of atropine poisoning include dry, burning mouth; difficulty swallowing; thirst; blurred vision; hot, dry skin; fever and tachycardia. Fever can spike to 109°F in infants. Urinary problems, confusion, mania, delirium, and psychotic behavior may continue for hours or days. With severe overdose, death can occur following circulatory and respiratory collapse.

Treatment

The treatment for atropine poisoning involves the administration of physostigmine or pilocarpine.

See also ALDICARB; ALDOMET; ALKALOIDS; ANTIHISTAMINES; BENZTROPINE; BETEL NUT SEED; CATAPRES; CHRISTMAS ROSE; CLIMBING LILY; COLOCYNTH; DEATH CAMAS; DIGITOXIN; FLY AGARIC; HENBANE; INDIAN TOBACCO; JIMSONWEED; MANDRAKE, AMERICAN; MUSCARINE; NIGHTSHADE, BITTERSWEET; NIGHTSHADE, DEADLY.

azalea See RHODODENDRON.

Bacillus anthracis This bacterium forms spores that can cause a serious disease called anthrax. _Bacillus anthracis_ is a zoonosis, which means it affects domestic and wild animals as well as humans. The fact that _B. anthracis_ forms spores makes it especially difficult to control because the spores can exist for decades in a dormant state until they find an environment favorable for rapid growth. The ability of the spores to survive extreme conditions for prolonged periods of time is one of the main reasons this bacterium has been used by terrorists.

Anthrax can appear in three different forms: cutaneous (skin), inhalational (lungs), and gastrointestinal. Most cases (95 percent) are cutaneous and they occur when the spores enter a cut or break on the skin when people handle products from infected animals. About 20 percent of untreated cases of cutaneous anthrax result in death, and deaths are rare if appropriate antibiotic therapy is initiated. Inhalational anthrax is usually fatal, and even with aggressive treatment about 50 percent of infected people die. It is contracted by breathing anthrax spores from infected animal products or, in the case of terrorism, by being deliberately exposed to the spores, as occurred in the United States in 2001 when anthrax spores were mailed to various postal facilities. The gastrointestinal form of anthrax appears after consumption of contaminated meat. Deaths typically occur in 25 to 60 percent of cases.

Symptoms

The range of symptoms differs depending on the type of anthrax that occurs. In skin anthrax, the first symptom is a small sore that develops into a blister, which then transforms into a painless ulcer with a black center. Other symptoms may include headache and malaise. A small percentage of cases becomes systemic and can be fatal. The warning symptoms of gastrointestinal anthrax are nausea, loss of appetite, bloody diarrhea, and fever, followed by stomach pain. Intestinal anthrax can become systemic and cause death. This form is rare in the United States. The most serious form is inhalational anthrax, which is marked by cold or flu symptoms followed by cough, chest discomfort, shortness of breath, muscle aches, and tiredness. Systemic infection has a mortality rate of nearly 100 percent. Symptoms for all three types of anthrax can appear within seven days of contact with the bacterium. For inhalational anthrax, symptoms can appear within a week or up to 42 days.

Treatment

To help prevent anthrax after exposure, antibiotic treatment (e.g., ciprofloxacin, levofloxacin, doxycycline, penicillin) combined with anthrax vaccine is critical and should be started immediately. Treatment after infection has occurred involves a 60-day course of antibiotics. After acute symptoms have appeared, antibiotics can kill the bacteria but will not affect the toxins that have formed. The effectiveness of treatment depends on the type of anthrax and how quickly treatment was initiated. Individuals may die within two to three days from respiratory failure, sepsis, and shock.

Prevention

An anthrax vaccine has been developed and is reportedly about 93 percent effective in preventing the disease. Immunization is not recommended for everyone. The Advisory Committee on Immunization Practices recommends the vaccine for the following people: those who work directly with the organisms in laboratories; those who work with imported animal furs or hides in areas where standards are not sufficient to prevent exposure to anthrax; people who handle potentially infected animal products in countries where incidence is high; and military personnel who are in areas with high risk for exposure to the organism. Pregnant women should be vaccinated only if absolutely necessary.

The immunization consists of three injections given two weeks apart, followed by three additional injections administered at six, 12, and 18 months. Annual booster injections are recommended thereafter.

Bacillus cereus   The *Bacillus cereus* bacteria multiplies in raw foods at room temperature, producing heat-resistant toxins most often found in steamed or refried rice. While occurrence is less common in the United States, it's likely that episodes are underreported because symptoms are so similar to other types of food poisoning. It's most commonly found in cereals (especially rice), vegetables, and pasta.

Symptoms
These bacteria produce two distinct types of food poisoning: The first features a short incubation period after eating tainted food (usually less than six hours), causing cramps and vomiting and occasionally a short bout of diarrhea. Almost 80 percent of patients with these symptoms who test positive for *B. cereus* poisoning have eaten steamed or refried rice at Chinese restaurants. The second type appears within eight to 24 hours after ingestion of tainted food and causes abdominal cramps and diarrhea with very little vomiting.

The illness is usually mild and self-limiting.

Treatment
There is no specific therapy beyond treating symptoms.

Prevention
Keep preparation surfaces clean, and don't allow leftovers to remain in the open air for long. Heat leftovers quickly, and eat them right away.

Bacillus thuringiensis (Bt)   A popular botanic insecticide, Bt is a species of bacterium sold in a variety of strains and it kills soft-bodied insects or those in their larval form. The most widely used strain kills larval caterpillars of many moths, including the gypsy moth, the cabbage moth, and the berry moth. Newly developed strains are aimed at beetle larvae (such as bean beetles and potato beetles), while others are aimed at borers. Some Bts from specialty stores combine the different strains into one superpesticide.

Bt will also kill some beneficial insects, but only in the soft-bodied larval stage. The Environmental Protection Agency (EPA) has declared Bt to be safe for humans and other mammals, birds, and fish. It is safe enough to be exempt from food residue tolerances, endangered species labeling, and groundwater restrictions.

See also BOTANIC INSECTICIDES; PESTICIDES.

BAL (2,3-dimercaptopropanol, dimercaprol, British anti-lewisite)   An antidote for mercury, copper, arsenic, gold, nickel, lead, and antimony poisoning, but less effective for silver poisoning. It may make iron, selenium, or cadmium poisoning worse, since BAL complexes act on the liver. It is best given as soon as possible following ingestion of the toxic substance.

baneberry *(Actaea)* **[Other names: black baneberry, cohosh, doll's eyes, European baneberry, herb-Christopher, necklaceweed, snakeberry, western baneberry]**   This plant of the buttercup family includes eight species of perennial herbs that grow less than 2 feet tall in richly wooded areas, boasting oversize leaves each with two or more leaflets. In warm weather (usually spring) this herb is adorned with distinct bunches of pearly white flowers at the tips of the stems. The fruit matures in late summer or early fall.

The white baneberry *(A. pachypoda* or *A. alba)* has snow-white fruit and is native to North America. The red baneberry or red cohosh *(A. rubra)* is another North American native and bears a red or ivory fruit. Cohosh, or herb Christopher *(A. spicata),* resembles *A. rubra* and has dark purple fruit sometimes used to make dye.

A. pachypoda thrives from Nova Scotia, Canada south along the east coast of the United States as far as Georgia, west to Missouri and north to Minnesota. *A. rubra* grows throughout Canada and the United States. *A. spicata* is cultivated in Canada and the United States.

Poisonous part
Only the red or white berries, foliage, and roots contain the unknown toxin, which is a fast-acting and deadly poison acting on the heart. The root is a violent purgative, irritant, and emetic. In mountain forests, the black berries are often confused with blueberries. While no loss of life has been reported in the United States, European children have died after eating baneberry fruit.

Symptoms
Prolonged contact with the skin causes skin rash. If the plant is eaten, symptoms begin within several hours to a few days, with excruciating pain and inflammation followed by blisters or open sores of the lips, tongue, mouth, and throat. Larger amounts of the plant cause vomiting streaked with bright-red blood; severe diarrhea and relentless abdominal cramps; excessive, blood-tinged urine; dizziness; fainting; and mental confusion or hallucinations. In critical cases, there are grand mal seizures.

Prognosis is guarded; often, the electrolytes and fluids of the body are depleted, and the kidneys and nervous system can sustain permanent damage if the symptoms are severe or prolonged. Death may follow if the poison is not cared for immediately.

Treatment
The irritating effects of this plant usually limit the amount ingested. Gastric lavage should be performed followed by the administration of milk or egg white as a demulcent. Renal function and fluid and electrolyte levels should be monitored.

Barbados nut *(Jatropha curcas)* **[Other names: curcus bean, kukui haole, physic nut, purge nut]** This small, spreading shade tree grows to about 15 feet and is found in southern Florida and Hawaii, Africa, Mexico, Asia, and Central and South America. Its flowers are small and green yellow, with three to five lobed leaves; it also produces a sticky sap. A resinous substance produced by insects feeding on the leaves is used to make a varnish for guitars. *Jatropha* is a genus of the spurge family found in both the Old World and New World, containing about 125 species of herbs, shrubs, and trees.

Unfortunately, while the seeds contained in the nut of this tree are extremely tasty, they contain more than 55 percent of an oil more potent than castor oil. In tropical areas the seeds are still used by folk healers, although they are quite dangerous.

Poisonous part
All parts of the Barbados nut contain the poison jatrophin, which is a harsh purgative. The poison kills by interfering with the synthesis of protein in intestinal wall cells. The seeds can be eaten if thoroughly roasted to remove the poison.

Symptoms
This plant is quickly fatal; within 15 to 20 minutes, symptoms appear: burning throat, bloating, dizziness, vomiting, diarrhea, drowsiness, leg cramps, difficulty breathing. May be fatal to children.

Treatment
Gastric lavage (unless there has been a great deal of vomiting already). Rehydration.

See also CORAL PLANT.

barbiturates A group of sedative drugs including pentobarbital (Nembutal), phenobarbital (Luminal or "downers"), secobarbital (Seconal or "reds"), thiopental (Pentothol), and amobarbital (Amytal), that work by depressing brain activity. Overdosing on barbiturates is a common cause of death from suicide. Because these drugs are highly addictive and often abused, their use today is strictly controlled. Overdose—particularly when used with alcohol—is common. The toxicity of a particular type of barbiturate depends on how quickly it is designed to act. All cause unconsciousness, and their effects depend in part on how well the liver metabolizes them.

Symptoms

Within 30 minutes (usually much sooner) sedation begins, followed by dizziness, headache, confusion, heart irregularities, low blood pressure, and then coma, which may last up to several days. While the toxicity level for barbiturates is high, they can be fatal in combination with alcohol.

Treatment

There are no direct antidotes to barbiturates. Barbiturates are quickly absorbed in the system, so gastric lavage needs to be performed no later than the first few hours after ingestion if treatment is to be effective. Even when it is performed quickly, however, often little of the drug is retrieved this way. This may be followed by repeated doses of activated charcoal. Fatality from barbiturate overdose ranges between 5 and 7 percent, but many people attempt suicide again using barbiturates. For this reason, follow-up mental health care is strongly recommended.

barium   While barium poisonings are not common, they are usually due to accidental contamination of food or a result of suicide. Water-soluble barium salts (barium acetate, carbonate, chloride, hydroxide, nitrate, sulfide) are extremely toxic, but the insoluble salt barium sulfate is not because it cannot be absorbed. The soluble barium salts are used in fireworks, depilatories, and rat poisons, and are used to manufacture glass and to dye textiles.

Symptoms

Within minutes to a few hours after ingestion, victims experience muscle weakness, followed by paralysis of the limbs and lungs, with additional heart problems. There may also be gastroenteritis with watery diarrhea, impaired vision, and central nervous system depression. However, victims usually remain conscious.

Treatment

Symptomatic treatment, with the administration of potassium chloride. Induce vomiting or perform gastric lavage; administer activated charcoal and a cathartic.

bee stings   For most Americans, a bee sting is a minor annoyance and can be fatal only if occurring in large numbers (hundreds in an adult). But between 1 million and 2 million Americans are severely allergic to the inflammatory substances in the venom of bees, wasps, hornets, and yellow jackets—which means they have been sensitized by the venom from a sting in the past so that a single subsequent sting could provoke a severe allergic reaction.

Bee stings cause three to four times more deaths in the United States than do snake bites, but the deaths are related to an individual's sensitivity, not the relative toxicity of any one insect poison. About 50 to 100 Americans die each year from bee stings. Since the bee venom toxicity is related to an individual's sensitivity and not to the venom itself, there is no bee antivenin available.

In the case of Africanized honey bees, it is often the large number of bee stings, as well as an individual's sensitivity, that causes death. Their venom is no more potent than that of native honey bees, but Africanized bees generally attack in great numbers and will pursue their prey long distances. They also will attack with little provocation, reacting to vibrations from a vehicle or noises, although many attacks occur when people disturb a hive. The first Africanized bee swarm in the United States was seen in October 1990. In July 1993, an 82-year-old man in Texas became the first person to die in the United States from Africanized honey bee stings after being stung more than 40 times.

While hornets and wasps usually do not attack unless their nest is threatened, yellow jackets are very aggressive and quick tempered. Of all the stinging insects, the most lethal is the wasp. The vicious hornet or yellow jacket (striped yellow and black) is so aggressive that it both stings and bites. Honeybees have round, smooth abdomens; bumblebees are two to three times larger than honeybees and have round, furry abdomens. Hornets, yellow jackets, and wasps have long, slender abdomens and are all usually striped yellow and black.

A bee sting activates the body's immune system, which releases antibodies that counteract the harmful effects of germs and toxins. However, some individuals release too much of this antibody, which can become life threatening.

Allergic reactions to bee stings, therefore, are more common in adults than in children because adults have had more of a chance to develop a serious allergy to the stings. Each subsequent sting usually results in a more serious allergic reaction in those already sensitized.

The severity of a sting also depends on where it is located on the body: A sting to the neck can affect breathing, and swallowing a bee can cause strangulation if the bee stings the inside of the throat.

Certain types of clothing can be good protection against a bee sting; white or light-colored clothing with a smooth finish is less likely to excite bees to attack. Leather is particularly irritating to bees, but they will also become disturbed with brightly colored, dark, rough, or wooly material. Bees also seem to become irritated over perspiration odors, perfumes, suntan lotions, and hair sprays.

To avoid being stung by bees, wasps, yellow jackets, and hornets, it is best to remain motionless and not to wave or swing your arms but to retreat slowly while protecting your face with your hands, or if possible to lie face down on the ground. An exception is an attack by Africanized honey bees or any colony of bees, in which case you should run and protect your head and face, which are the main targets of Africanized bees. If necessary, pull your shirt up over your head and seek shelter as quickly as possible.

Symptoms

When stung, allergic individuals experience soreness and swelling not only at the site of the sting but on other parts of the body as well. Symptoms in those allergic to bee stings include fever, chills, light-headedness, hives, joint and muscle pain, swelling of the lymph glands, and bronchial constriction. Other severe reactions include a sudden drop in blood pressure with loss of consciousness, difficulty breathing, shock and, occasionally, death within one hour. Multiple stings—30 or 40 insects—will cause a reaction even in an unsensitized individual, including chills, fever, vomiting, pulmonary edema, difficulty breathing, drop in blood pressure, and collapse.

Treatment

A bee will often leave its sting sac in the wound; thus to treat a sting, remove the stinger by scraping it away with a fingernail or the edge of a knife blade. Grasping it with tweezers will simply squeeze more venom into the wound. Wash the wound with soap and water and apply antiseptic and a cold compress; ice will help reduce swelling.

Pain and irritation can be relieved by applying a paste made from either baking soda and water, or meat tenderizer and water. The meat tenderizer, developed to break down meat protein, also neutralizes bee venom. For stings in the mouth or throat, give victim ice cubes to suck while seeking medical attention.

Those who have had a severe reaction should carry an emergency self-treatment kit, available only with a doctor's prescription, containing antihistamine tablets, alcohol swabs, and a preloaded syringe with epinephrine, which counteracts the allergic response of the sting. Diphenhydramine (Benadryl) can stop or slow symptoms, but it must be given immediately.

In addition, highly sensitized individuals may consider taking immunotherapy, but since this procedure carries a risk of anaphylactic shock, it should only be administered by a physician with access to epinephrine.

bellyache bush *(Jatropha gossypiifolia)* This annual found throughout the New World is a member of a large genus of shrubs or small trees with a three-sided seed capsule.

Poisonous part

The seeds are poisonous and contain a variety of toxins and cathartic oils. Ingestion of just one seed can be serious. The toxins inhibit protein synthesis in cells of the intestinal wall and may cause serious or fatal poisoning.

Symptoms

The onset of symptoms (nausea, vomiting, and diarrhea) occurs rapidly, unlike poisoning with other plants with toxic lectins.

Treatment

Treat symptoms; give fluids.

benzene This simple aromatic hydrocarbon is a common household solvent used as a cleaning agent for rubber, fats, grease paints, and lacquers and is a known carcinogen. Because of this, it has widely been replaced by toluene in many industrial products. It is no longer available for home or private use. Benzene is obtained from coke-oven gas or from petroleum, and it is highly toxic. Long-term exposure may lead to acute leukemia and aplastic anemia. Most cases of benzene poisoning are caused by skin contact or breathing fumes in poorly ventilated rooms; recent cases have been reported of fatalities following cleaning of tank cars. It may even occur after sniffing gasoline with a high benzene content.

Symptoms

Symptoms are caused by stomach irritation and benzene's depressive action on the body's central nervous system and bone marrow. Breathing these solvent fumes can cause headache, eye irritation, dizziness, visual disturbances, nausea, and euphoria; more toxic cases include tremors, delirium, unconsciousness, coma, and convulsions. In extreme cases, inhaling these fumes can be fatal.

Chronic cases of breathing benzene fumes cause a diminished production of all blood components and can lead to weakness, anorexia, and anemia, with abnormal bleeding. In cases of chronic poisoning, symptoms may not appear until months or years after contact—even after exposure to benzene has ceased.

Treatment

Call the poison control center before attempting any treatment. If fumes have been inhaled, get the victim into fresh air and give artificial respiration if needed. For skin contamination, rinse in running water for at least 15 minutes.

benzene hexachloride [Other names: gamma-hexane; 1,2,3,4,5,6-hexachlorocyclohexane; BHC; DBH; HCCH; HCH; trade name Streunex] This synthetic pesticide is found in a white crystalline, wettable powder, emulsion, dust, and solution in organic solvents. Both benzene hexachloride and lindane are moderately toxic when inhaled or absorbed and extremely poisonous if ingested. Disagreeable in odor, benzene hexachloride does not dissolve in water but is readily soluble in fats or oils and is therefore particularly dangerous if ingested after a fatty meal. Benzene hexachloride is widely used by veterinarians to combat fleas and ticks.

Symptoms

Benzene hexachloride affects the central nervous system and may cause liver and kidney damage. Symptoms appear within 30 minutes to three hours, although it may take as long as six hours before reactions appear. When benzene hexachloride is ingested, mucous membranes that touched the poison become irritated, followed by vomiting, diarrhea, and convulsions. Poisoning may be fatal, usually as a result of pulmonary edema. Bread tainted with HCH has sickened some people, including infants breastfed by women who have eaten the bread. Because benzene hexachloride is rapidly excreted by the body, chronic poisoning is unlikely.

Treatment

Symptomatic treatment.

benzodiazepines A class of drugs containing compounds that vary widely in their strength, duration, and clinical use. In general, they are given as muscle relaxants, to relieve short-term anxiety due to stress or trauma, to relieve the unpleasant delirium of alcohol withdrawal, and to help induce sleep. Fatalities from overdose of a benzodiazepine are rare, unless the drug is used with other central nervous system depressants (such as alcohol or barbiturates).

Benzodiazepines include Ativan (lorazepam), Centrax (prazepam), Dalmane (flurazepam), Librium (chlordiazepoxide), Serax (oxazepam), Tranxene (chlorazepate), and Valium (diazepam). Newer potent short-acting agents include Halcion (triazolam), Xanax (alprazolam), and Versed (midazolam). Rohypnol (flunitrazepam) is a benzodiazepine that is not legal in the United States but which is a drug of abuse, specifically as a date rape drug.

Symptoms

Most benzodiazepines are addictive, and all can be either taken by mouth or injected; a few are available as suppositories. In general, overdose symptoms include drowsiness, weakness, crossed eyes, double vision, uncoordination, and lassitude, followed by convulsions, coma, cyanosis, and breathing problems. Chronic abuse can produce a skin rash, stomach problems, headaches, and blurred vision. In all of these drugs, symptoms can appear within a few minutes to several hours. Respiratory arrest is more common with the shorter-acting drugs (Xanax, Versed, and Halcion).

Treatment

The administration of flumazenil (Mazacon) can quickly reverse a coma caused by benzodiazepine overdose.

See also DALMANE; DIAZEPAM; MIDAZOLAM.

benztropine (Cogentin) This is an antidote to many of the extrapyramidal side effects (wobbly gait, slurred speech, foaming at the mouth, forgetfulness, drooling, stiffness) sometimes seen with large doses of psychiatric drugs. It is pharmacologically similar to atropine.

See also ATROPINE.

benzylpiperazine [Street names include BZP, A2, Legal E, Legal X] First synthesized in 1944, benzylpiperazine was a potential antiparasitic drug that was later found to have both antidepressant and amphetamine-like properties, but it was never developed for the general market. Benzylpiperazine has become favored by drug abusers because of its amphetaminelike effects, and since 1996 it has been classified as a Schedule 1 controlled substance by the Drug Enforcement Administration.

Benzylpiperazine is usually taken orally as a powder, tablets, or capsules; it can also be smoked or snorted. Some abusers take it along with 1-(3-trifluoro-methyl phenyl)piperazine (TFMPP), a noncontrolled substance, in an effort to enhance its effects. Benzylpiperazine is sometimes used as a substitute for MDMA (methylenedioxymethamphetamine, or ecstasy) at raves because it reportedly causes arousal, euphoria, and a general feeling of well-being.

Symptoms

Benzylpiperazine produces a severe hangover effect after the drug wears off. Other side effects include dry mouth, urine retention, and dilated pupils. Effects of long-term use include confusion, irregular heartbeat, memory problems, and impotence, while typical overdose effects include psychotic episodes and seizures.

Treatment

Symptomatic. In New Zealand, where benzylpiperazine is legal, some manufacturers offer recovery pills, which contain vitamins and 5-HTP, which allegedly ease the hangover effect benzylpiperazine produces.

See also ECSTASY.

beryllium This hard, grayish metal is found naturally in coal, soil, mineral rocks, and volcanic dust. Beryllium compounds are mined and the beryllium is used in nuclear weapons and reactors, instruments, X-ray machines, mirrors, and aircraft and space vehicles. Beryllium ores are used to make ceramics for high-technology applications, while beryllium alloys are used in computers, sports equipment, automobiles, and dental bridges.

People who work in or live near beryllium industries have the greatest potential for exposure to the metal. Beryllium can harm the lungs if it is breathed in; the extent of the damage depends on the degree and length of exposure. Up to 15 percent of people who are exposed to beryllium on the job become sensitive to it and may develop chronic beryllium disease, an irreversible and sometimes fatal disease in which the lungs are scarred. Long-term exposure to beryllium can increase the risk of developing lung cancer.

The International Agency for Research on Cancer and the Department of Health and Human Services have determined that beryllium is a human carcinogen. The Environmental Protection Agency has categorized beryllium as a probable human carcinogen and estimated that lifetime exposure to 0.04 ug/m^3 beryllium can result in a one in 1,000 chance of developing cancer.

Beryllium enters the environment as dust from burning oil and coal and from industrial waste. The dust eventually settles on the earth and water, and the beryllium in industrial waste often ends up in waterways, where some of the compounds dissolve in water while most of them settle to the bottom.

Symptoms

People who develop chronic beryllium disease may be asymptomatic or begin with coughing, chest pain, shortness of breath, weakness, anorexia, and/or fatigue. The disease can also lead to right side heart enlargement and heart disease. Swallowing beryllium does not appear to cause effects in humans because only a minute amount of the metal is absorbed.

Treatment

Currently there is no cure for chronic beryllium disease, but treatment can help slow progression of the disease and prevent additional damage to the lungs. Immunosuppressive drugs such as prednisone are often prescribed because they help relieve symptoms while improving gas exchange between the lungs and the blood. Because prednisone can cause significant side effects, use of this drug should be discussed with a healthcare provider. Another option is oxygen therapy, which can be delivered via oxygen concentrators, compressed gas systems, or liquid systems, depending on the patient's needs. In serious circumstances, lung transplantation may be the only solution.

beta adrenergic blockers   These "beta blockers" slow the heart rate and reduce the force of the heart muscle's contraction and are used to treat high blood pressure, arrhythmias, angina, migraine headaches, and glaucoma. There are a wide variety of beta blockers, including Tenormin, Lopressor, Visken, and Inderal. People with asthma should not take beta blockers.

Symptoms

Unfortunately, the response to beta blockers varies from patient to patient, depending on overall health and other medications; it is possible to have a fatal reaction to even a normal dose. Ingestion of only two or three times the therapeutic dose should be considered to be potentially fatal for any patient. In addition, the sudden withdrawal of beta blockers can cause heart failure, especially in patients who have problems with the aorta. Many patients who overdose on beta blockers may also be taking other cardioactive drugs or have an underlying heart problem, both of which may worsen the effects of the overdose. Overdoses with beta blockers all have similar symptoms and toxicity ratings.

Treatment

Symptomatic treatment; perform gastric lavage (vomiting is not recommended because of the danger of seizures and coma). Administer activated charcoal and a cathartic. A glucagon bolus can be diagnostic and therapeutic as well. In severe cases of atenolol overdoses, hemodialysis may be useful; nadolol and sotalol are also reportedly removed by hemodialysis, while propranolol, metoprolol, and timolol are not. Hemodialysis should be considered only when treatment with glucagon and other pharmacotherapy are not successful.

betel nut seed *(Areca catechu)*   This poisonous seed is chewed for its narcotic effects by native peoples in central and southwestern Asia and South America, but too large an amount can be toxic.

Poisonous part

The seeds are considered extremely poisonous and contain the toxic alkaloid arecain and other poisons.

Symptoms

Within 20 minutes of ingestion, patients experience vomiting, diarrhea, difficulty breathing, impaired vision, convulsions, and death.

Treatment

Antidote is atropine.

birth control, botanical   From earliest times, people have searched for an herbal remedy for unwanted pregnancy; unfortunately, most plants capable of killing a fetus are also capable of killing the mother. The Amazon Indians chew the leaves of several jungle plants for contraceptive purposes, and the Chinese have used abortifacients since the ninth century.

According to Aristotle, oil from the cedar and olive prevent conception; in medieval times, onion juice smeared on the penis was supposed to work. Abortifacients over the centuries include thyme, rue, mugwort, ergot, iris, and pennyroyal; a chemical from the English yew was so widely used for abortion that the plant was known as the "bastard killer."

See also ERGOT; PENNYROYAL OIL; YEW.

birth control pills Medication containing progesterone or estrogen (or derivatives) used for the prevention of pregnancy. At present, they are not considered toxic when ingested accidentally by children.

bisphenol-A Also known as BPA, bisphenol-A is a controversial plastic chemical that may or may not pose a health hazard, depending on which research and/or researchers people choose to believe. Bisphenol-A, which is found in polycarbonate plastic and in epoxy resins, is used in a wide range of products, from water and baby bottles to the lining of metal products (including cans for food), a plastic coating for children's teeth to prevent cavities, refrigerator shelving, microwave ovenware, and eating utensils. It is also found in flooring, enamels and varnishes, adhesives, artificial teeth, nail polish, compact discs, and in parts of automobiles, tools, electrical appliances, and office instruments. High levels of bisphenol-A are known to disrupt hormone levels in the body.

There are two main views on the safety of bisphenol-A. One is that the plastic poses virtually no health threat. That is the opinion the European Food Safety Authority (EFSA) and the Food and Drug Administration took in summer 2008. The EFSA reviewed the research on bisphenol-A, much of which has been done on rodents, and concluded that bisphenol-A passes through the human body

much faster than it does in rodents and thus there is little chance that it can harm humans. This view conflicts with that of the U.S. government scientists at the National Toxicology Program (NTP), who said that based on results of studies done in rodents, there was concern about bisphenol-A because animal studies suggested low doses can cause changes in behavior and the brain, and that it may reduce birth weight and survival in fetuses. The NTP report initiated publicity which prompted questions among the general public about the safety of bisphenol-A and for some major retailers, including Wal-Mart, who decided to turn away baby bottles that contain bisphenol-A.

Other experts state that bisphenol-A poses at least a reasonable threat to health and thus should be banned, or, at the least, exposure should be severely limited. Canadian health officials, for example, announced their intention to ban the use of the chemical in baby bottles, and state and federal lawmakers have introduced legislation to ban the chemical's use in products made for children. As of August 2008, California and at least ten other states were considering bills to restrict use of the chemical. More than 6 billion pounds of the chemical are produced in the United States each year.

According to laboratory tests spearheaded by the Environmental Working Group in 2007, more than 50 percent of 97 cans of commonly eaten foods that were evaluated contained bisphenol-A. Ten percent of all canned food tested and 33 percent of infant formula tested contained enough BPA to expose a woman or infant to BPA levels more than 200 times the government's traditional safe level of exposure for industrial chemicals. Unfortunately, the government has not set safety standard limits for BPA in canned food, even though scientists have found exceedingly high levels in so many of these items. According to the Centers for Disease Control and Prevention, about 93 percent of Americans have traces of bisphenol in their urine.

black locust *(Robinia pseudoacacia)* [Other names: bastard acacia, black acacia, false acacia, green locust, pea flower locust, post locust, silver chain, treesail, white honey flower, white locust, yellow locust.] The towering locust tree can grow to be 80 feet tall and is found particularly in the eastern United States from Pennsylvania through Georgia, in the Smoky Mountains and the Ozarks.

Its compound leaves have a series of leaflets one inch long and a pair of woody thorns where the leaf stem emerges from the branch. The fragrant white flower clusters produce a flat, reddish brown fruit pod that remains over the winter months.

Poisonous part

The poison is a phytotoxin called "robin," a plant lectin (toxalbumin) that interferes with the synthesis of protein in the small intestine. It is particularly prevalent in the inner bark, seeds, and leaves.

Symptoms

Appearing within one or more hours, symptoms include nausea, vomiting, diarrhea, stupor, weak pulse, and gastroenteritis. Poisoning may be followed by shock, convulsions, and death, although these are uncommon.

Treatment

Gastric lavage; fluid and electrolyte level correction; oral administration of magnesium sulfate.

See also PHYTOTOXINS.

black snake, Australian *(Pseudeschis porphyriacus)*

The most common of the poisonous Australian snakes, the black snake has a blue-black body with a small head and a red belly and is found in marshy areas of Australia. Others in the same group include the spotted black snake *(P. guttatus)* and the mulga *(P. australis)*. Note: The Australian black snake should not be confused with the American black snake, a common—and nonpoisonous—snake.

Poisonous part

Its venom is a powerful anticoagulant.

Symptoms

Within 15 to 30 minutes symptoms appear: pain, swelling, a drop in blood pressure, confusion, slurring of speech, dilation of the pupils, strabismus (abnormal deviation of one eye in relation to the other), drooping of the upper eyelid, and muscle weakness. The respiratory muscles are affected last,

and respiratory muscle paralysis is the most common cause of death.

Treatment

Australian black snake antiserum should be used.

See also ANTIVENIN; SNAKES, POISONOUS.

black widow spider [Other names: button spider (South Africa), karakurt (Russia), katipo (New Zealand), malmignatte (Mediterranean).]

One of two species of poisonous spiders found in the United States, the black widow has a globe-shaped, shiny black body with a red or orange hourglass-shaped mark on its belly. On some spiders, there are several triangles or spots instead of the well-known hourglass shape. Male spiders, much smaller than the female, may have only a small, reddish dot on their belly and are not considered dangerous. Reluctant to bite humans, black widows are responsible for about three deaths in the United States each year. All six species of black widow are venomous, but none are usually fatal.

In the past, however, they were responsible for a number of deaths—particularly during swarms, recorded in Spain in 1833 and 1841 and in Sardinia in 1833 and 1839, when many people were bitten and some died. In addition, the Gosiute Indians of Utah mixed the venom of the black widow and the rattlesnake to coat their arrowheads.

Black widow spiders build their messy, tangled webs under or between rocks, under loose bark, around outdoor water faucets, and in woodpiles, garages, basements, garbage cans, and sheds. They also hide in cushions and under toilet lids, so that the most common and deadly bites are on the genitals. Although they are found throughout the United States and Canada, most inhabit warmer regions of the United States. They are also found in Mexico, Central America and the Antilles, and the western part of South America.

The brown widow *(L. geometrieus)* lives in the tropics and bears the same markings as the black widow, but it rarely bites humans.

Poisonous part

The venom of the black widow spider is a neurotoxin that acts on the nerve endings, destroying peripheral nerve endings and causing an ascending paralysis, usually affecting muscles in the thigh, shoulder, and back first.

Symptoms

The bite of a black widow is not extremely painful and may not be felt at all. There may be slight swelling and two tiny puncture marks at the wound site, and following the bite there is a dull, numbing pain increasing in intensity, peaking in one to three hours and continuing up to 48 hours. Within 10 to 40 minutes after the bite, the venom attacks the nerves, causing abdominal or chest muscles to become rigid and flu-like symptoms to appear. At the same time, there is stomach pain and muscle spasms in the extremities, along with difficulty in breathing and swallowing, chills, urinary retention, sweating, convulsions, paralysis, delirium, nausea, vomiting, drooping eyelids, headache, and fever. When death occurs, it is due to cardiac failure. Most victims recover without serious complications.

Treatment

Antivenin is available, but most people can be managed without using the equine-derived antivenin. However, it may be needed for elderly patients and children, who do not respond to more conventional therapy for high blood pressure, muscle cramps, or respiratory distress, or for pregnant women threatening premature labor. Apply an ice pack to the bite site and elevate the affected limb to heart level. Cleanse the wound and treat infection, give a tetanus shot if needed and monitor for at least six to eight hours. Muscle cramping may be treated with intravenous calcium or muscle relaxants; pain may be treated with morphine. Keep the victim warm and quiet and call a physician immediately.

bleach See ALKALINE CORROSIVES.

blister beetle Any of the more than 2,000 species of the insect family Meloidae, found throughout the Midwest and the eastern United States. These beetles secrete an irritating substance called can-

tharidin, collected from the European species *Lytta vesicatoria* (or Spanish fly). Powdered cantharidin is used as a topical skin irritant to remove warts and is also intensely irritating to the mucous membranes. Although Spanish fly has a reputation as an aphrodisiac, it is in fact deadly poisonous and often fatal.

Poisonous part

Blister beetle venom contains large amounts of cantharidin, which produces painful blisters and reddening when it comes in contact with the skin.

Symptoms

A large, painful blister with erythema following contact with the toxic substance secreted by the blister beetle.

Treatment

Ice packs to relieve pain; corticosteroid cream is helpful.

See also CANTHARIDIN.

bloodroot *(Sanguinaria canadensis)* This bitter-tasting perennial herb is considered to be very toxic and is found from southern Canada to Florida and as far west as Texas. It has shiny white poppy-like flowers that appear in early spring and when squeezed can produce a red juice. Bloodroot extract is used commercially as a dental plaque inhibitor. Bloodroot is usually found in woodlands and along fence rows.

Poisonous part

All parts of the plant contain the poison sanguinarine, which reduces the heart's action and muscle strength and is a nerve depressant. All parts are toxic when eaten; the red sap can cause a painful skin rash upon contact.

Symptoms

Appearing within one to two hours after ingestion, symptoms include violent vomiting, thirst, burning and soreness in the throat, heaviness of the chest, breathing problems, dilated pupils, faintness, and cardiac paralysis resulting in death.

Treatment

Gastric lavage and symptomatic treatment.

blowfish   See PUFFERFISH.

boomslang *(Dispholidus typus)*   Found in Africa, this is a dangerously venomous snake of the family Colubridae, the only rear-fanged colubrid that is dangerous to humans. Its venom is lethal in even the smallest quantities.

The boomslang lives in savannas throughout sub-Saharan Africa and easily blends into its surroundings, changing its skin and eye color, which makes it difficult to spot. When looking for prey, it can lie in a bush or tree, partly extended into the air for long periods of time. When provoked, the boomslang hisses and inflates its neck, showing the dark skin between the scales, and then strikes. However, it is normally a mild-mannered and placid snake that spends all its time in trees. It comes in two colors: a brownish gray and a vivid green.

Symptoms

Pain, swelling, hemorrhage, bleeding from nose and mouth, headache, vomiting, collapse, and death. The venom of the boomslang is fatal in tiny amounts.

Treatment

Antivenin is available.

See also ANTIVENIN; SNAKES, POISONOUS.

boric acid   This white, crystalline powder is used as an antiseptic and, in diluted amounts, to treat eye irritations. It is also used as a roach poison, food preservative and a buffer in talcum powder. The use of boric acid in large amounts on broken skin or mucous membranes is toxic. It is no longer added to baby powders, and the use of boric acid should be strongly discouraged in any products for infants.

While boric acid is fairly safe when used appropriately, it can be extremely dangerous and is toxic to all cells—especially those in the kidneys.

Symptoms

Primary symptoms are reddened, flaking skin, weight loss and hair loss, together with symptoms similar to those of toxic shock: fever, vomiting, dehydration, anuria, and convulsions.

Treatment

For ingestion, immediately perform gastric lavage followed by the administration of cathartics. For skin contamination, thoroughly wash the skin. Symptomatic treatment, including phenobarbital or diazepam to control convulsions.

See also BORON.

boron   This natural element is often combined with other substances to form compounds called borates. Borate compounds include boric acid, salts of borates, and boron oxide. Borates are used in industry to produce glass, fire retardants, cosmetics, photographic materials, soaps, cleaners, and wood preservatives. It is also used in leather tanning and high-energy fuel.

People are exposed to boron in food (primarily fruits and vegetables), in cosmetics and laundry products, and it is also widely distributed in ground water and surface water. Employees of borax mining and refining plants, as well as facilities where boric acid is manufactured, are also exposed to boron.

The Environmental Protection Agency (EPA) has determined that exposure to boron in drinking water at concentrations of 4 parts per million for one day or 0.9 parts per million for ten days should not cause any adverse effects in children. The Agency has also stated that a lifetime exposure to 1 parts per million of boron is not expected to cause any adverse effects.

Symptoms

Breathing moderate levels of boron in the workplace or when using certain products can result in productive cough and in irritation to the nose, eyes, and throat. Boron toxicity may cause rash, nausea, vomiting (may be blue-green in color), diarrhea, stomach pain, hypotension, and headache. Fever, hyperthermia, seizures, and tremors have also been reported. Ingestion of large amounts of boron can cause hair loss and damage to the brain, kidneys, liver, intestines, and testes, and can eventually lead to death. The acute toxic dose for adults is from 20 to 60 grams taken in a single dose, but infants have died after taking 5 grams, although others have survived after being given 9 grams of boric acid.

Some research indicates that boron increases blood levels of estrogen and testosterone as well as vitamin D2, calcium, copper, magnesium, and thyroxine (thyroid hormone), and that it reduces blood levels of insulin, phosphorus, and calcitonin.

Treatment

Symptomatic.

botanic insecticides Insecticides prepared from plant sources. Although many people choose "organic" botanic insect controls because they somehow seem safer than inorganic chemicals, they can still be poisonous. Because they have natural sources, botanic insecticides break down quickly in the environment and are consumed by soil microbes or—in the case of insect diseases—dissipate when there is no longer anything to infect. But they are still poisons; in fact, many of these compounds are extremely toxic—some more so than their manufactured "chemical" cousins. Most are deadly to a wide range of insects (both the "good" and "bad" insects); and some are toxic to birds, other animals, and humans. Botanic insecticides include nicotine, pyrethrin/pyrethrum, rotenone, neem, ryania, Bacillus thuringiensis (Bt), and sabadilla. Because they are derived from plants, contact with some of these (such as pyrethrins) can result in an allergic reaction.

See also BACILLUS THURINGIENSIS (BT); NICOTINE; PYRETHRIN; PYRETHRUM; ROTENONE.

botulin antitoxin The antidote to poisoning by the various strains of *Clostridium botulinum* (A, B, and E) that cause botulism. The antibodies bind and inactivate freely circulating botulin toxins, but they do not remove toxin that has already bound to nerve terminals and will not reverse paralysis that has already begun. Therefore, treatment within 24 hours of the onset of symptoms may shorten the course of the poisoning and may prevent total paralysis. Botulin antitoxin is not recommended in the treatment of infant botulism.

See also BOTULIN/BOTULINUM TOXIN; BOTULISM; BOTULISM, INFANT.

botulin/botulinum toxin The toxin produced by the single-celled botulinum bacterium; it is the most poisonous substance in the world—6 million times more toxic than rattlesnake venom. When ingested, it causes botulism, a form of food poisoning that can cause muscle paralysis and death.

Despite its deadly reputation, however, botulin is also used in small doses to treat various medical conditions and for cosmetic reasons. For decades it has been administered to manage uncontrollable blinking (blepharospasm), misaligned eyes (strabismus), and cervical dystonia, a neurological disorder that causes severe neck and shoulder muscle contractions. In 2002, botulin injections (Botox) were approved as a temporary treatment to minimize frown lines in the face, which it does by weakening or paralyzing certain muscles or by blocking certain nerves. These effects last about three to four months, after which a repeat treatment is needed. Side effects may include pain at the injection site, flulike symptoms, headache, and upset stomach.

botulism The most serious type of food poisoning, poisoning by the *Clostridium botulinum* toxin is rare and very deadly—two-thirds of those afflicted die, and the rest face a long recovery period. Botulism is more common in the United States than anywhere else in the world owing to the popularity here of home canning; there are about 20 cases of food-borne botulism poisoning each year. Botulism got its name during the 1800s from *botulus*, the Latin word for sausage, in the wake of poisoning from contaminated sausages.

The *C. botulinum* toxin is found in air, water, and food as inactive spores that are harmless—until the spores are deprived of oxygen, such as inside a sealed can or jar. If conditions are favorable, the spores will begin to grow, producing one of the most deadly toxins known to humans—6 million times more deadly than cobra venom.

Cases of botulism from commercially canned food are rare because of strict health standards enforced by the Food and Drug Administration, and most incidences of botulism occur during errors in home canning. Still, it is easy to prevent, since botulism is killed when canned food is boiled at 212°F for one minute or if the food is first sterilized by pressure cooking at 250°F for 30 minutes.

While the tightly fitted lids of home-canned food will provide the anaerobic environment necessary for the growth of botulism toxins, the spores will not grow if the food is very acidic, sweet, or salty, such as canned fruit juice, jams and jellies, sauerkraut, tomatoes, and heavily salted hams. Canned foods that are highly susceptible to contamination include green beans, beets, peppers, corn, and meat. Although the spores can survive boiling, the ideal temperature for their growth is between 78°F and 96°F. They can also survive freezing.

Even though botulism spores are invisible, it's possible to tell if food is spoiled by noticing if jars have lost their vacuum seal; when the spores grow, they give off gas that makes cans and jars lose the seal. Jars will burst or cans will swell. Any food that is spoiled or whose color or odor doesn't seem right inside a home-canned jar or can should be thrown away without tasting or even sniffing, since botulism can be fatal in extremely small amounts. Botulism can also occur if the *C. botulinum* bacteria in the soil enters the body through an open wound.

Symptoms

Onset of symptoms may be as soon as three hours or as late as 14 days after ingestion, they include nausea, vomiting, diarrhea, stomach cramps, weakness, blurred vision, headache, difficulty in swallowing, slurred speech, drooping eyelids, dilated pupils, and paralysis progressing to the respiratory muscles. The earlier the onset of symptoms, the more severe the reaction. Symptoms generally last between three and six days; death occurs in about 70 percent of untreated cases, usually from suffocation as a result of respiratory muscle paralysis. In infants, symptoms may go unrecognized by parents for some time until the poisoning has reached a critical stage. Infant botulism symptoms include constipation, facial muscle flaccidity, sucking problems, irritability, lethargy, and floppy baby syndrome.

Treatment

Prompt administration of the antitoxin (type ABE botulinus) lowers the risk of death to 25 percent. The Centers for Disease Control and Prevention in Atlanta, Georgia, is the only agency with the antitoxin, and it makes the decision to treat. Local health departments should be called first for this information. Emesis is indicated immediately following ingestion of food known to contain botulism toxin. But since emesis may not be complete and the disease can occur with a small amount of toxin, botulism may still develop. Patients with symptoms should not have lavage or an emetic. Enemas may be necessary. Patients are usually put on a respirator to ease breathing difficulties. In infant botulism, if symptoms are present, it is often too late to administer antitoxin, since the damage probably has already been done by the toxin. However, it is still possible to try.

See also BOTULIN ANTITOXIN; BOTULIN/BOTULINUM TOXIN; BOTULISM, INFANT.

botulism, infant   Unlike botulism in adults, which occurs after eating contaminated food, infant botulism is caused by the production of toxin produced by *C. botulinum* in the infant's intestinal tract. While it is believed that adults, children, and infants consume *C. botulinum* spores on a regular basis—since they are present in a wide variety of foods, house dust, etc.—for some reason the intestinal tracts of some infants under age one are susceptible to the spores. In particular, there appears to be a link between spores and honey; infants have died from eating honey contaminated with the spores, and for this reason, children under age one should never be fed honey.

Since researchers have not yet discovered why some infants appear to be susceptible to the botulism spores, parents are advised to keep rooms dust free and not to feed honey or corn syrups. Commercially prepared foods that are sterilized and contain low acid are botulism free. Research also suggests that mother's milk may also provide some immunological protection against infant botulism, although this has not yet been proven. A human-derived antitoxin is now available to treat infant botulism. Called Botulism Immune Globulin Intravenous (BIG-IV), it should be given as soon as possible after botulism is identified. Results of a five-year, double-blind, placebo-controlled trial found that infants who were treated with BIG-IV, when compared with controls, had a significant mean reduction in the length of the hospital stay, from 5.7 weeks to 2.6 weeks, as well as a reduced mean duration of stay in intensive care by 3.2 weeks, reduced use of mechanical ventilation by 2.6 weeks, and reduced use of tube or intravenous feeding by 6.4 weeks. Hospital costs were also significantly reduced. No adverse side effects were noted associated with use of BIG-IV.

See also BOTULIN ANTITOXIN; BOTULIN/BOTULINUM TOXIN; BOTULISM.

brewer's yeast   Once an antidote for thallium ingestion (found in depilatories and rat poison); it is no longer routinely used.

See also THALLIUM.

bromates (potassium bromate)   A corrosive poison once widely used (between the 1940s and the 1970s) in the neutralizer solutions of home permanent kits. While less toxic substances have now been substituted for products offered to consumers in the home, poisonings do still occur from products used by professionals. Bromates may still be found in commercial bakeries (bromate salts improve bread texture) and in the production of some types of explosives. They have been banned by many countries, including Canada and England.

Poisonous part

Bromate is usually found as a 3 percent solution with water and must be taken orally to be toxic. It becomes poisonous when the hydrochloric acid in the stomach turns the potassium bromate into hydrogen bromate, an irritating acid.

Symptoms

Within five to 20 minutes after ingestion, bromates can cause vomiting, collapse, diarrhea, abdominal

pain, lethargy, deafness, coma, convulsions, low blood pressure, kidney damage, and a skin rash.

Treatment

Gastric lavage or an enema, with solutions containing sodium bicarbonate; sodium thiosulfate is given intravenously as an antidote.

bromide   This former sedative was once found in over-the-counter products ranging from Bromo-Seltzer and Dr. Miles' Nervine, but today it is rarely used because of its potential toxicity. It can be found occasionally in well water and in some bromide-containing hydrocarbons. Because bromide affects not just the skin and stomach but the brain, and thus can cause a variety of aberrant behaviors, bromide exposure in the past was responsible for a number of admissions to psychiatric hospitals.

Symptoms

Nausea, vomiting, gastric irritation, lethargy, confusion, hallucinations, psychosis, weakness, stupor, coma, anorexia, constipation, and rashes.

Treatment

There is no specific antidote, but because bromide is excreted entirely by the kidneys, intravenous administration of sodium chloride will enhance elimination. Induce vomiting or perform gastric lavage if ingestion has been recent.

bronchial tube relaxers   Also called bronchial tube dilators, these drugs are used to alleviate asthma, bronchitis, and emphysema and to relieve spasms and tightness in the chest. They can be fatal if used in excessive amounts. Bronchial tube dilators also cause serious side effects if taken with or soon after another bronchial tube relaxer or decongestant pills or liquid. These drugs are dangerous when taken with antihypertensives, epinephrine and lithium. If taken with beta blockers, the effect of both drugs is diminished.

Symptoms

In large doses, bronchial fluid builds up and causes inflammation, pounding heartbeat, dizziness, nervousness, bad taste in the mouth, dry mouth, headache, insomnia, anxiety, tension, blood pressure changes, flushing, sweating, angina, and arm pain. Overdoses can cause convulsions, low potassium levels, hallucinations, serious breathing problems, fever, chills, vomiting, clammy skin, spike in blood pressure, and stroke.

Treatment

Administer oxygen and treat symptoms as needed.

brown recluse spider *(Loxosceles reclusa)* **[Other names: fiddleback or violin spider.]** The brown recluse is one of two species of poisonous spiders found in the United States and is by far the most dangerous of the spider family—ounce for ounce, its venom is more deadly than that of many poisonous snakes.

Native to Central and South America, the brown recluse is thought to have been inadvertently imported to the United States in crates of fruit and vegetables within the last 50 years. Since then, it has been making its way steadily north and westward and is now found ranging to Texas and Arkansas and as far north as Massachusetts.

Its brown or fawn-colored body is about a half inch long and has a dark, violin-shaped mark on its back. Although brown recluse spiders are sometimes found outdoors, most live in houses, spinning their webs in dark areas inside homes or outbuildings. They get their name from their habit of hiding in closets, dresser drawers, the folds of clothing, garages, attics, and sheds. Brown recluse spiders are not aggressive and will try to escape, not attack; but if trapped, they will bite. The venom of females is more deadly than that of males.

Symptoms

The bite of a brown recluse causes little pain, but within two to eight hours the pain will be severe and the area of the bite will become red. Any place on the skin the spider has bitten will necrose and die. Brown recluse venom contains a substance that is very destructive to tissue and causes a large, spreading sore that eventually turns into a blister, becoming dark and hard within four days. In some cases, this sore becomes star shaped and deep purple and within two weeks forms an open ulcer, although the venom does not necessarily kill. As this ulcer heals, it often becomes infected; in a very small percentage of victims the ulcer does not heal for an extremely long time.

The bite can also cause a range of systemic reactions, including fever, chills, weakness, nausea, vomiting, joint pain, and sometimes a generalized rash or reddish spots. Death, when it does come, usually occurs within the first 48 hours as a result of renal failure because of blood coagulation.

Treatment

There is no specific antivenin, although antivenin for other species of brown spiders of South America should give protection. Since this antivenin contains norepinephrine, administration of phentolamine may help head off swelling and necrosis. Antihistamines, muscle relaxants, and adrenocortical steroids may provide some relief. Exchange transfusion may be attempted. Immediate excision of the bite area may be the only way to prevent the massive necrosis caused by the brown recluse venom, although not all experts agree on this treatment. Most physicians will not touch the lesion until all destruction has been done, sometimes as long as 40 weeks after the bite. Skin grafts may be necessary to heal the ulcer. If the bite of a brown recluse is suspected, a physician should be called at once.

See also ANTIVENIN; SPIDER, POISONOUS.

brown snake *(Demansia textilis)* Found in Australia, the brown snake includes any of several species named for their primary color, ranging from light brown to dark green. This slender member of the cobra family can be about 7 feet long and is extremely bad tempered and poisonous. When threatened, it will rear and strike repeatedly. It is responsible for more deaths in Australia than any other snake. Brown snakes found in the Western Hemisphere are sometimes also called grass snakes, ranging from Canada to Honduras, and are harmless.

Symptoms

Symptoms can take up to 12 hours to appear and include abdominal pain, staggering gait, problems in swallowing, stiff jaws, respiratory distress, coma, cardiac failure, and death.

Treatment

Copperhead antivenin is used for this snakebite.
See also ANTIVENIN; COBRA; SNAKES, POISONOUS.

brown spider   See BROWN RECLUSE SPIDER.

bryony (*Bryonia dioica, B. alba* or *B. cretica*)   Also called the devil's turnip or British mandrake, bryony is considered to be very toxic (fewer than 40 berries will kill an adult). A common climbing plant in public gardens with pretty red berries and black and yellow seeds, bryony blooms in the summer and is found in England, Wales, and other northern countries. The entire plant has a foul-smelling milky juice, and its fleshy white roots can be mistaken for turnips or parsnips. When the berries are distilled, the resulting beverage can cause abortions. Medically, it can be used as a diuretic.

Poisonous part

Roots and berries contain the poisons glycoside, bryonin, and bryonidin.

Symptoms

Within several hours after ingestion, victims experience burning mouth, nausea, vomiting, diarrhea, convulsions, paralysis, and coma; death follows because of respiratory arrest. The juice can also irritate the skin and cause a rash.

Treatment

Perform gastric lavage, while keeping the victim warm and quiet. Replace fluids and monitor electrolyte levels, and provide pain medication as needed.
See also GLYCOSIDE.

buckeye *(Aesculus)* [Other names: conquerors, horse chestnut, fish poison.]   These trees—consisting of about 13 species—have white, pink, yellow, and red clusters of flowers and compound leaves. The seed pod is leathery, with glossy brown seeds bearing a brown scar. The trees are found in the central and eastern temperate zones to the Gulf Coast and California and in parts of Canada.

Poisonous part

Flowers, nuts, sprouts, and twigs are toxic and contain a mixture of cytotoxic saponins known as aescin.

Symptoms

Because the saponins are not well absorbed, poisoning is generally not fatal unless as a result of frequent exposure. In addition, the unpleasant taste usually prohibits ingestion in large enough quantities to kill. Generally, symptoms are limited to severe gastroenteritis, inflammation of mucous membranes, depression, weakness, and paralysis. However, there have been reports of fatalities among children.

Treatment

Gastric lavage, general treatment for gastroenteritis, with fluid and electrolyte replacement and administration of oral magnesium sulfate.
See also SAPONIN.

bushmaster *(Lachesis muta)* One of the larger and most dangerous South American pit vipers is the bushmaster, which is found in tropical forests from Costa Rica to the Amazon Basin. The longest venomous snake in the New World (it can grow up to 12 feet long), the bushmaster can be either tan or pink with dark diamond markings, and while this snake is rarely seen, its bite is potentially lethal.

The bushmaster is the only American pit viper that lays eggs.

Symptoms

Within a very short time, victims begin bleeding from the gums, nose, and eyes and experience chills, fever, sweating, falling blood pressure, convulsions, and death. In cases of a severe bite, the victim will also experience swelling above the elbows or knees within two hours.

Treatment

Death from heart failure is unavoidable unless antivenin is given quickly.
See also ANTIVENIN; PIT VIPERS; SNAKES, POISONOUS.

buttercup *(Ranunculus)* [Other names: bassinet, blister flower, butter-cress, butter daisy, butter-flower, crowfoot, devil's claws, figwort, goldballs, goldweed, horse gold, hunger weed, lesser celandine, pilewort, ram's claws, St. Anthony's turnip, sitfast, spearwort, starve-acre, water crowfoot.]   Annual or perennial herbs that grow in wet, moist, or swampy places throughout the United States and Canada. They range in height from a few inches to 3 feet tall, with yellow, red, or white flowers.

Poisonous part

The sap and roots are toxic and contain protoanemonin, a direct irritant and vesicant of the skin and mucous membranes.

Symptoms

After ingestion, symptoms include severe pain, swelling, and blisters in the mouth, followed by bloody diarrhea and painful abdominal cramps. The toxin, which affects the central nervous system, also causes systemic symptoms including dizziness and sometimes convulsions.

Treatment

Because of the intense pain following ingestion, large amounts of this plant are generally not eaten. If this is the case, gastric lavage is recommended followed by the administration of demulcents (such as milk); give plenty of fluids and monitor kidney function.

cadmium Found in sulfide ores (together with zinc and lead), cadmium is used in electroplating, as a pigment and stabilizer in plastics, in soldering and welding and in nickel-cadmium batteries. Solder made of cadmium used for water pipes, and cadmium pigments in pottery, can contaminate water and acidic food.

Symptoms

Cadmium fumes and dust are at least 60 times more toxic than other forms, causing chemical pneumonitis and pulmonary edema and hemorrhage, in addition to coughs, wheezing, headache, and fever. Symptoms appear within 12 to 24 hours after inhalation. Ingested cadmium, on the other hand, affects the gastrointestinal tract and the kidneys, causing nausea, vomiting, cramps, diarrhea, and death as a result of shock or acute kidney failure. The kidney damage is irreversible.

Treatment

There is no evidence that chelation therapy is effective. In cases of inhalation poisoning: Monitor blood and general condition; remove the victim from exposure and give supplemental oxygen if necessary. For ingestion: Treat fluid loss; perform gastric lavage but do not induce vomiting because cadmium salts are an irritant; and administer activated charcoal (but do not give cathartics in the presence of diarrhea).

caffeine This alkaloid is one of the most widely consumed drugs in the United States and is contained in a wide variety of products, including coffee, chocolate, medications, and over-the-counter stimulants.

In one recent study, about 30 percent of Americans said they drank between five and 10 cups of coffee a day, resulting in a daily dose of 500 to 600 milligrams of caffeine daily.

Caffeine can be found naturally in kola nuts, cocoa beans, tea leaves, and coffee beans. This white, odorless, crystalline powder was first extracted from plants in 1820. Caffeine is quickly absorbed orally, rectally, and through the skin and is rapidly metabolized and excreted. At one time, it was often combined with aspirin and phenacetin in a wide range of prescription and over-the-counter medications, and it is still included today in many analgesics, stimulants, and cold preparations available without a prescription.

It is believed that caffeine affects the synthesis and release of catecholamines (especially the stress hormone norepinephrine), and after ingestion, it quickly disperses throughout all organ systems, crossing both the blood-brain barrier and the placenta. At high doses, it affects blood vessels, breathing, the brain, and the spinal cord.

In newborns, however, the metabolism of caffeine is markedly delayed, which contributes to caffeine toxicity in infants exposed to the substance.

Symptoms

Caffeine toxicity can be chronic or acute, but despite its extreme popularity, few deaths have been recorded. The acute lethal dose of caffeine in adults may be as low as 6 grams, although the dose is much lower for children. One gram can cause symptoms of toxicity.

Chronic "caffeinism" is caused by constantly consuming products containing caffeine, such as colas and chocolates. The effects might include headache, indigestion, insomnia, restlessness,

AMOUNTS OF CAFFEINE IN COMMON PRODUCTS

Source	Amount*	Dose
Beverages		
Brewed coffee	85–120 mg	cup
Instant coffee	60–100 m	cup
Cola**	25–60 mg	glass
Tea	30–75 mg	cup
Cocoa	6–42 mg	cup
Decaffeinated coffee	2–6 mg	cup
Medications		
Migraine drugs	50–100 mg/dose	
Analgesics	15–40 mg/dose	
Cough/cold	15–125 mg/dose	
Over-the-counter stimulants	65–250 mg/dose	

* Approximation based on range gathered from several sources
** Caffeine-containing colas only

nervousness, confusion, tremors, constipation, fever, and sensory disturbances.

Toxic symptoms can appear in adults after one gram of oral caffeine. Victims of caffeine toxicity often complain of irregular heartbeat and nervousness, together with sleeplessness, excitement, and mild delirium. In severe cases of overdose, symptoms include loss of consciousness, rapid heartbeat, irregular heart rhythms, seizures, and caffeine-induced psychosis. A number of deaths have reportedly occurred following caffeine-induced seizures. There have also been cases in which caffeine has worsened the symptoms of persons already suffering from schizophrenia or manic-depression. The most widespread and chronic symptom of caffeine is a severe headache upon withdrawal, although the reason behind this is not known.

Treatment

Gastric lavage, with supportive and symptomatic treatment including withholding further caffeine. To control seizures, diazepam and phenobarbital can be administered. Cardiac evaluation is essential, as death is most commonly due to arrhythmia. Specific treatment may be necessary.

calcium   Necessary for the normal function of a wide variety of enzymes and organ systems in the body, calcium is used in the treatment of poisoning by fluoride, oxalate, phosphate, or the intravenous anticoagulant citrate. It is also helpful in the treatment of muscle cramping or rigidity following black widow spider bites. Calcium overdose can cause kidney stones, constipation, and calcium deposits in the body. Recommended upper limits is 2,500 milligrams a day.

See also BLACK WIDOW SPIDER; FLUORIDE; OXALATES; PHOSPHATE ESTERS.

calcium EDTA   This chelating agent is used in the treatment of acute and chronic lead poisoning and may also be helpful to treat poisoning with manganese, zinc, chromium, nickel, or heavy radioisotopes. It is not effective in the treatment of mercury, gold, or arsenic poisoning.

See also ARSENIC; LEAD POISONING; MERCURY.

calcium oxalate   See OXALATES.

California mussel *(Mytilus californianus)*   These mollusks become poisonous to eat because of feeding on toxic one-celled animals called dinoflagellates.

See also DINOFLAGELLATE; PARALYTIC SHELLFISH POISONING; SHELLFISH POISONING.

camphor   This respiratory aid and mild local anesthetic is found in mothballs and liniments; the related compound camphorated oil (a 20 percent solution of camphor in oil) is highly toxic but was banned by the Food and Drug Administration in 1982. Both the ingestion of camphor and the prolonged inhalation of camphor vapors can be toxic. Because of its strong medicinal odor, camphor is included in a large number of over-the-counter products. Camphor is rated as very toxic, with a lethal dose of 50 to 500 milligrams per kilogram. According to the Food and Drug Administration, in 1979 alone there were 768 cases of camphor poisoning and more than 20 fatalities. All of these fatalities were the result of either a child accidentally ingesting a product not labeled as toxic that was intended for topical use, or the accidental substitution of a camphor-containing medicine instead of the proper drug (most commonly, camphor for castor oil or cod liver oil).

Symptoms

Appearing within 15 to 60 minutes after ingestion or prolonged vapor inhalation, symptoms include headache, excitement, a feeling of warmth, clammy skin, weak pulse, nausea, vomiting, burning in the mouth and throat, and delirium. Camphor can also be smelled on the breath. Twitching and muscle spasms may be followed by convulsions and circulatory failure.

Treatment

Gastric lavage followed by administration of activated charcoal via tube. Vomiting is not induced because of the danger of seizures. Valium may be used to control convulsions; hemodialysis may help eliminate the drug from the body.

campylobacteriosis *Campylobacter* was first recognized in the 1970s as a cause of campylobacteriosis, the so-called traveler's diarrhea. Linked to raw and undercooked poultry, unpasteurized milk, and untreated water, this common foodborne illness causes an estimated 4 million infections and 1,000 deaths every year. While the illness can be uncomfortable and even disabling, deaths occur primarily among those with impaired immune systems, the very young, or the very old. In one of the best-known outbreaks during the 1980s, more than 3,000 residents in Bennington, Vermont, became ill with diarrhea when their town's water supply was contaminated with the rod-shaped bacterium. The disease may also spread throughout child-care centers.

The most common source of infection is contaminated poultry (one-third to half of all raw chicken on the market is contaminated). Consumers get sick when they eat undercooked chicken, or when the organisms are transferred from the raw meat or raw meat drippings to the mouth. It also can survive in undercooked lamb, beef, or pork, in water, and in raw milk.

Symptoms

Symptoms begin between two to 10 days and may last up to 10 days; they include fever, headache, and muscle pain followed by sometimes-bloody diarrhea, abdominal pain and nausea, fatigue and body aches. The infection can be fatal. The Centers for Disease Control and Prevention estimates 100 people die of the disease each year.

Diagnosis

The infection is diagnosed by culturing a stool sample.

Treatment

Unless antibiotics are taken at the very beginning of the illness they won't alleviate symptoms, although they will shorten the infectious period. Without treatment, stool is infectious for several weeks, but three days of antibiotics will eliminate the bacteria. For mild cases, rest and fluids should be sufficient. Young children are usually given antibiotics (usually erythromycin) as a way of reducing the risk of passing the infection on to other children.

Complications

Occasionally infection may provoke meningitis, urinary tract infections, reactive arthritis, or a paralyzing neurologic illness called Guillain-Barre syndrome.

Prevention

Avoid unpasteurized milk or untreated water from mountain streams or lakes.

cantharidin A powder obtained from the blister beetle, cantharidin is used to remove warts and is extremely irritating to the mucous membranes. Nicknamed "Spanish fly," it is popularly believed to be an aphrodisiac; it is in fact a deadly poison that is responsible for many fatalities. When ingested, Spanish fly is highly toxic.

Symptoms

Ingestion of Spanish fly causes burning in the throat and sloughing of the upper gastrointestinal tract. Kidney failure can occur, and death often follows.

Treatment

Dilute with four to eight ounces of water. Do not induce emesis. Treatment is also supportive; hemodialysis may be necessary if the kidneys fail, and treatment of the throat injury is similar to that for lye ingestion. Also, treat gastrointestinal bleeding.

See also BLISTER BEETLE.

cantil snake *(Agkistrodon bilineatus)* Also called a Mexican moccasin, this pit viper is a brightly colored and extremely dangerous snake found in the low regions of the Rio Grande all the way to Nicaragua. Related to the cottonmouth (or water moccasin), this snake has a yellow or red tail that contrasts with the dull appearance of the rest of the body.

Pit vipers seem to be extremely highly evolved for capturing, killing, and eating fairly large, warm-blooded prey, with retractable hollow fangs in the front of the upper jaw. The fangs can be folded back and then positioned forward as the mouth opens to strike. The pit viper's name comes from the heat-sensitive pits located on each side of the head between the nostril and the eye, which are used to locate its prey.

Seriousness of the bite depends on a wide variety of variables, including the snake's size (usually the larger, the more venomous) and whether the snake is hungry or alert. The angle of the bite and its depth and length also affect the seriousness of the bite. In addition, the size of the victim can be important (children and infants are at greater risk), and the health of the victim at the time of the bite will also affect the outcome. Persons with diabetes, hypertension, or blood coagulation problems and the elderly are particularly sensitive to snake venom, and menstruating women may bleed excessively following the bite of a pit viper. Several cases of miscarriage have been reported when pregnant women have been bitten.

Finally, the location of the bite itself is crucial to its seriousness; venomous snake bites on the head and trunk are twice as serious as those on the extremities, and bites on the arms are more serious than those on the legs.

Poisonous part

The venom of the pit vipers is a mixture of proteins that acts on a victim's blood. Even snakes that appear to be dead by the side of the road have been reported to bite. The size of the snake can give an idea of its potential dangerousness and can be judged by the distance between the fang marks. Fang marks less than 8 mm would be a small snake; between 8 and 12 mm indicates a medium-size snake, and more than 12 mm suggests a large venomous snake. Even snakes that have been "defanged" can be dangerous, since all snakes grow new fangs from time to time.

Symptoms

Swelling, internal bleeding, changes in red blood cells; central nervous system symptoms sometimes include convulsions, psychotic behavior, muscle weakness, and paralysis. In addition, there are general systemic symptoms of fever, nausea, vomiting, diarrhea, pain, and restlessness. Tachycardia and bradycardia can develop, and kidney failure has been reported.

Treatment

Within the first 30 to 45 minutes after the bite of a pit viper, apply a venous tourniquet a few inches above the bite, loosening it every 15 to 30 minutes and reapplying it above the level of progressive swelling. Keep the victim quiet, lying down to decrease metabolic activity (which affects the spread of the venom). The wound area (especially if it is an arm or leg) should be kept lower than the heart. Within 30 minutes, trained individuals can incise the wound area and apply suction. Antivenin is available but should be administered within four hours; antivenin is rarely helpful if given more than 12 hours after the bite. Tetanus prophylaxis is advisable; other treatment might include blood transfusions, intravenous fluids, treatment for convulsions, and antihistamines to control itching. In addition, broad-spectrum antibiotics may be administered, since snakebites are notorious for becoming infected. If antivenin has not been administered (or was given hours after the bite), sloughing of the skin around the bite is common. Some individuals may be sensitive to the antivenin, so skin testing is advised.

While certain anecdotal reports in the popular press have reported that some individuals become immunized after many bites of the pit viper, scientifically controlled attempts to develop immunity in human beings have failed.

See also ANTIVENIN; PIT VIPER; SNAKES, POISONOUS.

carbamate A group of synthetic pesticides made up of carbon, hydrogen, oxygen, and nitrogen. They include carbaryl, chlorpropham, carbofuran, aldicarb, pirimicarb, bufencarb, isolan, maneb, propoxur, thiram, Zectran, zineb, and ziram.

Symptoms

Generally, poisoning signs and symptoms may include headache, dizziness, nausea, diarrhea, blurry vision, constricted pupils, slowed heart rate, excessive sweating and salivation, inability to walk, chest discomfort, muscle twitching, incontinence, unconsciousness, and seizures.

Treatment

Atropine is the antidote for most carbamate poisonings.

See also CARBARYL; ORGANOPHOSPHATE INSECTICIDES.

carbaryl (Sevin) This derivative of carbamic acid ($H_2N\text{-}COOH$) is used as an herbicide, insecticide, and medicinal agent and is one of the carbamates, a relatively new class of contact insecticides that supplement the organophosphates.

Symptoms

Carbaryl poisoning resembles parathion intoxication, although it is much less toxic. Symptoms include nausea, vomiting, abdominal cramps, diarrhea, excess salivation, sweating, lassitude, weakness, tightness in the chest, blurring of vision, eye pain, loss of muscle coordination, slurred speech, muscle twitches, breathing problems, blue skin, incontinence, convulsions, and coma. Death occurs from respiratory arrest and paralysis of the respiratory muscles. It is an eye and skin irritant and does not accumulate in the tissues. It is poisonous through ingestion or skin absorption.

Treatment

Give atropine immediately; some reports suggest atropine is dangerous in the presence of anoxia (loss of oxygen); correct cyanosis (blueness of skin) before giving atropine. Give oxygen, artificial respiration as needed. Perform gastric lavage or administer syrup of ipecac if vomiting is not prompt.

Wash contaminated skin with soap and water (or 95 percent ethyl alcohol). Irrigate affected eyes with water or saline. Administer isotonic saline to counteract dehydration and electrolyte imbalance.

See also CARBAMATE; ORGANOPHOSPHATE INSECTICIDES.

carbolic acid See PHENOL.

carbon monoxide A colorless, odorless, poisonous gas that is produced by the incomplete combustion of solid, liquid, and gaseous fuels. Appliances fueled with gas, oil, kerosene, or wood may produce carbon dioxide. If these appliances aren't installed, maintained, and used properly, carbon monoxide may accumulate to dangerous levels.

Carbon monoxide is also found in the exhaust of internal-combustion engines, including car engines. Common sources include gas cooking ranges, hot water heaters and dryers, wood- or coal-burning stoves and fireplaces, oil burners, and kerosene heaters. Gas water heaters and dryers and oil burners must have stacks that direct the carbon monoxide outside. Wood-burning stoves and fireplaces must have chimneys that vent the gas outside. Unvented kerosene heaters spread carbon monoxide gas indoors; therefore, a window must always be open slightly when you use a kerosene heater. Cooking with a charcoal grill in an enclosed area also releases carbon monoxide; for this reason, such grills should never be used indoors.

More than 20,000 people in the United States are treated yearly in hospital emergency rooms for carbon monoxide poisoning; this number is believed to be low, since many people mistake the symptoms for the flu or are misdiagnosed and never get treated.

Symptoms

Breathing carbon monoxide causes headaches, dizziness, weakness, sleepiness, nausea, vomiting, confusion, and disorientation. At very high levels, the level of the gas in the blood rises, leaving the patient confused and clumsy. Loss of consciousness and death soon follow. Symptoms are particularly dangerous because the effects often are not recognized, since the gas is odorless and some of the symptoms are similar to the flu or other common illnesses. Breathing low levels of the chemical can cause fatigue and increase chest pain in people with chronic heart disease; indeed, it has sometimes caused fatal heart attacks.

Some people are particularly susceptible to carbon monoxide, including unborn babies, infants, and people with anemia or a history of heart disease.

Treatment

It's essential to get the victim into fresh air right away, and then call for help. If the victim isn't breathing (or is breathing irregularly), perform artificial respiration. Keep the victim warm and quiet to prevent shock. Medical personnel can give oxygen (often with 5 percent carbon dioxide and sometimes under pressure). A physician should be consulted to check for long-term effects, even if the victim seems to have recovered.

Prevention

Dangerous levels of carbon monoxide can be prevented by proper appliance use, maintenance, and installation. A qualified service technician should check a home's central and room heating appliances (including water heaters and gas dryers) each year. The technician should look at the electrical and mechanical components of appliances, such as thermostat controls and automatic safety devices. In addition,

- chimneys and flues should be checked for blockages, corrosion, and loose connections;
- individual appliances should be serviced regularly;
- kerosene and gas space heaters (vented and unvented) should be cleaned and inspected to make sure they operate properly;
- new appliances should be installed and vented properly;
- adequate combustion air should be provided to assure complete combustion;
- the room where an unvented gas or kerosene space heater is used should be well ventilated, and doors leading to another room should be open to insure proper ventilation; and

- an unvented combustion heater should never be used overnight or in a room where someone is sleeping.

Although carbon monoxide can't be seen or smelled, there are tangible signs that might indicate a problem: visible rust or stains on vents and chimneys, appliances that make unusual sounds or smells, or an appliance that keeps shutting off.

One of the best ways to prevent carbon monoxide poisoning is to install carbon monoxide detectors that meet the requirements of Underwriters Laboratories (UL) standard 2034. Detectors that meet the UL standard measure both high carbon monoxide concentrations over short periods of time and low concentrations over long periods of time. Detectors sound an alarm before the level of carbon monoxide in a person's blood becomes dangerous. Detectors that meet the UL 2034 standard currently cost between $25 and $100.

Since carbon monoxide gases move evenly and fairly quickly throughout the house, a CO detector should be installed on the wall or ceiling in sleeping areas but outside individual bedrooms.

In addition, there are inexpensive cardboard or plastic detectors that change color and do not sound an alarm and have a limited useful life, since they require someone to look at the device to determine if the gas is present. Since carbon monoxide can build up rapidly while a family sleeps, these devices would not sound an alarm to awaken people.

carbon tetrachloride   A colorless, volatile liquid with a characteristic odor, this once-common household solvent is used to clean metals, in dry cleaning, and to remove oil, grease, wax, and paint. An ingredient in fire extinguishers and insecticide sprays, it is also used in the manufacture of Freon propellants and refrigerants. Consumers can no longer buy carbon tetrachloride; it is available only for industrial or commercial use. This dangerous chemical can cause liver and kidney damage if inhaled or drunk.

Symptoms

Breathing these solvent fumes can cause headache, eye irritation, dizziness, visual disturbances, and nausea. In extreme cases, inhaling these fumes can be fatal. If this chemical is drunk, symptoms include headache, nausea, pain in the abdomen, and convulsions.

Treatment

Victim should vomit unless unconscious or having convulsions. If fumes were inhaled, the victim should be taken into fresh air and given artificial respiration if necessary. Skin contamination should be treated with running water for at least 15 minutes. Drinking large amounts of this substance has been reported to be fatal in 90 percent of cases, but with early intervention prognosis is good.

carbutol   See BARBITURATES.

cardiac glycosides   One of the toxic glycosides in the plant kingdom that affect the heart, cardiac glycosides remain one of the major therapies for congestive heart failure. There are more than 400 different types, but the most common is digitalis, which is found in the foxglove *(Digitalis purpurea)* and other "digitoxins" (similar to digitalis) found in *Nerium oleander* and the lily family.

Most cardiac glycosides come from the figwort, lily, and dogbane families. In therapeutic amounts, they will act directly on the heart to increase the force of contractions and decrease the heartbeat—but no one knows how.

Symptoms

Overdoses produce nausea, dizziness, blurred vision, and diarrhea. It is suspected that there is a relationship between the cardiac glycosides and plant toxicity. Poisonous plants containing cardiac glycosides include pheasant's-eye, dogbane, lily of the valley, foxglove, and oleander.

Treatment

Treatment may include administration of activated charcoal, gastric lavage, an electrocardiogram, and blood tests to check digitalis, potassium, and magnesium levels. An antidote (sheep-derived digoxin antibody Fab fragments) is effective against some plant cardiac glycosides and should be considered in life-threatening complications, such as hyperka-

lemia, high-degree heart block, cardiac arrest, and ventricular dysrhythmias.

See also FOXGLOVE; GLYCOSIDE; LILY OF THE VALLEY; OLEANDER.

carneum   A variety of chrysanthemum used in the production of the botanic insecticide pyrethrum.

See also BOTANIC INSECTICIDES; PYRETHRUM.

Carolina horse nettle *(Solanum carolinense)* [Other names: ball or bull nettle, ball nightshade, sandbriar, tread softly.]   This member of the Solanum family grows from Nebraska to Texas, east to the Atlantic and in extreme northern Ohio, southern Ontario, and southern California. It is a member of a very large genus with 1,700 species, most of which have not been evaluated toxicologically.

Poisonous part

Human poisoning is usually attributed to immature fruit, which contains the toxin solanine glycoalkaloid.

Symptoms

While there is little danger of fatal poisoning in adults, children may ingest a fatal amount of this plant. Symptoms appear several hours after ingestion and include gastric irritation, scratchy throat, fever, and diarrhea (solanine poisoning is often confused with bacterial gastroenteritis).

Treatment

The same general supportive care that would be given in gastroenteritis cases; fluid replacement may be required.

cascabel   See RATTLESNAKE, CASCABEL.

cassava *(Manihot esculenta)* [Other names: bitter cassava, juca, manioc, manioc tapioca, sweet potato plant, yuca.]   Found in the tropics, this is a tuberous edible plant of the spurge family and is cultivated for its roots, from which cassava flour, breads, tapioca, laundry starch, and alcoholic beverages are made. It is believed that cassava was once cultivated by the Maya in the Yucatán. Tapioca is the only cassava product on sale in northern markets.

If improperly prepared and cooked, cassava can cause poisoning to those who eat it, although there is no danger if it is prepared properly. Cassava meal and tapioca are made from the tuberous plant, but the plant must be heated and the poison dissolved out before the plant is edible. The two kinds of cassava (bitter and sweet) are often confused, but the bitter variety is more poisonous. Both require careful preparation.

Cassava appears in many varieties, with usually large fan-shaped leaves very much like the castor bean. The varieties range from low herbs to tall, slender trees and are found in dry areas as well as along riverbanks in Guam, Hawaii, the West Indies, Florida, and the Gulf Coast states.

Poisonous part

Cyanogenetic glycosides (linamarin and lotaustralin) are broken down in the body to produce hydrocyanic acid; they occur in different amounts in most varieties. The roots are the most poisonous, although the leaves also contain variable amounts. Primitive people were able to remove the poison by grating, pressing, and heating the tubers. The poison amygdalin in the juice breaks down into hydrocyanic acid, which can cause cyanide poisoning and has been used for darts and arrows.

Symptoms

Experts differ as to how rapidly death can occur, with times ranging from within minutes to hours. Symptoms can include nausea, respiratory problems, twitching, staggering, convulsions, coma, and death.

Treatment

Gastric lavage followed by a 25 percent solution of sodium thiosulfate.

castor bean *(Ricinus communis)* **[Other names: African coffee tree, castor oil plant, gourd, koli, man's motherwort, Mexico weed, palma Christi (from the shape of its leaves, resembling Christ's hand), steadfast, wonder tree.]** This is considered by some sources to be the most dangerous plant in the United States. It is the source of castor oil and is also used as a mosquito repellent and a cathartic. Castor bean is grown for commercial and ornamental use in the United States and the tropics and has become naturalized in Florida, along the Gulf and Atlantic coasts, in southern California, and in Hawaii.

A member of the spurge family, castor bean is a large annual that grows up to 15 feet high and has hollow stems that bear blue-green leaves up to three feet across. It produces bronze-red clusters of flowers in June followed by spiny seed pods containing plump seeds; the pods are often removed because of the highly toxic content concentrated in their seeds.

Early Americans made a laxative from the beans. Native to Africa, the plant is now naturalized throughout the tropics. *R. communis* is the only species in its genus, but there are hundreds of varieties.

Poisonous part

All parts of the plant (especially the seeds) contain the poison ricin, a plant lectin (toxalbumin) that is one of the world's most toxic substances. While the toxic mechanism of ricin is not well understood, it is thought that it inhibits the synthesis of protein in the intestinal wall. Small amounts of castor oil are also present in the seeds. If the beans are swallowed whole, the hard seed coat prevents absorption and therefore inhibits poisoning, but two to six beans can be fatal if well chewed. In a child, one or two seeds can be fatal.

Symptoms

Usually developing after several hours, symptoms include a burning sensation in the mouth, throat, and stomach, nausea, vomiting, severe bloody diarrhea, abdominal cramps, dulled vision, convulsions, trouble in breathing, paralysis, and death from within hours up to 12 days. One to six well-chewed seeds may be fatal to a child. Castor beans can also induce labor.

Treatment

There is no known antidote for ricin poisoning, so treatment is primarily supportive and symptomatic. Perform gastric lavage immediately, with bismuth subcarbonate or magnesium trisilicate to line the stomach. Fluids and electrolytes must be monitored. Administration of activated charcoal can be successful, since charcoal binds ricin well.

Catapres (clonidine) One of a group of antihypertensive drugs designed to lower blood pressure, Catapres is considered to be supertoxic in either its tablet or injectable form. Once it is administered to control blood pressure, an abrupt withdrawal of the drug can precipitate a dangerous spike in blood pressure, psychosis, hyperexcitability, irregular heartbeats, and death.

Symptoms
Within 30 minutes after ingestion, an overdose causes slow heartbeat, drowsiness, stomach upset, rash, low blood pressure, depressed breathing, coma, and heart failure.

Treatment
Atropine is administered, while monitoring the cardiorespiratory system and kidney function.

See also ANTIHYPERTENSIVE DRUGS.

catfish *(Siluriformes)* Related to carp and minnows, the catfish gets its name from the four to five long whiskers on the upper jaw; many also have spines in front of the dorsal and pectoral fins that may cause painful stings, especially by young catfish. There are about 2,500 species of catfish in about 30 families mostly living in fresh water, although a few live in the sea. Those who make their homes in fresh water are found throughout the world and are generally bottom swimmers, scavenging on animal or vegetable matter during the night. Catfish stings are common and can be very painful; they are usually the result of handling the fish while removing it from hook or net. While most varieties cause only a painful sting, the venom of one species, *Plotosus lineatus* (found in the Indo-Pacific), can be lethal.

Symptoms
While death is rare, the sting of the catfish causes an immediate severe stinging or throbbing pain, which may stay at the site of the wound or spread throughout the body and last for several hours or days. There may be redness and swelling at the site of the sting, and the area may become numb.

Treatment
Flush the wound with fresh or salt water, and then soak the affected area in hot water or put hot compresses on it. The water should be very hot (122°F), so that the heat will deactivate the poison. Continue applying hot water for 30 minutes to an hour. These common stings often become infected, and removal of the barb is essential. X-rays can determine whether the barb has actually been removed; if not, the wound should be opened and the spine taken out. Both antibiotics and tetanus prophylaxis are indicated.

centipedes While small centipedes from temperate zones are harmless, the larger varieties found in the tropics can cause pain by injecting venom through their claws. The biggest is the giant centipede *(Scolopendra gigas)*, which ranges from the Southern United States to the West Indies. Centipedes are found in loose soil and leaf litter and under stones and may not have 100 feet—despite their name.

Poisonous part
These insects inject toxic substances into the skin from a pair of hollow jaws that act like fangs. The venom is relatively weak. The giant centipede is the only one in the United States dangerous to humans.

Symptoms
Generally a mild inflammation at the wound site with mild swelling of the lymph nodes. The bite of the giant centipede causes inflammation, swelling and redness and systemic symptoms that fade within five hours.

Treatment
Apply cool compresses at wound site; for the bite of the giant centipede, use cool saline compresses with painkillers or sedatives as required.

charcoal, activated   This substance, which absorbs a wide variety of toxins and renders them ineffective, is an indispensable part of any first aid kit. Activated charcoal is made from coal, lignite, or waste from paper manufacturers, and soft organic material like vegetables. It is used to prevent the absorption of toxins in the gastrointestinal tract within a few minutes of administration.

Activated charcoal can be effective with most chemicals and is considered one of the best, cheapest, and most practical emergency antidotes. For maximum effectiveness, activated charcoal should be administered within the first hour of poison ingestion. The sooner it is given, the more poison it is capable of absorbing.

According to some reports, the recommended dosage of activated charcoal is 30–50 grams in four ounces of water for children and 50–100 grams in 8 ounces of water for adults—a dose far larger than those included in most home poison kits.

Activated charcoal will inactivate syrup of ipecac and should not be given at the same time. It should be administered only after vomiting has been successfully induced. It is nontoxic and is inert if aspirated, and there are contraindications to its use. It is not used when a neutralizing agent is administered by mouth (such as to treat iodine ingestion or mercury, iron, strychnine, nicotine, or quinine poisoning).

In addition, it is not used when a patient is vomiting blood, nor is it effective with certain heavy metals such as iron salts or lithium. Activated charcoal is also poorly effective with products involving alcohol and petroleum distillates and is contraindicated after ingestion of strong acids or strong alkalies. It should not be given if analysis of gastric contents is necessary, or if the contents need to be viewed (to tell the color or number of pills, etc.).

Caution:

Giving artificial charcoal too fast usually causes vomiting.

See also IPECAC SYRUP.

charcoal briquettes   A type of compressed fuel intended for outdoor use in charcoal grills and hibachis. However, in enclosed areas with little ventilation, the burning charcoal releases fatal amounts of carbon monoxide gas. At least 40 fatalities have been reported in recent years because of the indoor use of such charcoal in campers, trailers, tents, boats, apartments, and other enclosed areas.

See also CARBON MONOXIDE.

chelating agent   Chemicals used to treat poisoning by metals such as arsenic, mercury, lead or iron, these agents combine with the metal to form a less poisonous substance, which is then more quickly excreted in the urine. Penicillamine is a common chelating agent as is EDTA (ethylene diamine tetraacetic acid), which is FDA-approved for treatment of lead poisoning.

The word *chelate* is derived from the Greek *chele*, which refers to the claw of a lobster; this describes the pincerlike binding ability of metal ions.

See also ARSENIC; LEAD POISONING; MERCURY.

cherries, wild and cultivated *(Prunus)*   Although the cherry tree is widely cultivated for its fruit, the pits and leaves of the tree are poisonous.

Poisonous part

The pits contain cyanogenic glycosides (amygdalin), a substance that, when eaten, releases hydrocyanic acid.

Symptoms

Some hours may pass before symptoms appear, since the glycosides are not released until they are hydrolyzed in the gastrointestinal tract. When they do appear, symptoms include shortness of breath, vocal cord paralysis, abdominal pain, muscle twitches, vomiting, lethargy, sweating, and weakness. In severe poisoning, symptoms progress to seizures, unconsciousness, stupor, and coma.

Treatment

Gastric lavage (if conscious) followed by a 25 percent solution of thiosulfate. If the victim is unconscious, acidosis is corrected and shock treated, together with the administration of oxygen and a cyanide antidote.

See also CYANOGENIC GLYCOSIDES.

cherry pit   See PRUNUS.

children and poisons   Every year in the United States, about 10 million cases of poisoning occur. Eighty percent of these cases involve a child under the age of five years. Poisoning among children typically occurs because of curiosity, an inability to read warning labels, a desire to imitate adults, and inadequate supervision by adults. Despite the staggering high number of poisonings in children, only about 50 children die each year from a toxic substance, a number that is tragic yet remarkable.

Medications for children

Children can be poisoned if they have access to a medicine cabinet or other place where medications have been stored, but it is also possible for them to be poisoned if they are given the wrong type or amount of medicine. Follow these safe-medicine guidelines at all times:

- Follow medicine label directions carefully to avoid accidental overdoses.
- If anything about label directions on your child's prescription medicines seems different, unusual or odd, CALL THE PHARMACIST IMMEDIATELY. Do not assume that a mistake is impossible.
- Never give your child medicine in the dark. Many medicine bottles look alike in dim light. Take the time to be sure you are dispensing the correct medication.
- Know your child's current accurate weight; weight affects dosage.
- Do not substitute a kitchen teaspoon for a measuring teaspoon when giving medicine.
- Properly dispose of unused and outdated medications.
- Do not use prescription medication for anyone other than the person it was prescribed for.
- Never refer to medicine as "candy" to a child.
- Avoid taking your medicine in front of your child, since youngsters like to imitate grown-ups.
- When you are using medicine or giving it to someone else, never let young children out of your sight, even if that means taking them along to answer the phone or the door.

Just because you can buy medicine without a prescription does not mean that the medicine is safe if taken in overdose. The painkiller acetaminophen is one of the most commonly misused medications during childhood. Because it's been available over the counter for years and is sold in a variety of dosage formulations, most parents feel very comfortable in giving acetaminophen for pain or fever. However, studies have found that many parents give too much of the drug too often. In fact, it is not uncommon for parents to give their children adult dosages, which can lead to significant liver disease and even death.

While acetaminophen is the nonprescription drug most often given in error, parents also make mistakes with other over-the-counter products, including cold medications, antihistamines, and cough suppressants.

Medicine cabinet safety

The key to keeping the home safe from poisons is to go room by room and poison-proof the whole place. The best starting point is probably the bathroom medicine cabinet, where most people store all the family's medications. (Actually, the bathroom is the worst place to store medicine; the moist, warm environment tends to change or degrade the chemicals.) Follow these guidelines to make sure your medicines are stored safely:

- Keep pills in their original containers.
- Always close and put away the container as soon as you are finished using it.
- Always keep medicines out of sight and out of reach of children.
- To prevent toddlers or kids from getting into cabinets, consider buying a "cabinet lock" for the medicine chest.
- Always use child-resistant caps.
- Remember that child resistant does not mean childproof. To be legally designated as "child resistant," the container must take more than five minutes for 80 percent of five-year olds to open (which means that 20 percent can get into it in less time).

- Never keep medicine on a countertop or bedside table.
- Clean out the medicine cabinet from time to time, and throw out all unneeded medicine once the illness it treated is over. Pour contents down the drain or the toilet and rinse out the container before throwing away.
- Never assume that children will not take or could not have taken a medication because it tastes bad to you.
- Never assume that children will not take or could not have taken a medication because it is too big for them to swallow.
- Be especially careful about medicine in handbags and suitcases, which may be left unprotected around the house.

Toxins, in infants and toddlers

The most important thing to remember is this: *babies are not tiny adults.* Because babies have a low body weight, a very small amount of a potentially harmful substance can have a toxic effect. Another factor is that infants and young children grow rapidly, and so any chemicals to which they are exposed can be incorporated into their body tissues in high amounts. Compounding this problem is that infants and toddlers have immature intestines, liver, and kidneys—the organs responsible for detoxifying substances—as well as a nervous system (including the brain) that is extremely vulnerable to environmental toxins.

Although parents need to be extremely careful about exposing their children to toxic substances, some items are considered to be nontoxic to children unless they are ingested in very large amounts. That is not to say that these substances will not cause some symptoms; however, they are generally nontoxic to children. These nontoxic substances are listed in the accompanying table.

Nontoxic Substances
antacids
antibiotics
aquarium products
baby oil
birth control pills
blackboard chalk
bubble bath
candles
caps for a cap pistol
castor oil
cosmetics
dehumidifying packets
denture adhesive
deodorants
diaper rash ointment
dry cell batteries
eye makeup
fabric softener
glycerin
graphite (in "lead" pencils)
hand creams and lotions
kaolin
lanolin
lauric acid
lipstick
modeling clay
multivitamins (without iron or fluoride)
nail polish
petroleum jelly
putty
shaving cream
soaps
stearic acid
tallow
teething rings
watercolor paints

Poison in toys

Toxic children's toys have become a critical issue in recent years, and the Consumer Product Safety Commission (CPSC) has recalled millions of toys believed to contain dangerous amounts of lead paint or other toxic substances. In April 2006, it was reported that there was lead in children's necklaces that had been shipped from China and sold in the United States at Dollar General stores from January 2003 through December 2005 for one dollar apiece. In June 2007, the CPSC recalled 1.5 million Thomas and Friends wooden railway toys that contained lead paint. In September 2007, Mattel recalled 675,000 Barbie Accessory toys because of high levels of lead paint. In November 2007, a toy called Aqua Dots, imported from China, consisted of beads that had a chemical coating on them. When the beads were ingested, the chemical metabolized into gamma hydroxybutyrate, a date rape drug, with the potential to cause unconsciousness, seizures, drowsiness, coma, and death. No deaths were associated with ingesting the beads, but most of the affected children were hospitalized.

See also LEAD.

chinaberry *(Melia azedarach)* [Other names: African lilac tree, bead tree, China tree, false sycamore, hog bush, Indian lilac, Japanese bead tree, paradise tree, Persian lilac, pride of China, pride of India, Texas umbrella tree, West Indian lilac, white cedar.] Found in the southern United States from Virginia to Florida west to Texas, in Hawaii, the West Indies, and Guam, the chinaberry tree grows as high as 50 feet, with 2-inch-long serrated leaves and fragrant purple flower clusters. The yellow fruit contains up to five smooth black seeds.

Poisonous part

Fruit and bark contain tetranortriterpene neurotoxins and unidentified gastroenteric toxins; toxicity varies considerably depending on the concentration of toxin in the plant.

Symptoms

Following a fairly long latency period, symptoms include faintness, confusion, stupor, vomiting, and diarrhea, which can lead to shock. Breathing problems may be followed by convulsions, paralysis, and, very rarely, death. While six to eight fruits can be lethal to a child, human exposures in the United States are generally limited to severe gastroenteritis.

Treatment

Replace fluids and electrolytes, give activated charcoal, and treat symptoms. Kidney and liver function should be monitored. There is no antidote.

chinchonism A syndrome produced by overdose of quinine, salicylates, and cinchophen, consisting of ringing in the ears, hearing and balance problems, blurred vision, photophobia, headache, nausea, vomiting, diarrhea, flushed skin, sweating, fever, and skin rash.

See also CINCHOPHEN; QUININE; SALICYLATES.

chloral hydrate The well-known "Mickey Finn" or "knockout drops" popularized in the detective fiction of the 1930s, chloral hydrate is the oldest prescription sleeping pill available today. It was introduced in 1862 as a derivative of chloroform and quickly became a popular drug of abuse during those years; it is one of five sedative-hypnotic drugs introduced before 1900.

Symptoms

A central nervous system depressant, chloral hydrate in therapeutic doses produces drowsiness within 30 minutes after ingestion, followed by a sound sleep within an hour. Unlike with other sedatives, under normal conditions there is rarely a hangover afterward. However, doses larger than 2 grams can cause poisoning, and the reported fatal dose is between 5 and 10 grams. The toxicity of chloral hydrate does vary considerably but in general acts in three ways: depressing the central nervous system, corroding the skin and mucous membranes, and affecting some major organs. Ingested in large amounts, chloral hydrate causes sleepiness, confusion, clumsiness, slow and shallow breathing, weakness, low blood pressure, cyanosis, and a deep coma within 30 minutes of ingestion. It may be fatal in a few hours—or even sooner, as a result of respiratory collapse. In addition, there may be kidney and liver damage.

Chloral hydrate can also cause chronic poisoning, resulting in a skin rash, confusion, dizziness, drowsiness, depression, and a wide range of behavioral abnormalities, including irritability, poor judgment, and a general lack of interest in personal appearance.

Chloral hydrate is radiopaque, and diagnosis of overdose can be confirmed with an abdominal X-ray.

Treatment

There is no known antidote to chloral hydrate poisoning. Treatment is similar to poisoning with other narcotics: gastric lavage (only if begun soon after ingestion, because of this drug's rapid absorption in the gastrointestinal tract). Since onset of action is so rapid, induced vomiting could be dangerous. Afterward, administer activated charcoal and provide demulcents (such as milk). Provide supportive treatment (including oxygen). Hemodialysis may also be effective.

chloramine gas   A deadly gas that results from the combination of ammonia and cleaners containing hypochlorite salts. For this reason, two different types of household cleansers should never be mixed.

Symptoms
Breathing these fumes can cause headache, eye irritation, dizziness, visual disturbances, and nausea.

Treatment
Remove victim from contaminated air; observe for breathing problems.

Chloramine-T (sodium *p*-toluenesulfochloramine) This drinking water disinfectant and deodorant contains 12 percent chlorine, which is slowly released on contact with water; as a solution, it is used as a mouthwash. It is also used to remove odor from cheese.

Symptoms
It is believed that this compound works by transforming chloramine-T into a derivative of cyanide, resulting in cyanosis, respiratory failure, collapse, and frothing at the mouth. Death follows within a few minutes. It is suspected of causing rapid allergic reactions in hypersensitive victims.

Treatment
Gastric lavage, followed by the administration of sodium nitrate and sodium thiosulfate. Patients who survive 24 hours are expected to recover.

chlorate poisoning   Chemicals used in some defoliant weed killers and in industries to make dyes, explosives, or matches can cause kidney, liver, and intestinal damage and can be fatal in small doses, especially in children.

Symptoms
Ulcers in the mouth, abdominal pain, and diarrhea.

Treatment
If spilled onto skin or eyes, wash off immediately with water. If ingested, seek medical help immediately. Methylene blue is effective only if given in the very early stages. Otherwise, gastric lavage, exchange transfusion, bicarbonate infusion, hemodialysis, and heparin are suggested.

chlordane (1,2,4,5,6,7,8,8 octachloro-4,7-methano-3a,4,7,7a-tetrahydroindane; chlordan octachloro-tetrahydro methano indane) [Trade names: CD-68, Dowklor, Octa-Klor, Ortho-Klor, 1068, Toxichlor, Velsicol 1068.]   One of a group of synthetic organochlorine pesticides, chlordane is a viscous liquid with a chlorine odor ranging from colorless to amber. Introduced in 1945, use and commercial production have been prohibited in the United States and many other countries since 1988, because it does not disperse in the environment but instead accumulates in biological systems.

It dissolves in both water and fat and is available as a powder, dust, emulsion concentrate and a concentrated solution in oil. Skin absorption is rapid, but reports of human poisonings are limited.

Symptoms
Chlordane is a fairly quick acting chemical and less toxic than similar pesticides, but still toxic; violent convulsions appear suddenly within 30 minutes to three hours after ingestion. The first 12 hours are the most dangerous, and death—if it is likely to occur—will usually take place within this time frame. It is possible, however, that a person will live up to 20 days after ingestion before finally succumbing. Other symptoms include liver damage and congestion in the brain, lung, heart, and spinal cord. The estimated lethal oral dose of chlordane in an adult is 3–7 grams. It has been implicated in acute blood abnormalities.

Treatment

There is no specific antidote. Perform gastric lavage, but do not induce vomiting because of the risk of sudden onset of seizures; administer activated charcoal and a cathartic. Irregular heartbeat may respond to propranolol. If convulsions last for some time, recovery is unlikely.

See also CHLORINATED HYDROCARBON PESTICIDES.

chlorinated hydrocarbon pesticides This group of insect-fighting chemicals was once widely used in agriculture and malarial control programs around the world from the 1940s through the 1960s, However, environmental contamination has led to their disfavor; DDT and chlordane, for example, are banned from commercial use because they do not disperse in the environment and because they accumulate in biological systems. Some have been shown to cause cancer in humans, including chloroform, vinyl chloride, aldrin, chlordane, dieldrin, heptachlor, lindane, toxaphene, and carbon tetrachloride. Instead, organophosphates (such as malathion and diazinon) have more or less replaced the chlorinated hydrocarbons, since they control insects, are biodegradable and (according to their manufacturers) do not contaminate the environment.

The most highly toxic of the group are aldrin, dieldrin, endrin, and endosulfan; moderately toxic are chlordane, DDT, heptachlor, kepone, lindane, mirex, and toxaphene; slightly toxic are ethylan (perthane), hexachlorobenzene, and methoxychlor.

As a group, these insecticides interfere with the transmission of nerve impulses throughout the body (especially the brain), causing behavior changes, involuntary movements and depressed respiratory system. They may also cause liver or kidney damage and may also be carcinogenic. In general, the route of poisoning is through the skin (especially with aldrin, dieldrin, and endrin).

Symptoms

Soon after these chemicals are ingested, symptoms of nausea and vomiting appear followed by confusion, tremor, coma, seizures, and respiratory depression. There have been reports of delayed and recurrent seizures and irregular heartbeat.

Treatment

There is no specific antidote for chlorinated hydrocarbon poisoning. Treat symptoms and perform gastric lavage, but do not induce vomiting. Then administer activated charcoal and a cathartic.

See also CHLORDANE; DDT; DIELDRIN; ENDRIN; LINDANE; MIREX.

chlorine This yellow-green gas with an irritating odor is widely used to manufacture chemicals, as a swimming pool disinfectant and cleaner, and as a bleach. Chlorine and chlorine-containing compounds are also found in table salt (sodium chloride), plastics (polyvinyl chloride), aerosol propellants (chlorofluorocarbons), and pesticides, as well as throughout the body in all nerve and muscle tissues.

Chlorine was also used briefly as a chemical weapon during World War I, but it was subsequently replaced by other chemicals. Current toxic exposures come from accidental spills and the improper use of household products. A derivative of chlorine's derivative, hypochlorite, is found in most household bleaches in solutions of 3 to 5 percent; adding ammonia to this hypochlorite solution may release chloramine, which can cause unconsciousness, especially if the area is small and unventilated. However, a person would need to be in the fumes for more than an hour for serious problems to develop. Adding an acid to hypochlorite solution releases chlorine gas.

A natural chemical element and a gas at room temperature, chlorine is easily liquefied under pressure. Pure chlorine rarely occurs in nature, except in volcanic eruptions—and even then, the quantities released are small.

Accidental spills or leaks of chlorine gas during transport or storage are the greatest exposure hazard today; in the event of such a spill, whole neighborhoods or towns may be evacuated. Chlorine and hydrochloric acid rank first and third respectively in causing injuries and deaths from large accidents involving industrial chemicals, although the actual number of incidences is small.

Symptoms

When in contact with moist tissue (such as the eyes and upper respiratory tract), chlorine gas is a strong irritant and causes corrosive injury; aqueous solutions of chlorine also cause corrosive injury to eyes, skin, and gastrointestinal tract. Inhaling chlorine gas causes immediate burning of eyes, nose, and throat, with coughing and wheezing. More serious poisoning results in croupy cough, hoarseness, and upper airway swelling to the point of obstruction. In quite severe cases of poisoning, pulmonary edema may result. Skin or eye contact with either the gas or the concentrated solution causes corrosive burns. Ingestion of 3–5 percent hyperchlorite solution is not particularly serious, causing an immediate burning in the mouth and throat but no further injury. More concentrated solutions may result in serious esophageal and gastric burns, together with drooling and severe throat, chest, and abdominal pain and with perforation of the esophagus or stomach.

There is a slight increase in the risk of bladder cancer and possibly colon and rectal cancers in longtime users of chlorinated water supplies.

Hypochlorite in bleach is a corrosive substance that can damage skin, eyes and other membranes. According to poison control centers, a high number of children each year accidentally swallow laundry bleach, although relatively few fatalities are reported (probably because of the vomiting that bleach causes). However, damage to the esophagus and stomach can occur.

Treatment

While many experts recommend administration of corticosteroids in an attempt to limit esophageal scarring, this treatment is unproven and may be harmful in those with perforations or serious infection. For the inhalation of chlorine gas, give humidified supplemental oxygen, and observe for signs of upper airway obstruction. Treat symptoms. For ingestion of hyperchlorite solution greater than 10 percent (or with symptoms of corrosive injury), check for serious esophageal or gastric injury with a flexible endoscope. A chest X-ray will also reveal a perforated esophagus.

For contaminated skin and eyes, flush exposed skin with water; irrigate eyes with water or saline. For ingestion of hypochlorite solution, immediately give water or milk by mouth. Do not induce vomiting; perform gastric lavage after concentrated liquid ingestion. Do not use activated charcoal, since it may interfere with the endoscopist's view.

See also CHLORINE GAS.

chlorine gas This yellow-green gas is used in the manufacture of plastics, purified water, cloth, and paper and usually causes poisoning after a leak in a storage tank. The damage following exposure to chlorine gas depends on its concentration, duration of exposure and the water content of the exposed tissue, but it is capable of causing rapid and extensive tissue destruction. Chlorine gas is 30 times more toxic to cells than hydrochloric acid.

Symptoms

Skin contact causes severe burns; inhalation of gas at greater than three to six parts per million causes conjunctivitis, keratitis, sore throat, burning chest pain, and coughing. A moderate exposure causes immediate, severe irritation of the mucous membranes of the nose, throat, and eyes, with a distressing cough. Excessive exposure results in a severe, productive cough, difficulty in breathing, and cyanosis. There may be prolonged vomiting, restlessness and anxiety, followed by lack of oxygen and heart attack.

Treatment

Remove the victim from the environment. Wash eyes with saline after the application of topical anesthesia. Burns should be washed with saline; hospitalization may be necessary. Bronchodilators and humidified oxygen will alleviate breathing problems, together with the administration of steroids.

See also CHLORINE.

chlorobenzene derivatives These chemicals are a type of synthetic organic insecticide and include DDT, TDE, DFDT, DMC, neotrane, ovotran, and dilan. They are soluble in fat (not water), and according to reports, the amount of these chemicals present in the body fat of individuals in the United States is higher than in Canada, England, France, and the former West Germany. In those preparations that are still legally available, the commercial solutions are sold in dry mixtures or in solutions of one or more inorganic solvents (kerosene, benzene, etc.), which are also toxic in themselves.

Symptoms

These compounds affect the central nervous system and result in restlessness, irritability, muscle spasm, tremor, and convulsions followed by depression, collapse, and breathing problems due to respiratory failure. Absorption through the skin or by inhalation causes eye, nose, and throat irritation, blurred vision, pulmonary edema, and skin problems. Chronic poisoning symptoms include loss of weight, liver, and kidney damage, and disturbances of the central nervous system.

Treatment

Gastric lavage followed by saline cathartics. Avoid all fats and oils (including milk), since they increase the rate of absorption of chlorinated hydrocarbons. Administer phenobarbital sodium for tremors, and barbiturates for convulsions, and provide oxygen if necessary. If the skin has come in contact with these insecticides, wash with soap and water immediately to head off skin problems and systemic absorption. Remove contaminated clothing.

See also DDT; INSECTICIDES.

chloroform (trichloromethane) This chlorinated hydrocarbon solvent is used in the production of Freon and as a solvent in the chemical and pharmaceutical industries; it is a direct central nervous system depressant.

It was discovered independently and simultaneously in 1831 in Germany, France, and the United States, and accounts of its abuse were reported in the United States in that same year. Dentist Horace Wills, the first person in the United States to use nitrous oxide in surgery, died from complications resulting from his own chronic chloroform abuse. Chloroform was introduced as an anesthetic during surgery in 1847; it became so popular that Queen Victoria knighted its discoverer, Dr. James Simpson, after he delivered her eighth child.

However, as other anesthetics were discovered and the number of overdoses of chloroform rose, its medical use lost favor. It has since been abandoned

because of the toxic effects on the liver, which can progress to fatal cirrhosis. In addition, about 10 percent of the population have a genetic response to chloroform that results in an uncontrolled high fever (above 110°F) during or after anesthesia.

Chronic low levels of the chemical may still be found in some municipal water supplies.

Symptoms

In addition to its effects on the central nervous system, chloroform may also cause heartbeat irregularities and damage the liver and kidneys. Chloroform is also toxic to the fetus and is a suspected carcinogen. Ingestion or inhalation causes a mild to moderate systemic toxicity, including headache, nausea, vomiting, confusion, and drunkenness followed by coma, respiratory arrest, and heartbeat irregularities. Kidney and liver failure may be discovered up to three days after exposure.

Treatment

If skin or eyes have come in contact with chloroform, remove affected clothing and wash with soap and water; irrigate eyes with tepid water or saline. If inhaled, remove the victim from the area and give oxygen. If ingested, perform gastric lavage, but do not induce vomiting (chloroform is rapidly absorbed and may depress the central nervous system). Administer activated charcoal and a cathartic; provide supportive treatment. Acetylcysteine may help prevent kidney and liver damage.

See also ANESTHETICS, GASEOUS/VOLATILE.

chlorthion See ORGANOPHOSPHATE INSECTICIDES.

choke cherry pit See *PRUNUS.*

Christmas rose (Helleborus niger) Also called black hellebore or winter rose, this very poisonous plant of the buttercup family is found in the northern United States and Canada and blooms from late fall through early spring—often in the snow. Its groups of evergreen leaflets resemble fingers on a hand; its flowers are white to pinky green and appear during Christmas in milder climates. The

Christmas rose is found in damp, shady places and is closely related to the later-blooming Lenten rose (*H. orientalis*).

Poisonous part

All parts of the plant contain the digitalis-like glycosides helleborin, hellebrin; and the direct irritants saponins and protoanemonin.

Symptoms

Within 30 minutes after ingestion, the poison will blister the mucous membranes in the mouth, with abdominal pain, severe diarrhea, vomiting, and death from cardiac arrest. The amount ingested will determine the length of time between ingestion and the appearance of symptoms; generally, poisoning symptoms include conduction defects and sinus bradycardia.

Treatment

Amyl nitrate, strychnine, and atropine are often used as cardiac and respiratory stimulants. Perform gastric lavage or induce emesis, and activated charcoal may be given repeatedly.

See also BUTTERCUP; GLYCOSIDE; SAPONIN.

chromium This silver metal is used by electroplaters, welders, lithographers, and metal or textile workers and can be toxic by skin contact, inhalation, or ingestion.

Poisonous part

Trivalent chromium compounds (chromic oxide, chromic sulfate) and chromate salts of lead, zinc, barium, bismuth, and silver do not readily dissolve in water and, because they are poorly absorbed, are not very toxic. Hexavalent compounds (chromium trioxide, chromic anhydride, chromic acid, and dichromate salts) do dissolve in water and are more easily absorbed by the lungs, gastrointestinal tract, and skin. Some of the hexavalent compounds are also carcinogenic.

Symptoms

Skin/eyes: contact with the skin may cause severe burns; contact with the eyes can cause serious corneal injury. There have been reports of fatalities after skin contact causing only 10 percent burned surface area, because the skin burns enhance absorption. Inhalation: symptoms (which may appear several hours after exposure) include upper respiratory tract irritation, wheezing, and pulmonary edema. Ingestion: there may be immediate gastroenteritis, with massive fluid and blood loss leading to shock and kidney failure. Other symptoms include hepatitis and cerebral edema. Serious poisoning has occurred from ingesting as little as 500 mg of hexavalent chromium.

Treatment

Treat symptoms; chelation therapy is not effective. Skin/eyes: wash exposed area with soap and water (for eyes, flush with tepid water or saline). Inhalation: give supplemental oxygen if necessary. Ingestion: (of hexavalent compounds) ascorbic acid may be administered; give milk or water to dilute corrosive effects, and perform gastric lavage, but do not induce vomiting because of the potential for corrosive injury. Administer activated charcoal.

ciguatera Ciguatera poisoning occurs after eating any of more than 300 species of fish that may contain a type of toxin undetectable by inspection, taste, or smell. The fish are toxic at certain times of the year when they ingest a specific type of plankton that contains "ciguatoxin." Ciguatoxin is an odorless, tasteless poison that can not be destroyed by either heating or freezing.

Ciguatoxin is usually found in larger coral-reef fish, including barracuda, snapper, amberjack, surgeon fish, sea bass, and grouper. Other species of warm-water fish, such as mackerel or triggerfish, may also be contaminated. Not all fish of a given species or from a given locality will be toxic at the same time.

Ciguatera occurs most often in the Caribbean islands, Florida and Hawaii, and the Pacific Islands. Recent reports recorded 129 cases over a two-year period in Dade County, Florida, alone. It appears to be occurring more often, probably because of the increased demand for seafood around the world and its recurrence in edible fish. Experts believe this type of poisoning is underreported because it is usually not fatal and symptoms don't last long.

Isolated instances of ciguatera poisoning have occurred along the eastern United States coast, from south Florida up to Vermont. Hawaii, the U.S. Virgin Islands, and Puerto Rico also report sporadic cases.

Poisonous part

The toxin involved in this type of poisoning is ciguatoxin, which is found in greatest concentration in internal organs.

Symptoms

There are both stomach and neurologic symptoms, with a curious type of sensory reversal, so that picking up a cold glass would cause a burning hot sensation. Other symptoms include a tingling sensation in the lips and mouth followed by numbness, nausea, vomiting, abdominal cramps, weakness, headache, vertigo, paralysis, convulsions, and skin rash. Coma and death from respiratory paralysis occur in about 12 percent of cases. Subsequent episodes of ciguatera may be more severe. Ciguatera is usually self-limiting and subsides within several days.

Complications

Sometimes, the neurological symptoms may persist for weeks or months. Occasionally, symptoms have lasted for several years, or patients have relapsed. These relapses may be associated with alcohol or dietary changes. Rarely, death occurs from breathing or heart failure.

Treatment

Some experts suggest pralidoxime chloride is an effective antidote. Other treatment is supportive.

Prevention

The only way to prevent this infection is to avoid tropical reef fish, since there is no easy way to routinely measure the toxin in any seafood product before eating.

See also DINOFLAGELLATE; SHELLFISH POISONING.

cimetidine (Tagamet) An ulcer-healing drug related to antihistamines, cimetidine was first introduced in 1976. It reduces the secretion of hydrochloric acid in the stomach and helps heal gastric and duodenal ulcers and heals inflammation of the esophagus.

Symptoms

On rare occasions, an overdose (or even a therapeutic dose) produces a toxic psychosis within a few hours of ingestion, with confusion, disorientation, agitation, and hallucinations. Symptoms will usually clear within 24 hours.

Treatment

Treat symptoms of agitation with gastric lavage; barbiturates may be used cautiously to control central nervous system stimulation.

See also ANTIHISTAMINES.

cinchophen A painkiller used to treat gout, it is available in both oral and injectable form. Cinchophen carries the risk of liver damage, which makes its use in the treatment of gout dangerous.

Symptoms

Appearing between six and 12 hours after ingestion, symptoms include gastrointestinal irritation, anorexia, diarrhea, vomiting, high fever, delirium, convulsions, coma, and death.

Treatment

Treatment is the same as with salicylate poisoning (induce vomiting or perform gastric lavage followed by activated charcoal and a cathartic).

clematis Many different species of this popular and quite beautiful flowering climber can be found throughout Canada and the north temperate United States.

Poisonous part

The whole plant is poisonous and contains the toxin protoanemonin, which irritates both the skin and the mucous membranes.

Symptoms

Ingestion causes intense pain, blistering, and inflammation in the mouth and throat together with excess salivation, bloody diarrhea, abdominal cramps, dizziness, and, in severe cases, convulsions and mental confusion.

Treatment

Usually, the immediate pain upon chewing leaves or flowers limits the amount of toxin ingested. In cases of large amounts of poisoning, gastric lavage should be performed and demulcents administered. Kidney function should be monitored.

climbing lily *(Gloriosa rothschildiana; G. superba)*

Also called glory lilies, climbing lilies have striking bright crimson and yellow flowers with finger-like petals and lance-shaped leaves tipped with tendrils. They are primarily cultivated in the southern United States, the West Indies, and Hawaii.

Poisonous part

The entire plant contains the toxin colchicine, especially the fleshy, tuberous roots.

Symptoms

Immediately after ingestion, the victim experiences burning pain in the mouth and throat with intense thirst followed by nausea and vomiting. Within two hours, abdominal pain and severe diarrhea develop, which may lead to shock. There is sometimes kidney damage. Because colchicine is not readily excreted, illness can last for some time.

Treatment

Give fluids, and monitor blood pressure and kidney function. Administer atropine and painkillers.

Clostridium botulinum

Clostridium botulinum The deadliest known type of food poisoning is botulism, which is caused by the *Clostridium botulinum* toxin, the most poisonous substance in the world. In fact, the fearsome reputation of botulism is well deserved, since two-thirds of botulism victims die. Those who survive face a long recovery period. The bacteria's resistance to heat makes the spores an important cause of poisoning in improperly cooked or canned foods. While still fairly uncommon, botulism occurs more often in the United States than anywhere else in the world due to the popularity of home-canning; there are about 20 cases of foodborne botulism poisoning in the United States annually.

See also BOTULISM.

Clostridium perfringens

Clostridium perfringens This type of bacteria, a close cousin of *C. botulinum*, can produce a dangerous toxin that multiplies quickly in reheated foods, which is why it's known as the "cafeteria germ." It's often found in foods served in large amounts, such as in school cafeterias and hospitals, left in inadequately heated steam tables or at room temperature. It exists in undercooked beef, meat pies, stews, burritos, tacos, enchiladas, and reheated meats or gravies made from beef, turkey, or chicken. Once eaten, the bacteria produce a toxin in the digestive tract about six hours later; however, a large amount of the bacteria must be eaten in order to cause illness.

This type of food poisoning is very common in the United States, with an estimated 10,000 cases occurring each year, according to the U.S. Centers for Disease Control and Prevention. Outbreaks have been often traced to restaurants, caterers, and cafeterias that don't have adequate refrigeration facilities. Most cases go unreported.

Symptoms

Symptoms appear suddenly (within eight to 24 hours after eating) and include severe cramps and abdominal gas pains followed by a 24-hour bout of watery diarrhea. There may be nausea but usually no vomiting or fever. While usually a mild illness, it can be dangerous to infants and the elderly, who may become dehydrated. A person can get this illness more than once, but a patient is not infectious.

Diagnosis

A test can detect the presence of the bacterium. The bacteria will also grow on a culture plate in a lab from either the food or a stool sample.

Treatment

Drink small sips of clear fluids or electrolytes to replace what is lost. If you are dehydrated, seek medical help.

Prevention

The bacteria produce spores, a dormant form of bacteria that isn't killed by cooking. However, the spores can't reproduce into bacteria at temperatures below 40°F or above 140°F. Therefore, keep hot foods hot and cold foods cold and don't keep reheating and reusing leftovers for several meals.

clove cigarettes   See PHENOL.

cobra   A large group of highly poisonous snakes of the family Elapidae, most of which expand the neck ribs to form a hood. Most species of cobras are found in warm regions of Africa and are favorites of snake charmers. Cobra bites are fatal between 10 and 50 percent of the time, depending on the species; if untreated, they can be fatal within minutes to several hours.

Cobras that are found in the East have fang openings facing forward, enabling the snake to spit. Snakes that spit their venom usually direct the poison at the victim's eyes at distances of up to more than 7 feet; the venom can cause temporary or permanent blindness unless promptly washed out.

These snakes live in holes in the ground, and while they can climb into a shrub looking for food, they are usually seen underfoot. They are considered fairly placid, preferring to flee rather than fight. An angry cobra surprised in its hole will hiss loudly; if disturbed in the open, it will turn and face its victim, inflating its hood and looking very fierce. However, its striking range is limited, and it will often strike with its mouth closed in the hope of discouraging an attacker.

Included in the cobra family are the Indian or Asian cobra, the Egyptian or African cobra, the ringhals, the black-necked cobra, and the tree cobra. Those of the cobra family without hoods include the blue krait, pama, black mamba, green mamba, taipan, death adder, tiger snake, Australian black snake, brown snake, eastern coral, Arizona coral, African coral, black-banded coral, and the Brazilian giant coral.

Symptoms

The venom of a cobra snake is a toxin chemically different from that of other snakes; some suggest it may contain a cardiotoxin. Within 15 to 30 minutes symptoms appear: pain, swelling, a drop in blood pressure, confusion, slurring of speech, dilation of the pupils, strabismus (deviation of the eye), drooping of the upper eyelid, and muscle weakness. The respiratory muscles are affected last, and respiratory muscle paralysis is the most common cause of death. The venom from this snake family is twice as toxic as strychnine and nearly five times more toxic than the venom of a black widow spider.

Treatment

The specific antiserum for the type of cobra involved should be used.

cobra, black-necked   See COBRA, SPITTING.

cobra, Egyptian *(Naja haje)*   Most likely the asp of ancient history and of Cleopatra's suicide, the Egyptian cobra is dark with a narrow hood. It inhabits much of Africa, in the savanna and sometimes near water, and has also been seen in a few small areas in Saudi Arabia. Also known as the African cobra, it is quiet but inquisitive and highly aggressive when restrained. It is considered small but can grow as long as 6 feet.

Cobras live in holes in the ground, and while they can climb into a shrub if they have to, it is unusual to see them anywhere but on the ground. These snakes will hiss if threatened in their holes, but if threatened in the open, they will pack their coils around themselves, spread their hoods and turn to face the enemy.

Symptoms

Within 15 to 30 minutes symptoms appear: pain, swelling, a drop in blood pressure, and confusion followed by death if the poison spreads to the respiratory muscles.

Treatment

Antivenin is available, but only the specific antiserum for the type of cobra involved should be used; victims are often tested for sensitivity before being treated.

See also ANTIVENIN; SNAKES, POISONOUS.

cobra, Indian *(Naja naja)*   Also known as the Asian cobra, this favorite of snake charmers kills many thousands of people each year. It is commonly found in paddy fields and urban areas of southern Asia, Indonesia, Taiwan, and the Philippines. In India, the species has a black-and-white spectaclelike mark on a very wide hood; in other locations, the Indian cobra has a ring or bar on its hood. Growing up to 6 feet long, it is generally inoffensive but highly aggressive when restrained; it is active at dusk and during the night. When confronted by an aggressor, it rears up the front of its body and inflates its hood, standing its ground. Its venom is highly neurotoxic; it is fatal so often because it comes into populated areas to seek out rats.

Symptoms
Pain radiating from the wound, swelling, numbness, drooping eyelids, difficulty in speaking, weakness, respiratory distress, blindness, convulsions, and death.

Treatment
Antivenin is available, but only the specific antiserum for the type of cobra involved should be used; victims are often tested for sensitivity before being treated.

See also ANTIVENIN; SNAKES, POISONOUS.

cobra, king *(Ophiophagus hannah or Naja hannah)*
The world's largest venomous snake, the king cobra (or hamadryad) is found in forests and areas of rural agriculture from southern China to the Philippines and Indonesia. This huge snake can grow as long as 18 feet; when angered, it raises its head and can stand as tall as a person. A normally quiet snake, the king cobra is highly dangerous when aroused; its bite is lethal about 10 percent of the time. It spreads a small hood, and while adult snakes have a dull color with no markings, young snakes sport a black skin with narrow chevrons of pale yellow on buff.

King cobras are often found in pairs, which may be the origin of the ancient belief that a person who kills a king cobra will be pursued and killed by its mate, intent on revenge.

King cobras are the most intelligent and curious of snakes and in captivity will watch any activity going on outside their cage. They are rarely kept in zoos outside of the tropics, however, because they are selective feeders, existing entirely on other species of snakes.

Symptoms
Within 15 to 30 minutes symptoms appear: pain, swelling, a drop in blood pressure, and confusion followed by death if the poison spreads to the respiratory muscles.

Treatment
Antivenin is available, but only the specific antiserum for the type of cobra involved should be used; victims are often tested for sensitivity before being treated.

See also ANTIVENIN; SNAKES, POISONOUS.

cobra, spitting *(Naja nigricollis)*   This nervous and aggressive cobra is widely found throughout Africa, except in the extreme south and the Sahara. It is one of the cobras that can eject venom at a victim's eyes at distances of up to more than 7 feet; the venom can cause temporary or permanent blindness unless promptly washed out. Also called the black-necked cobra, this snake prefers to spit and rarely bites. The sprayed venom is harmless to unbroken skin.

Symptoms
The venom of a cobra snake is chemically different from the venom of other snakes. Within 15 to 30 minutes symptoms appear: pain, swelling, a drop in blood pressure, and confusion followed by death if the poison spreads to the respiratory muscles.

Treatment
The specific antiserum for the type of cobra involved should be used, and victims are often tested for sensitivity before being treated.

See also ANTIVENIN; SNAKES, POISONOUS.

cocaine   One of the most popular of the abused drugs in America today, cocaine is an alkaloid of the coca plant grown on the slopes of the Andes, where it has been cultivated for thousands of years. The oval leaves that provide cocaine and 13 other alkaloids are picked four times a year, and the 4-foot-high bushes continue to produce the leaves for up to 30 years. After the leaves arc harvested, they are dried (sometimes in the sun or in a fire) and then packed for shipment. Cocaine has many uses as a medicine, and is especially valuable as a local anesthetic. As a solution of one of its acid salts, cocaine has long served as a topical anesthetic in the eye and on mucous membranes, but it is not commonly used in clinical medicine today. It is, however, still used in veterinary medicine.

Indians throughout the Andes chew coca leaves at an early age and continue the habit through their lifetime. Cocaine was first extracted from the leaves of the coca bush in Germany more than 100 years ago, and the kick obtained from sniffing the white powder was soon recognized. Indeed, cocaine was enthusiastically recommended by many medical authorities, including Sigmund Freud, who believed it could cure alcoholism and promote sexuality. Sir Arthur Conan Doyle, another cocaine adherent, popularized it further by making his character Sherlock Homes a sniffer and needle abuser of the white powder.

In the United States, a soft drink developed in 1886 by an Atlanta druggist contained a touch of cocaine and caffeine from the African cola nut, becoming famous as Coca-Cola; under pressure from the U.S. government in 1903, however, all cocaine was removed from the beverage. Coke's removal of the drug kicked off a federal crackdown on the use of cocaine, and beginning in 1906 a series of laws placed it under strict federal regulation.

Cocaine may be sniffed ("snorted"), smoked, or injected; combined with heroin and injected, it is called a "speedball." Addicts prefer to inject it intravenously for the brief but intense elation that it induces. Similar to amphetamine in some of its action, cocaine even in a large oral dose dissipates quickly (usually within two to three hours).

"Crack" (the "freebase" form of cocaine) is made by dissolving cocaine salt in solution and extracting the freebase form with a solvent, such as ether. Heat is often applied to hasten solvent evapora-tion. Cocaine sold as a street drug may also contain caffeine, phenylpropanolamine, ephedrine, or phencyclidine.

Cocaine is a local anesthetic and a central nervous system stimulant, with an intoxication resembling an amphetamine "high." It is well absorbed in the body, and smoking or injections can produce the maximum effects within a few minutes. Oral or nasal application may take up to 30 minutes. Its toxicity varies greatly from one individual to the next and is also affected by the presence of other drugs in the system. Still, the oral lethal dose is described as about 1 gram in adults, but some addicts are reported to have consumed as much as 10 grams in one day, reflecting an acquired tolerance. The method of use also affects toxicity; injecting or smoking cocaine may produce such rapid high levels in the brain or heart that convulsions or heart attack may occur, while the same dose ingested or snorted may produce only a feeling of euphoria.

Symptoms

Cocaine can be toxic to both the central nervous and the cardiovascular systems. Symptoms include anxiety, agitation, delirium, psychosis, muscle rigidity, hyperactivity, seizures, and coma. Chronic cocaine use causes weight loss, insomnia, and paranoid psychosis. In addition, symptoms may include fatal heart irregularities, severe hypertension, stroke, coronary artery spasm, heart attack, chronic heart disease, shock, and kidney failure. Death is usually caused by a sudden fatal heart irregularity, seizure, brain hemorrhage, or multiple organ failure. Other symptoms can occur from snorting or smoking cocaine, including chest pain, nasal septal perforation, and skin ulcers ("coke burns").

Treatment

There is no specific antidote. Provide symptomatic treatment; after cocaine ingestion, perform gastric lavage but do not induce vomiting because of the risk of seizures. Administer activated charcoal and a cathartic. For those who have ingested large packets of cocaine in an attempt to smuggle or hide the drug, give repeated doses of activated charcoal and consider whole gut lavage (otherwise, laparotomy and surgical removal may be necessary).

codeine (methylmorphine) This narcotic pain-killer is a naturally occurring alkaloid of opium (from the poppy plant) used in medicine as a cough suppressant and narcotic analgesic drug. It was first synthesized from morphine (an opium derivative) in 1832; although it can be extracted directly from opium, most of the codeine used in drugs is produced from morphine. When taken over a long period of time, codeine may be habit-forming.

Supertoxic, it is used to treat mild to moderate pain and can also be used as an antidiarrheal. It is found in combination with a wide range of other drugs, such as acetaminophen, aspirin, caffeine, and cough suppressants. Because of its value as a cough suppressant, it had been included in a number of cough medicines in the past. But because they were available to those who experimented with drugs, codeine was removed from many of these products. However, more than 40 prescription cough medicines still contain codeine.

Nearly transparent, it has no odor and a bitter taste and is sold as either a powder or liquid. In some forms it is a Schedule II drug (a strictly controlled drug considered by law to have a high potential for abuse), and psychological dependence can develop fairly rapidly, but it is not a major drug of abuse.

Symptoms

Within 20 minutes after ingestion, victims will begin to feel sleepy, giddy, and clumsy, with a slow heartbeat; overdoses can lead to excitability, breathing problems, coma, and death.

Treatment

Naloxone is the antidote; other symptoms are treated as they appear.

See also ALKALOIDS; NALOXONE.

Cogentin See BENZTROPINE.

coliform bacteria The common microorganism *Escherichia coli* (or *E. coli*) that is found in the intestines of humans and other animals; in the gut the bacteria do not cause disease, but a high concentration of the bacteria in drinking water supplies or aquatic ecosystems is often an indicator of pollution.

colocynth *(Citrullus colocynthis)* Also known as bitter apple or bitter cucumber, this extremely toxic bitter fruit is native to the Mediterranean but can also be found in Central America.

Poisonous part

The toxic fruit contains colocynthin, which is used as an insecticide, purgative, and abortifacient.

Symptoms

Within several hours of ingestion, symptoms of bloody diarrhea appear, followed by cramps, headache, kidney failure, and death. Those who live more than two days will most likely recover.

Treatment

Administer milk to relieve stomach irritation and atropine to minimize gastric secretions, plus medication for pain.

comfrey *(Symphytum officianale)* [Other names: gum plant, healing herb, knitbone, nipbone.] Once a popular tea herb found in every herbalist's garden and used to aid digestion and promote healing, comfrey has been shown to be poisonous by recent studies, although the findings are considered by some to be controversial.

Naturalized throughout North America and native to Europe and Asia, comfrey is a hardy perennial with a stout, brown-black root (from which the plant gets its nickname, "slippery root") and blue, yellow, white, or red tubular flowers appearing in May and June. It grows to about 3 feet high and has coarse, hairy egg-shaped leaves; its fruit of black nuts can be seen in August. It is found along stream banks and in rich soils of moist meadows.

As early as 400 B.C. comfrey was used to stop heavy bleeding and to treat bronchial problems. Its popularity as a treatment for broken bones gave the plant its name, a derivative from the Latin *conferta* ("to grow together"). In the 19th century during the Irish potato famines, the plant was seen as a solution to world hunger by Englishman Henry Doubleday, who founded an association still in existence today to promote the plant's use.

While remedies derived from the roots have been prescribed since the early 1500s for everything from tumors to burns and gangrene, in the early 1970s darker reports about this herb's character began to surface: a weed containing pyrrolizidine alkaloids fell into some wheat being harvested in Afghanistan. When the farmers and their families ate the bread made from the contaminated wheat, 25 percent of the 7,200 villagers developed liver ailments within two years.

Poisonous part

Recent studies show the roots and leaves of all varieties contain potentially dangerous compounds called pyrrolizidine alkaloids, which have caused liver tumors in animals. While comfrey leaves (from which tea is brewed) have only one-tenth the alkaloid concentration as the root, several teas on the market contain both root and leaves. In other comfrey products, such as comfrey-pepsin tablets (called "digestive aids"), comfrey root is a primary ingredient.

Symptoms

In 1976 and 1985 there were two cases of pyrrolizidine-alkaloid poisoning in humans, probably from drinking comfrey tea. One recent study found that rats fed a diet that was 8 percent comfrey developed liver cancers within six months; another showed that certain alkaloids in comfrey cause chronic liver problems in rats.

Treatment

Physicians suggest that since comfrey tea won't cure illness and may damage the liver, it is wise to avoid this herb until researchers perfect an accurate test for alkaloid levels in comfrey leaves.

See also HERBS, UNSAFE.

compound 1080 Also known as sodium fluoroacetate and used as a rat poison, this is one of the most toxic substances known; fluoroacetic acid is no longer sold in the United States because of its danger, but fluoroacetate is still available.

Fluoroacetate blocks cell metabolism, and as little as 1 mg is enough to cause serious symptoms. The effects of fluoroacetate poisoning are similar to those of cyanide and hydrogen sulfide, although they take longer to develop.

Symptoms

Within a few minutes to several hours after ingestion, symptoms appear, including nausea, vomiting, diarrhea, metabolic acidosis, agitation, confusion, seizures, coma, respiratory arrest, and heartbeat irregularities. Death results from respiratory failure due to pulmonary edema or ventricular fibrillation.

Treatment

There is no antidote. Perform gastric lavage but do not induce vomiting, since seizures may occur as early as 30 minutes after ingestion. Administer activated charcoal and a cathartic.

See also CYANIDE; HYDROGEN SULFIDE.

cone shell *(Conus)* These highly toxic stinging shells are found on or around coral reefs in warm waters, and although prized by collectors for their bright, spotted shells, they have caused several human deaths. Cone shells are tiny (only one to three inches long) members of the enormous mollusk family, with a cone-shaped shell with wavy stripes or an irregular pattern. The more than 70 different species in this family of toxic marine snails can fire a barbed harpoonlike device from a slit in their shell to obtain food and protect against predators.

There are three main types of cones—those that eat worms, mollusks, or fish. Of all the cones, the fish-eating varieties are most dangerous to humans; they have teeth strong enough to pierce cloth.

Cones live in warm waters of barrier reefs in the Indo-Pacific, Australia and the Mediterranean, southern California and New Zealand. Some of the most common include the geography cone *(C. geographus)*, striated cone *(C. striatus)*, and the tulip cone *(C. tulipa)*.

Poisonous part

The cone shell uses its sting to secrete a neurotoxin that competes for acetylcholine in the body, and can be fatal within 15 minutes.

Symptoms

Pain, swelling, numbness or tingling, dizziness, blurred vision, difficulty swallowing, weakness, ataxia, breathing problems, paralysis, coma, and death.

Treatment

There is no known antidote. Contact medical help immediately; flush the wound with fresh- or salt water, and then soak the affected area in hot water or put hot compresses on it. The water should be very hot (122°F), so that the heat will deactivate the poison. Continue applying hot water for 30 minutes to an hour. Have the victim lie still with the stung part immobile and lower than the heart. Tie a flat strip of cloth around the stung arm or leg two to four inches above the sting. It should be snug but loose enough to allow a pulse farther out on the limb. Check periodically and loosen if necessary, but do not remove it. If swelling reaches the band, tie another band two to four inches higher up and remove the first one. Generally, victims recover within 48 hours.

coniine   The most important of the six alkaloids found in all parts of *Conium maculatum* (poison hemlock), a plant widely found throughout the United States and Europe. The whole plant exudes a foul odor (similar to cat urine or mice) at least in part attributable to the volatile coniine. Prolonged inhalation of the odors is said to cause a narcosis. The toxic potential of coniine has been known since earliest times and was presumably instrumental in the death of Socrates.

See also ALKALOIDS; HEMLOCK, POISON.

copperhead, Australian *(Denisonia superba)*   A poisonous snake of the cobra family found in Tasmania and along the coasts of southern Australia. About 5 feet long, this copperhead is usually copper or reddish brown. Although dangerous, it is unaggressive when not disturbed.

Symptoms

The venom of a cobra snake is a toxin chemically different from that of other snakes; some suggest it may contain a cardiotoxin. Within 15 to 30 minutes symptoms appear: pain, swelling, a drop in blood pressure, confusion, slurring of speech, dilation of the pupils, strabismus (abnormal deviation of one eye in relation to the other), drooping of the upper eyelid, and muscle weakness. The respiratory muscles are affected last, and respiratory muscle paralysis is the most common cause of death.

Treatment

Antivenin is available, but only the specific antiserum for the type of cobra involved should be used; victims are often tested for sensitivity before being treated.

See also ANTIVENIN; SNAKES, POISONOUS.

copperhead snake *(Agkistrodon contortrix)*   Also called highland moccasin, this species of copperhead is a member of the Viperidae family and one of several unrelated snakes that get their name from the reddish color of the head. The *Agkistrodon* variety is the North American copperhead, a venomous species found in swampy, rocky, and wooden regions of the eastern and central United States. It is considered a pit viper because of the characteristic small sensory pit between each eye and nostril.

Usually less than three feet long, the copperhead is a pink or red snake with a copper-colored head with reddish brown hourglass-shaped crossbands on its back. While many bites are reported, the venom of this snake is relatively weak and rarely fatal. The copperhead has retractable hollow fangs in the front of the upper jaw that can be folded back and then positioned forward as the mouth opens to strike.

Seriousness of the bite depends on a wide variety of variables, including the snake's size (usually the larger, the more venomous) and whether the snake is hungry or alert. The angle of the bite and its depth and length also affect the seriousness of the bite. In addition, the victim's size (children and infants are at greater risk) and health at the time of the bite will also affect the outcome. People with diabetes, hypertension, or blood coagulation problems and the elderly are particularly sensitive to snake venom, and menstruating women may bleed excessively following the bite of a pit viper. Several cases of miscarriage have been reported when pregnant women have been bitten.

Finally, the location of the bite itself is crucial to its severity; venomous snake bites on the head and trunk are twice as serious as those on the extremities, and bites on the arms are more serious than those on the legs.

Poisonous part

The venom is a mixture of proteins that acts on a victim's blood, and even snakes that appear to have been killed by the side of the road have been reported to bite. The size of the snake can give an idea of its potential dangerousness and can be judged by the distance between the fang marks. Fang marks less than eight millimeters apart suggests a small snake; eight to 12 millimeters indicates a medium-size snake and more than 12 mm suggests a large venomous snake. Even snakes that have been "defanged" can be dangerous, since all snakes grow new fangs from time to time.

Symptoms

Swelling, internal bleeding, and changes in red blood cells; central nervous system symptoms include convulsions and sometimes psychotic behavior, muscle weakness, and paralysis. In addition, there are general systemic symptoms of fever, nausea, vomiting, diarrhea, pain, and restlessness. Slow or rapid heartbeat can develop, and kidney failure has been reported.

Treatment

Within the first 30 to 45 minutes after the bite, apply a venous tourniquet a few inches above the bite, loosening it every 15 to 30 minutes and reapplying it above the level of progressive swelling. Keep the victim quiet, lying down to decrease metabolic activity (which affects the spread of the venom). The wound area (especially if it is an arm or leg) should be kept lower than the heart. Within 30 minutes, trained individuals can incise the wound area and apply suction. Antivenin is available but should be administered within four hours; antivenin is rarely helpful if given more than 12 hours after the bite. Tetanus prophylaxis is advisable; other treatment might include blood transfusions, intravenous fluids, treatment for convulsions, and antihistamines to control itching. In addition, broad-spectrum antibiotics may be administered, since snakebites are notorious for becoming infected. If antivenin has not been administered (or was given hours after the bite), sloughing of the skin around the bite is common.

See also ANTIVENIN; PIT VIPER; SNAKE, POISONOUS.

coprine A water-soluble substance found in the wild mushroom *Coprinus atramentarius* and a few other less common species of the same genus. Its metabolites inhibit the liver enzyme acetaldehyde dehydrogenase. If even small amounts of ethanol (alcohol) are consumed within several days after eating the mushroom, acetaldehyde accumulates in the blood, causing illness. In the absence of alcohol, however, *C. atramentarius* is a safe, edible mushroom.

See also INKY CAP; MUSHROOM POISONING.

coral plant (*Jatropha multifida*) This plant is so poisonous that even a small amount—just one seed—can be toxic for a small child. This large, attractive plant is often kept as a houseplant despite its toxicity. It has large, deeply lobed circular leaves and coral-red flowers that bloom most of the year, and its yellow fruit has one seed in each of its three sides. It is a member of a large genus of shrubs or small trees with a three-sided seed capsule, found throughout the Western Hemisphere.

Poisonous part

Seeds and perhaps other parts of the plant contain the poison jatrophin, which interferes with protein synthesis in the intestinal wall. The coral plant also contains a plant lectin (toxalbumin) and cathartic oils that are toxic. Ingestion of just one seed can be serious. The plant lectin inhibits protein synthesis in cells of the intestinal wall and may cause serious or fatal poisoning.

Symptoms

The onset of symptoms (nausea, vomiting, and diarrhea) occurs rapidly, unlike poisoning with other plants with toxic lectins.

Treatment

Give fluids and provide supportive treatment.
See also BARBADOS NUT; BELLYACHE BUSH.

coral poisoning A cut from a coral reef may seem innocuous and is often ignored by visitors to the temperate waters where coral reefs are found. Because coral abrasions always contain pieces of animal protein and bits of coral material, even the slightest scratch may become infected, turning into a nasty ulcer that recurs for many years.

In addition to the true corals, there is also a "hydroid" coral, or stinging coral (also called fire coral), which is important to the formation of reefs. Its exoskeleton is made up of calcium carbonate, which is covered with tiny pores and is found off the Florida Keys and in the Caribbean.

Symptoms

Immediately after coming in contact with the coral, the victim exhibits welts, itching, and burning at the wound site. The wound may weep and form wheals. Stinging coral causes burning pain on contact.

Untreated, a coral cut—which looks innocuous enough at first—can within days become an ulcer that continuously sloughs off and is surrounded by a painful swelling. This ulcer can be incredibly painful—much more so than it looks—and can be quite disabling. If the wound is on the legs, the victim may be unable to walk for months. Generalized symptoms can include enlargement of local lymph glands, fever, and malaise. Relapses are common and occur without warning.

Fire coral scrapes often result in bleeding that helps remove the toxin but may be severe enough to require direct pressure on the wound to control blood loss.

Treatment

Ideally, antiseptics should be applied as soon as a person gets the smallest coral cut. Cleanse with soap and water, dry and clean with alcohol, dry again, and rinse with hydrogen peroxide. In severe cases, the person should be put to bed with the wound elevated and given kaolin poultices, antibiotics, and antihistamines.

coral snake There are about 65 species of this strongly patterned snake, a member of the cobra family—and all are dangerous. While true coral snakes are found primarily in the tropics, similar forms can also be found in Asia and Africa. In addition, there are two varieties of coral snakes found in the United States, the only species of Elapidae that are native here. They are the eastern coral snake *(Micrurus fulvius)* and the Arizona coral *(Micruroides euryxanthus euryxanthus)*. Although coral snakes rarely bite when handled, the venom of some of them is capable of killing a person. The largest genus *(Micrurus)* ranges from the southern United States to Argentina. Other coral snakes include the African coral *(Aspidelaps lubricus);* the black-banded coral *(Micrurus nigrocinctus)* found in Central America; and the often-fatal Brazilian giant coral *(M. frontalis),* found in southern South America.

Poisonous part

Strikingly colored, coral snakes have alternating red and black bands separated by narrow yellow or white rings. Their grooved fangs are fixed to the front part of the upper jaw and cannot be folded back, unlike the vipers and pit vipers. This is one of the snakes for which an old rhyme can sometimes be useful to differentiate poisonous from nonlethal varieties. Old folk rhymes hold that it is possible to tell the difference between harmless and deadly coral snakes by the stripes—deadly varieties have red stripes next to yellow ones. There are several versions of these rhymes: "Red on yellow, kill a fellow; red on black, okay Jack" or "Red touching yellow, dangerous fellow."

Symptoms

Numbness at bite, headache, facial swelling, sore throat, skin hypersensitivity, drooping eyelids, photophobia, vomiting, rapid heartbeat, backache, irritability, and death. Some species of coral snakes have a venom that breaks down the red blood cells and frees the hemoglobin, which then appears in urine.

Treatment

Antiserum is available for some species, but not for all. There is antivenin for the eastern coral snake; there is no antivenin for the Arizona coral snake.

See also ANTIVENIN; ANTIVENIN, CORAL SNAKE; SNAKES, POISONOUS.

coral snake, Arizona *(Microruoides euryxanthus euryxanthus)* Also known as the Sonoran coral, this is one of two coral snake species found in the United States. A rare variety of coral snake, it has a potent bite but rarely strikes humans. Found in the southwestern United States deserts, it is quite small and rarely seen, coming out from its underground retreat only at night—usually after a warm rain. When disturbed, it buries its head in its coils and raises and exposes the bottom of its tail.

Several harmless snakes look very similar in color to the coral snakes, and it is important to be able to tell the difference. The Arizona coral has wide red and black bands separated by yellow rings, all almost the same width.

Poisonous part

The venom of the coral snakes contains a deadly neurotoxin that can be fatal and is believed to block the uptake of acetylcholine at the receptor sites. Their small, nonmovable fangs are not as efficient as those of vipers, and so this snake must hold on to its victim for a longer period of time in order to inject its venom.

Symptoms

Symptoms appear within one to five hours, although occasionally it takes even longer. Early signs are systemic and include slurring of speech, dilation of the pupils, strabismus (eye movement), drooping of the upper eyelid, and muscle weakness. The respiratory muscles are affected last, and respiratory muscle paralysis is the most common cause of death in coral snakebites.

Treatment

Antivenin is available; should it be inaccessible, it may be possible to maintain life by intensive life support measures through the period of acute respiratory muscle paralysis. The poison is metabolized after about four days, symptoms fade and recovery is usually complete in those who survive.

coral snake, eastern *(Micrurus fulvius)* Also called a harlequin snake, this fairly small non-hooded member of the cobra family is found in North Carolina and Missouri to northeastern Mexico in moist, dense vegetation near ponds or streams and in hardwood forests, pine flats, rocky hillsides, and canyons. While common, this nocturnal snake is rarely seen and prefers burrowing at night.

About 30 inches long, the eastern coral snake has wide bands of red and black separated by narrow yellow rings, and the head is completely black from the end of its blunt nose to just behind the eyes. The red rings are sometimes spotted with black. The eastern coral can be confused with the harmless scarlet snake and the scarlet king snake.

One of the few snakes that make a warning noise as they strike, the eastern coral has been heard to produce a succession of popping noises by drawing air at its vent and then expelling it.

Symptoms

The bite of the eastern coral snake is unlikely to be fatal unless there is a prodigious amount of venom or the bite is in a particularly vulnerable place. Symptoms appear within one to five hours, although occasionally it takes longer. Early signs are systemic and include slurring of speech, dilation of the pupils, strabismus (abnormal deviation of one eye in relation to the other), drooping of the upper eyelid, and muscle weakness. The respiratory muscles are affected last.

Treatment

Antivenin is available.

See also ANTIVENIN; ANTIVENIN, CORAL SNAKE; SNAKES, POISONOUS.

corn cockle *(Agrostemma githago)* Native to Europe but introduced in America, the annual is tall and gray, with purple pin petals and pink flowers, and is occasionally grown as an ornamental. The milled seeds of this noxious weed may be found in flour.

Poisonous part

The entire plant is poisonous (active ingredient is githagin and saponin glycosides), but the seeds are particularly deadly—especially if ground up with flour or cereal.

Symptoms

Frequent ingestion of small amounts causes a chronic disease resulting in pain, prickling and burning of the lower extremities, and increasing paralysis. Symptoms may appear within 30 minutes to an hour after ingestion and include dizziness, diarrhea, respiratory distress, vomiting, headache, sharp pain in the spine, coma, and death.

Treatment

Gastric lavage and treatment of symptoms.

corticosteroids Used principally as an anti-inflammatory agent, these drugs are used to treat arthritis, bursitis, certain skin diseases, adrenal gland insufficiency, thyroiditis, some cancers, asthma, and other disorders. Though normally not highly toxic, they pose a serious danger to those with allergies or gastrointestinal tract disease, peptic ulcers, or poor heart function. Treatment is the same as that for general anti-inflammatory drugs.

See also ANTI-INFLAMMATORY DRUGS.

cortinarius mushrooms The members of the *Cortinarius* genus of mushrooms, once thought to be harmless, are deadly poison—almost as poisonous as the *Amanita* genus of mushrooms. A little more than a cup of the cooked mushrooms can be fatal. Found in central Europe, the mushrooms have caps ranging from blue violet (which can be eaten) to those of brown or red (deadly); they get their name from the veil that sometimes covers the gills of young mushrooms.

Poisonous part

The mushroom contains the poison orellanin, which damages the liver and kidneys.

Symptoms

Symptoms do not appear until three days to two weeks after ingestion; by then, the victim develops excessive thirst and may drink several liters of fluid a day. By this time, the liver and kidneys usually have been irreversibly damaged. Other symptoms may include nausea, headache, muscular pains, and chills.

Treatment

Gastric lavage, if performed immediately after ingestion. In general, the only treatment once symptoms appear are kidney and liver transplants.

See also MUSHROOM POISONING; MUSHROOM TOXINS.

cottonmouth snake See WATER MOCCASIN.

Coyotillo *(Karwinskia humboldtiana)* A small tree or shrub that grows in Texas, New Mexico, and Mexico, and reaches a height of up to 24 feet. Its small green flowers bloom during the summer, and its black to brown fruit matures around October. The plant is toxic to humans as well as to cattle, hogs, goats, sheep, and fowl.

Poisonous part

The leaves and fruit are poisonous and contain polyphenolic compounds.

Symptoms

Chronic ingestion may cause ascending paralysis; weakness occurs after a latent period of several weeks; paralysis may progress for a month or more. The neurological picture is similar to that of Guillain-Barré syndrome or other polyradiculoneuropathies.

Treatment

Supportive. If victims survive respiratory paralysis, they will recover completely.

crack cocaine   See COCAINE.

creosote   Creosote is the name used for a variety of products that are mixtures of many chemicals; those products include wood creosote, coal tar creosote, coal tar, and coal tar pitch. Creosotes don't occur naturally in the environment; they are created by high-temperature treatment of woods (wood creosote) or coal (coal tar creosote), or from the resin of the creosote bush (creosote bush resin).

Coal tar creosote is the most common form of creosote in the workplace and at hazardous waste sites in the United States; it is referred to by the U.S. Environmental Protection Agency (EPA) as "creosote." This thick, oily liquid is typically amber to black in color and is a distillation product of coal tar. It has a burning, caustic taste. Coal tar creosote is the most widely used wood preservative in the United States; it is applied to preserve and waterproof wood for log homes, railroad ties, telephone poles, marine pilings, and fence posts. It's also a restricted-use pesticide and is used as an animal and bird repellant, insecticide, animal dip, fungicide, and pharmaceutical agent for the treatment of psoriasis. About 300 chemicals have been identified in coal tar creosote, but there may be as many as 10,000 other chemicals in the mixture.

Wood creosote ranges in color from clear to yellow; it's a greasy liquid with a characteristic smoky odor and sharp burned taste. The major chemicals in wood creosote are phenol, cresols, and guaiacol. This type of creosote has been used as a disinfectant, a laxative, and a cough treatment; it is rarely used today in the United States but is still used as an expectorant and a laxative in Japan.

Coal tar and coal tar pitch are the by-products of the high-temperature treatment of coal to make coke or natural gas; they are usually thick, black or dark brown liquids or semisolids with a naphthalene-like odor. Coal tar products, which have a sharp, burning taste, are found as ingredients in medicines used to treat skin diseases such as psoriasis and in insecticides, animal dips, and fungicides.

Coal tar creosotes, coal tar, and coal tar pitch are similar in composition; the major chemicals in them that can cause harmful health effects are polycyclic aromatic hydrocarbons, phenol, and cresols. Creosotes and coal tars are complex mixtures that contain primarily condensed aromatic ring compounds or phenols.

Coal tar creosote components dissolved into water move through the soil to eventually reach and enter groundwater, where they may persist; once in the water, biodegradation may take months. Biodegradation in soil can take months for some components of coal tar creosote, or much longer for others.

No federal criteria have been set for creosote levels in water, and there are no air standards. In 1978, the EPA initiated a special review of creosote based on its cancer-causing reputation; as a result, it did not ban the substance but proposed a set of regulations intended to reduce exposure. Creosote is listed as a hazardous air pollutant in the 1990 Clean Air Act, requiring the EPA to set emission standards and is on the EPA community right-to-know list. Creosote is also a restricted-use pesticide, meaning that it may be applied only by certified applicators.

The Consumer Awareness Program recommends against using creosote-treated wood products in proximity to food, animal food, and public drinking water. People are advised not to burn creosote-treated wood, and applicators must wear protective clothing, special face masks or goggles, respirators, and gloves. If creosote is used on wood that will touch bare skin (such as in playground furniture or outdoor furniture), two coats of urethane or shellac sealer must be applied. A sealer should also be applied to treated wood used in areas where inhalation exposure may occur, such as in barns and stables.

Symptoms

The International Agency for Research on Cancer and the EPA have determined that coal tar creosote probably causes cancer in humans. The EPA has determined that coal tar pitch is a human carcinogen; it classified coal tar creosote as a carcinogen in the 1992 Toxic Release Inventory (TRI).

Cancers of the skin and scrotum have been linked to long-term exposure to low levels of these chemical mixtures, especially through direct contact with skin during wood treatment or manufacture of coal tar creosote-treated products, or in coke or natural gas factories. Cancer of the scrotum in chimney sweeps has been associated particularly with prolonged skin exposure to soot and coal tar creosote.

Eating food or drinking water contaminated with a high level of creosotes may cause burning in the mouth and throat, as well as stomach pains. Brief exposure to large amounts of coal tar creosote may result in a rash or severe irritation of the skin, chemical burns of the surfaces of the eye, convulsions, mental confusion, kidney or liver problems, unconsciousness, or even death.

Longer exposure to lower levels of coal tar creosote, coal tar, or coal tar pitch by direct contact with skin or by exposure to the vapors from these mixtures can also result in sun sensitivity and cause damage to skin, such as reddening, blistering, or peeling. Longer exposures to the vapors of the creosotes, coal tar, or coal tar pitch can also cause irritation of the respiratory tract.

Treatment

If the victim is alert, give a slurry of activated charcoal and perform careful gastric lavage if there are no deep burns in the mouth or pharynx. AVOID ADMINISTRATION OF ALCOHOL. Remove contaminated clothing, and blot up liquid on skin (caregiver should wear gloves). Wash exposed areas of the skin, and give morphine for pain. Sodium bicarbonate may ease symptoms; give oxygen as needed and monitor vital signs.

See also PHENOL.

crocus   See MEADOW SAFFRON.

croton *(Croton tiglium)*   Also known as mayapple, this supertoxic plant is native to Southeast Asia and now also grows in the southwestern United States. Croton oil in alcohol is also known as a "Mickey Finn."

Poisonous part

Seeds and extracted oil from the plant are deadly.

Symptoms

Skin contact results in immediate blistering and irritation, which can last up to three weeks. If the seeds or oil are ingested, symptoms appear within 10 to 15 minutes and include burning pain in the mouth and stomach, bloody diarrhea, kidney and liver damage, nausea, vomiting, fast heartbeat, coma, and death.

Treatment

Vomiting and gastric lavage are ineffective. Give fluids orally along with intravenous infusion to correct electrolyte imbalance; treat symptoms.

cryptosporidiosis   One of the more recently discovered types of food poisoning, cryptosporidiosis is a reportable disease caused by a protozoan called *Cryptosporidium parvum*. The invisible microbe infects cells lining the intestinal tract; it was not identified as a cause of human disease until 1976.

In 1993, a waterborne outbreak in Milwaukee sickened about 400,000 people. *Parvum* has been associated with diarrhea outbreaks in child-care centers throughout the country. In 1994, 302 cases were reported to the New York state health department.

Today it is a major threat to the U.S. water supply. Able to infect with as few as 30 oocysts, *Cryptosporidium* has been found in untreated surface water as well as in swimming pools, wading pools, hot tubs, ice cubes, fruits and vegetables, lakes, rivers, day-care centers, and hospitals.

Experts estimate that 2 percent of the population in North America is infected and that 80 percent of the population has had an infection in the past. In the United States, many outbreaks are never identified, and the number of cases that occur each year aren't well documented. Some immunity follows infection, but the degree to which this immunity occurs is not clear.

This parasite lives its entire life within the intestinal cells; it produces worms that are excreted in feces. These infectious worms can survive outside the human body for long periods of time, passing into food and drinking water, onto objects, and spread from hand to mouth.

Because it is transmitted by the fecal-oral route, the greatest risk occurs in those infected people who have diarrhea, those with poor personal hygiene, and diapered children. It's also found in contaminated water, vegetables fertilized with manure, unpasteurized milk, or any food touched by an infected food handler.

Symptoms

Between one and 12 days after infection, victims experience watery diarrhea together with stomach cramps, nausea and vomiting, fever, headache, and loss of appetite. However, some people with the infection don't experience any symptoms at all. Healthy patients usually suffer with symptoms for only about two weeks.

Diagnosis

The infection is diagnosed by identifying the parasite during examination of the stool. If cryptosporidiosis is suspected, a specific lab test should be requested, since most labs don't yet routinely perform the necessary tests.

Treatment

The Food and Drug Administration has approved nitazoxanide for treatment of diarrhea caused by *Cryptosporidium* in people who have a healthy immune system. Most people who have a healthy immune system will recover from the infection without treatment. Affected individuals should drink plenty of fluids to prevent dehydration. Young children and pregnant women may be more susceptible to dehydration, and rapid loss of fluids from diarrhea may be life-threatening to infants. People who have a compromised immune system are at greater risk for more severe and prolonged illness. The effectiveness of nitazoxanide is not certain in this population.

Complications

People with an impaired immune system may have a severe and lasting illness; the resulting chronic diarrhea in this group may be fatal. Invasion of the lungs in these patients also may be fatal.

Prevention

Unfortunately, chlorine does not kill the protozoan; drinking water must be filtered to eliminate it. Many municipal water supplies do not have the technology to provide this filter. To prevent further transmission, hands should be washed often before and during food preparation, especially after changing diapers or working around young children. Infected people should not prepare any food that will be eaten raw. Fruits and vegetables should be thoroughly washed before eating. Cattle are a source of infection, so consumers shouldn't drink unpasteurized milk or untreated, unfiltered water in other countries.

cube jellies   See JELLYFISH.

curare *(Strychnos)*   A centuries-old extract from the bark and juices of trees in Central America *(Strychnos toxifera),* it has been used as a poison for arrows and for blowgun darts in Central and South America. Curare is a skeletal-muscle relaxant drug, one of the alkaloid family of organic compounds.

It is used in medicine today as an auxiliary to general anesthesia (frequently with cyclopropane), especially in abdominal surgery. Curare acts as a neuromuscular blocking agent that produces flaccidity in striated muscle. Used by South American Indians against enemies and animals, curare is now widely available in the United States as a drug, where it is used to stop normal breathing and allow the patient to be placed on a respirator in order to treat the lungs.

Poisonous part

All parts of the *S. toxifera* plant contain tubocurarine, a drug that interferes with muscle contractions by interfering with the action of the neurotransmitter acetylcholine. Curare is harmless if swallowed. Its poison is activated only if injected or administered intravenously.

Symptoms

Almost immediately, curare affects the muscles of the toes, ears, and eyes, then those of the neck and limbs followed by muscles important for breathing. Death comes as a result of respiratory paralysis.

Treatment

There is no treatment or antidote, since curare works so quickly.

cyanide [**Other names: hydrogen cyanide (prussic acid), potassium cyanide, sodium cyanide.**] The various forms of cyanide (gas, salts) can be swallowed, inhaled, or absorbed through the skin, and it is one of the most rapidly acting poisons known. The inhalation of cyanide in its extremely volatile form called hydrocyanic acid (or prussic acid) can be fatal in just a few minutes. Hydrocyanic acid occurs naturally in a large variety of seeds and pits (such as peach, apricot, apple, plum, etc.) and has many industrial uses.

In addition, many other plants have cyanogenic glycosides that have a similar effect, although they take longer to act. These amygdalin-containing fruit seeds include choke cherries, cassava beans, and bitter almonds.

Hydrogen cyanide is found in fumigants, insecticides, rat poisons, metal polish, and electroplating solution and has also been used in gas chambers. Potassium cyanide and sodium cyanide are both white solids smelling faintly of bitter almonds. Certain cyanides irritate the eyes so powerfully that they have been used in some types of tear gas. In the household, cyanide can be found in many products from silver polish to rat poison.

Symptoms
Cyanide prevents the body's red blood cells from absorbing oxygen by interfering with the body's enzymes. When the cells can't get oxygen, they produce a rapid progression of symptoms; a person who swallows or smells too much cyanide can lose consciousness, fall into convulsions, and die within 15 minutes. Mortality from cyanide may be as high as 95 percent.

Treatment
Call poison control before attempting any treatment, which must be rapid. Do not induce emesis. An antidote kit (containing amyl nitrite perles and intravenous sodium nitrite and sodium thiosulfate) is available. The longer the patient can be kept alive the better the prognosis, since the body can neutralize cyanide by combining it with sulfur compounds to form inactive sulfocyanates. A new fast-acting antidote (within three minutes) was discovered by researchers at the University of Minnesota Center for Drug Design and Minneapolis

VA Medical Center in 2007 and was slated to enter human clinical trials within three years.

See also CHERRIES, WILD AND CULTIVATED; CYANOGENIC GLYCOSIDES; *PRUNUS*.

cyanogenic glycosides A toxic glycoside (a compound found in plants that contains sugar) that gives off hydrocyanic acid and other cyanide compounds when exposed to acids and enzymes in the digestive tract. When this hydrogen cyanide is produced by cyanogenic glycosides, it interferes with the level of oxygen in the blood and causes the blue skin coloring common in cyanide poisoning. Cyanogenic glycosides are found in apricot, cherry, and peach pits, and apple seeds, but they are released only if the pits of seeds are ground and eaten; if swallowed whole, they cause no harm because of the hard outer shell covering.

See also CHERRIES, WILD AND CULTIVATED; CYANIDE; PRUNUS.

cyclohexane hexachloride   See LINDANE.

cyclopropane A flammable general anesthetic not widely used today because of its high cost and explosive nature. Cyclopropane works by depressing all functions of the central nervous system.

Symptoms
When given in large amounts, this anesthetic will stop breathing with possible damage to heart, liver, and kidneys. Symptoms include stupor, unconsciousness, and respiratory paralysis. Convulsions may follow.

Treatment
Symptoms will disappear once the anesthetic is removed. Keep warm, provide CPR if required. Stabilize blood pressure.

See also ANESTHETIC, GASEOUS/VOLATILE.

Cyclospora A one-celled organism, *Cyclospora* causes symptoms similar to *Cryptosporidium* and led to illness in hundreds of residents of at least a dozen states in a 1995 outbreak. Like *Cryptosporidium, Cyclospora* pollutes water and taints food. The infection (cyclosporiasis) is spread from the fecal-oral route, both from person to person and via tainted water or food.

The United States has battled several cyclospora epidemics which began in the spring of 1996 and one included an outbreak in the 11 states east of the Rocky Mountains that caused 1,000 people to get sick from contaminated raspberries. Another raspberry-related outbreak affected 54 people at a wedding reception in Philadelphia in 2000. Since the infection is fairly new, experts believe many cases are simply not diagnosed or reported. Doctors must specifically request testing for *Cyclospora;* it is not detected by routine lab tests.

Some cases have been traced to contaminated strawberries, others to raspberries or mixed fruit. In other cases, experts can't find the original source of the infection.

Symptoms

One to two weeks after infection, symptoms of diarrhea, nausea and vomiting appear, together with fever and stomach pain. Symptoms may be intermittent over the course of the disease, which can last for several weeks. While rarely fatal, untreated diarrhea can cause severe dehydration, which can be a serious health threat to very young children, very old people, and people with faulty immune systems. If not treated, symptoms may last for a few days to a month or more.

Diagnosis

Special lab tests can identify the parasite in stool, which may require specimens collected over several days.

Treatment

A combination of two antibiotics, trimethoprim and sulfamethoxazole, can control the infection; otherwise, rest and plenty of fluids.

Prevention

Wash hands often, especially if you change diapers or work around young children. Thoroughly wash fruits and vegetables before eating. Infected people should not prepare food that is eaten raw. Certain areas of high infection should boil water for one minute before use. The organism doesn't appear to be killed by iodine or chlorine and can even elude filtration systems. The only thing that kills this parasite is boiling the water in which it lives.

daffodil (Narcissus) [Other names: jonquil, white narcissi]   The creamy or yellow flowers of the daffodil can be seen throughout temperate North America. This spring-flowering bulb has been recorded in history as early as the second century B.C. and is extremely popular today in gardens. Daffodils have a trumpet-shaped center against star-shaped petals, with the trumpet often being a contrasting color. The plant stands around 2 feet tall with five-inch blooms. There are about 50 species of daffodil and more than 13,000 hybrids.

Poisonous part

The leaves, berries, stems, and roots all contain toxic compounds, but the most potent concentration is found in bulbs, also referred to as rhizomes or corms. The flowers are not toxic. Poisonous substances are alkaloids, including masonin and homolycorine. Most poisonings occur in children who eat the leaves, bulbs, or stems. During World War II, starving cattle in the Netherlands were fed daffodil bulbs when feed supplies dwindled, and the animals were fatally poisoned. Bulbs should be kept in a secure place away from food areas, where they may be mistaken for onions, and clearly marked.

Symptoms

Alkaloids may cause dizziness, abdominal pain, diarrhea, and nausea. Convulsions and death may occur if enough of the plant has been consumed. Some people who handle daffodils commercially, especially florists and flower growers, frequently experience daffodil dermatitis ("daffodil itch"), which occurs when they make contact with the sap of the bulbs and stems.

Treatment

Induce vomiting and administer copious amounts of fluids; introduce activated charcoal and treat symptoms.

Dalmane (flurazepam)   An anticonvulsant and a muscle relaxant used to relieve anxiety, Dalmane is not as strong as Valium (diazepam) but is still considered toxic. This is a drug often chosen for suicide when combined with alcohol. It reacts negatively with other anticonvulsants, antidepressants, antihistamines, antihypertensives, oral contraceptives, disulfiram, erythromycins, monoamine oxidase (MAO) inhibitors, narcotics, sedatives, sleeping pills, and tranquilizers.

Symptoms

Within 10 to 20 minutes of ingestion, patients become groggy and fall into sleep, dropping further into unconsciousness if a large dose has been taken. Withdrawal psychosis is also possible.

Treatment

Gastric lavage; increase oxygen while maintaining blood pressure.

See also DIAZEPAM.

dantrolene   This drug is used in the treatment of the very high fevers common in anesthesia overdose. It is not, however, a substitute for other means of controlling temperature such as sponging and fanning. Dantrolene is a muscle relaxant that may cause diarrhea, muscle weakness, and, sometimes kidney damage.

daphne *(Daphne)* **[Other names: bois joli, copse laurel, dwarf bay, February daphne, flax olive, lady laurel, spurge flax, spurge laurel, spurge olive, wild pepper, winter daphne, wood laurel.]** One of the oldest plants recognized as a poison, daphne is found throughout the British Isles, the northeastern United States, and eastern Canada. It is widely planted as an ornamental and is sometimes kept indoors as a flowering houseplant. This unusually fragrant rounded shrub has clusters of purple or white flowers that grow in the spring before the leathery leaves appear. Fruits are scarlet or yellow with a pit. Of all the daphne species, the *Daphne mezereum* variety is the most deadly, although all species are considered poisonous.

Poisonous part

All parts of this plant are poisonous, especially the berries, bark, and seeds; berries of *D. mezereum* are bright red; those of *D. laureola* are green, then blue and finally black when fully ripe. Poisonous substances are the glycoside daphnetoxin and mezerein, an irritating, blistering resin. This plant is considered particularly dangerous to children.

Symptoms

Symptoms appear in 45 minutes to several hours and include swelling and blistering of the lips, salivation and problems in swallowing, burning and ulceration in the digestive tract, stomach pain, vomiting, bloody diarrhea, weakness, convulsions, shock, coma, and death. Just a few berries can be fatal to a child. This plant may also cause systemic damage to the kidneys.

Treatment

Gastric lavage with caution, since the mucous membranes may have been damaged as a result of this poison. Victims often go into shock after poisoning with daphne.

Darvon See NARCOTICS.

datura See JIMSONWEED.

DDT **(dichlorodiphenyltrichloroethane)** One of a group of chlorinated hydrocarbons, this insect-fighting chemical was once widely used in agriculture and malarial control programs around the world. It was developed in Switzerland in the early 1940s and was found to be much more effective than previous insecticides and became an important weapon in fighting insect-transmitted diseases. Unfortunately, some insects have adapted to the poison and are resistant to its effects. However, because of its toxicity, it was banned in the United States in 1973 because it does not disperse in the environment but accumulates in biological systems. It is still used in some other parts of the world.

This broad-spectrum insecticide dissolves easily in oil and therefore builds up in fatty tissue; eating animals that have consumed DDT—or even that have eaten others that have consumed DDT—will poison anyone who eats the meat.

While it can be inhaled or absorbed through the skin, the most common means of human exposure is by eating DDT-contaminated food. In fact, inhaling the dust or coming in contact with the solution is rarely harmful to humans unless the person is wearing some sort of oily insect repellent that would aid absorption. However, toxic doses are possible if the skin contact area is large or the exposure lengthy.

Symptoms

DDT affects the central nervous system, causing muscle weakness, excitability and convulsions, with tremor, confusion, headache, numbness of the tongue, lips and face, and vomiting. Twitchings begin in the face and proceed in rising strength to involve all muscles. In fact, attacks resemble the convulsions of strychnine poisoning, since they can be set off by light or noise. Respiratory arrest and heart attack are followed by death.

Chronic poisoning causes weight loss, headache, loss of appetite, nausea, eye irritation, weakness, and increasing tremors followed by convulsions, coma, and death.

Contact with the eyes may cause temporary blindness. People who work with DDT may also experience a gradual sensitization and allergic reactions to the chemical.

Treatment

If convulsions continue for some time, recovery is not likely. Treat symptoms, and perform gastric lavage, but do not induce vomiting. Administer activated charcoal and a cathartic. Stimulants (such as epinephrine) may induce heart attack; administer anticonvulsants (such as Valium) to control convulsions.

See also CHLORINATED HYDROCARBON PESTICIDES.

deadly cort See GALERINA MUSHROOMS.

death camas *(Zigadenus venenosus)* **[Other names: alkali grass, black snake root, hog's potato, mystery grass, poison sego, sand corn, soap plant, squirrel food, water lily, wild onion.]** One of the lily family and often mistaken for an onion, the death camas is found throughout North America (especially the extreme southeast) and Alaska and Canada.

Leaves are grassy and long and narrow—up to two feet tall—and at the top, the stem has a branched cluster of greeny white to yellow flowers. The plant's bulb looks like an onion, but does not have an oniony odor.

Poisonous part

Fresh leaves, stems, bulbs, and flowers are poisonous, but the seeds are particularly deadly. Poisons include zygacine, veratrine and zygadenine, protoveratridine, iso- and neogermidine. While cattle are usually poisoned by death camas, it is possible for humans to be poisoned as well.

Symptoms

Symptoms appear within one hour and include burning of the mouth, vomiting, thirst, weakness, slow heartbeat, staggering, paralysis, convulsions, coma, and death.

Treatment

There is no antidote, but gastric lavage should be performed if the victim has not vomited. Fluids and the administration of atropine or ephedrine may also be required.

death cap/death cup *(Amanita phalloides)* One of the deadliest members of the *Amanita* genus of mushrooms, the death cap or death cup is found in woods or their borders and is responsible for most of the fatalities associated with mushroom poisoning. It has a green or brown cap and appears in summer or early fall. Some experts also include the destroying angel as part of the *Amanita phalloides* group.

Poisonous part

This deadly mushroom contains peptide toxins, phalloidin and two amanitins that damage cells throughout the body within six to 12 hours after ingestion. The toxins are not affected by drying, cooking, or boiling in water.

Symptoms

First symptoms are caused by the action of the amatoxins on the intestine, but this is not responsible for the ultimate outcome. Twelve hours after ingestion, symptoms include violent abdominal pain, vomiting, bloody diarrhea, loss of fluid, and intense thirst. A latency period follows, up to five days, but by then the toxins have damaged the liver, kidneys, and central nervous system. There is a decrease in urinary output and a drop in sugar levels in the blood, which leads to coma and—more than 50 percent of the time—death.

Treatment

During the first phase, give fluids and monitor electrolytes; urine flow should be maintained, and repeat doses of activated charcoal may be given. If management is successful, the victim will recover within one week. Various strategies have been tried to treat this type of mushroom poisoning in Europe, including massive doses of vitamins, corticosteroids, sex hormones, high-dose glucose, penicillin G, and thioctic acid. None of these has been proven effective.

See also AMANITA MUSHROOMS; MUSHROOM POISONING.

decongestants A range of drugs used to relieve nasal congestion, they work by constricting blood vessels in the nose, which reduces swelling. They are used to treat sinusitis, allergies, and acute upper respiratory infections.

Decongestants include phenylpropanolamine (PPA), phenylephrine (PHE), ephedrine (EPH), and pseudoephedrine (PEP); all but PPA are available over the counter as nasal decongestants and cold preparations that usually contain antihistamines and cough suppressants as well. Combinations of these drugs with caffeine are sold on the street as amphetamine or cocaine substitutes.

Many of these drugs react negatively with other drugs. Patients sensitive to epinephrine, ephedrine, terbutaline, or amphetamines may also be sensitive to drugs such as PPA.

In November 2000, the Food and Drug Administration (FDA) issued a public health warning to consumers, advising them to stop using any medications that contained PPA, as research showed there was a risk of hemorrhagic stroke associated with its use. The FDA also asked drug manufacturers to discontinue the marketing and sales of over-the-counter medications that contained PPA, and stores across the United States pulled these drugs from their shelves.

Symptoms

Poisoning with products containing PPA, PHE, and EPH may provoke symptoms after ingesting just two or three times the recommended dose. PEP is slightly less toxic (symptoms occur with four to five times recommended dose).

Patients taking monoamine oxidase (MAO) inhibitors may be extremely sensitive to these drugs, developing severe high blood pressure after ingesting even less-than-recommended doses.

The most serious symptom of these drugs is severe high blood pressure, together with hypertensive complications of headache, confusion, seizures, and stroke. In fact, intracranial hemorrhage may occur in even normal, healthy young people after only a slight rise in blood pressure. The high blood pressure caused by PPA and PHE occurs together with slow heartbeat, while EPH and PEP usually cause high blood pressure with rapid heartbeat.

Using antihistamines or caffeine may increase the high blood pressure with PPA and PHE. PPA may also cause heart attack and stroke.

Treatment

There is no specific antidote. Give symptomatic treatment; monitor vital signs and electrocardio-gram. Do not use beta blockers to treat high blood pressure without first giving a vasodilator (phentolamine or nitroprusside), for they will worsen the high blood pressure. Do not induce vomiting because of the danger of worsening the high blood pressure. Perform gastric lavage if the victim has ingested the drug within 30 to 60 minutes or has taken a large dose. Administer activated charcoal and a cathartic.

deferoxamine This specific chelating agent is used in the treatment of iron overdose, particularly in the presence of shock, acidosis, severe gastroenteritis, leukocytosis, and high blood sugar. It binds to the circulating free iron, and both are excreted in the urine, turning it an orange-pink color. Deferoxamine is also sometimes used to determine the presence of free iron in the body by administering the chelating agent and then looking for the characteristic pinkish rose color of the urine.

See also IRON IN DRUGS AND SUPPLEMENTS.

Demerol See MEPERIDINE; NARCOTICS.

Depakene See VALPROIC ACID.

derrin See ROTENONE.

derris The powdered root of various species of the botanical genus *Derris,* used as an insecticide. It is also used to kill fish without damaging the food supply, enabling game fish to be introduced into the same body of water. The toxic principles of derris include rotenone.

Symptoms

When absorbed through the skin, derris root may cause dermatitis. It is also more toxic than its rotenone and rotenoid content would suggest; it is believed this discrepancy may be due to the presence of other toxic agents in the derris powder. Absorption and toxicity are enhanced by olive oil.

Treatment

Symptomatic and supportive, including removal of the material from the skin and gastrointestinal tract. Oily cathartics should not be used, since absorption may be increased by their use.

See also ROTENONE.

destroying angel (*Amanita bispongera* [smaller death angel], *A. ocreata, A. verna* [fool's angel] and *A. virosa* [destroying angel or death angel]) A mushroom of the poisonous *Amanita* genus, the destroying angel (and its close relatives, named above) are extremely deadly, with a 90 percent fatality rate and no known antidote.

The fool's angel is the most common; it is relatively smaller than the others and chalky white. The destroying angels have a large white body and are found in forests during wet periods in summer and autumn. Experts disagree as to the classification of these related mushrooms, which is why they are listed together here. These amanitas are found in the mid-Atlantic states to Florida and west to Texas and are found in dry pine woods, although the smaller death angel can also be found in wooded lawns, especially near oak trees.

Poisonous part

The main poisons found in these mushrooms are the slow-acting amanitin and the fast-acting phalloidin. Amanitin causes most of the symptoms, and phalloidin causes degeneration in kidney, liver, and heart muscles. These mushrooms are deadly; one or two cooked mushrooms can be fatal, and there exists a report that one-third of one raw cap has killed a child.

Symptoms

After these mushrooms are eaten, there are typically no symptoms for six to 15 hours—and sometimes as long as two days. Symptoms begin suddenly with severe abdominal pain, nausea, vomiting, and diarrhea, followed by extreme abdominal pain, excessive thirst, violent vomiting, urinary problems, weakness, jaundice, convulsions, coma, and death. Severe dehydration eventually results in cardiac arrest. Death occurs within two days of ingestion of a large amount of mushrooms, but more generally it may take up to three days of remissions followed by repeated, more acute attacks. Death occurs in 50 to 90 percent of cases. Recovery can take up to one month.

Treatment

There is no known antidote, although some victims survive if given a liver transplant. Gastric lavage is also instituted. Animal studies suggest that early treatment with penicillin G, silibinin, or cimetidine may partially protect against liver injury. Treat fluid and electrolyte loss to head off massive circulatory collapse.

See also AMANITA MUSHROOMS; MUSHROOM POISONING.

dextromethorphan Found in many over-the-counter cough and cold medicines, dextromethorphan is frequently involved in poisonings with children, although fatalities are rare. Dextromethorphan is also frequently combined with antihistamines, decongestants, or acetaminophen. It is a popular choice for cough suppressants because it works as well as codeine but is not addictive.

Symptoms

Toxicity depends on other ingredients in the particular product that was ingested. Mild overdoses cause ataxia, clumsiness, restlessness, and sometimes visual and auditory hallucinations. More serious overdoses produce stupor, coma, and breathing problems, especially if alcohol has been ingested at the same time. In addition, persons taking monoamine oxidase inhibitors who ingest a normal dose of dextromethorphan may experience high blood pressure and very high fever.

Treatment

Mild overdoses require only supervision; in more severe cases, the drug naloxone has reported to be an effective antidote in some cases, but not in others. Induce vomiting or perform gastric lavage; administer activated charcoal and a cathartic.

DFP   See NARCOTICS.

diarrheic shellfish poisoning Although this type of diarrhea-causing shellfish poison has not been confirmed in the United States, the organisms that produce the poison are found in U.S. waters and an outbreak has been confirmed in eastern Canada. DSP is associated primarily with mussels, oysters, and scallops.

Symptoms

This type of shellfish poisoning begins within 30 minutes to two or three hours, depending on the amount of tainted shellfish eaten. Symptoms (nausea, vomiting, diarrhea) may last as long as two or three days, but recovery is complete with, no aftereffects and the disease is not usually life threatening.

Treatment

No treatment is necessary.

diazepam (Valium) One of the group of benzodiazepines used in the treatment of anxiety or agitation caused by hallucinogenic drug overdose; to control seizures because of convulsant drug overdose; and to relax excessive muscle rigidity and contractions following strychnine poisoning or the bite of the black widow spider.

See also BENZODIAZEPINES; BLACK WIDOW SPIDER; STRYCHNINE.

dieffenbachia *(Dieffenbachia)* [Other names: dumb cane, dumb plant, mother-in-law's tongue, tuft root.] This extremely common plant has been used indoors as an attractive foliage houseplant for hundreds of years, but it can cause mouth pain if ingested and can be fatal in large amounts.

There are a number of dieffenbachia species, including *D. amoena, D. bausei, D. candida, D. exotica, D. maculate,* and *D. seguine.* Dieffenbachia belongs to the family Araceae, which also includes other ornamental plants such as the jack-in-the-pulpit, philodendron, pothos, and calla lily.

These shade-loving plants have bright green oblong leaves and can grow quite tall, with fleshy stems as much as an inch thick. They may be found in outdoor gardens in southern Florida and Hawaii.

Dieffenbachia's toxic qualities have been known for a long time; in the past, slaves were punished by rubbing their mouths with dieffenbachia, and there are reports that the Nazis experimented with this plant in concentration camps during World War II.

Poisonous part

All parts of this plant (including the sap) contain potent irritants including proteolytic enzymes, raphides of calcium oxalate, and other, unknown toxins. The calcium oxalate raphides in this plant are really sharp crystals that puncture tissue; it is possible that the plant contains enzymes that attack cells through the punctures. The mechanisms behind its ability to cause systemic poisoning as well as localized irritation are not known.

Symptoms

All varieties of dieffenbachia contain a range of potent irritants that can cause serious tissue damage to eyes, skin, and mucous membranes. Chewing a leaf from this plant causes almost immediate, intense pain, blistering and burning of the mouth and tongue, excess salivation, swelling of the tongue and throat, and difficulty in swallowing. Pain and swelling may persist for several days and leave damaged tissue behind. Because of the immediate pain upon ingestion, poisoning with large amounts of the plant is unlikely; however, in this event the toxins can swell the throat tissue, blocking the airway and leading to death. Some sources report that dumb cane can also cause systemic poisoning resulting in nausea, vomiting, and diarrhea and damage to internal organs. The name "dumb cane" comes from its tendency to paralyze vocal cords.

Treatment

Pain and swelling in the mouth will slowly fade even without treatment, although cool liquids (such as milk or Popsicles) and painkillers may help. Perform gastric lavage, and give antihistamines for local swelling.

See also PHILODENDRON.

dieldrin [Trade names: Compound 497, HEOD, Octalox.] A highly toxic chlorinated hydrocarbon pesticide used against potato beetles, corn pests, and rape plant parasites. Its manufacture in the United States was banned in 1974 under the Environmental Protection Agency (EPA) Fungicide and Rodenticide Act, although it is still produced for use in Holland.

Dieldrin is highly soluble in fat, where it accumulates in humans or animals until a toxic level is reached. It can be inhaled, absorbed, or ingested and is particularly dangerous when heated, as it can give off very toxic chloride fumes.

Symptoms

Within 20 minutes to 12 hours dieldrin produces headache, dizziness, nausea, vomiting, sweating, excitability, irritability, convulsions, coma, and death.

Treatment

There is no specific antidote. Perform gastric lavage but do not induce vomiting because of the risk of sudden onset of seizures; administer activated charcoal and a cathartic. Irregular heartbeat may respond to propranolol.

See also CHLORINATED HYDROCARBON PESTICIDES.

digitalis A group of drugs used as a heart medicine that are purified from the seeds and leaves of the common foxglove plant *(Digitalis purpurea).* Digitalis strengthens and slows contractions of the heart and restores circulation in persons with congestive heart failure. It also slows the rate of ventricular contraction in those with atrial fibrillation. In small doses, digitalis can strengthen a weak heart and slow down a rapid heartbeat; in large doses, however, it can be fatal by dangerously slowing down heart function. The most commonly used drugs in this group are digoxin and digitoxin.

The active principles in digitalis include a group of steroids called cardiac glycosides. Dosage must be measured with extreme care, since the lethal dose is only three times the effective dose.

Symptoms

Overdose is evident with both gastrointestinal and neurologic problems, including anorexia, nausea, vomiting, diarrhea, depression, visual disturbances, fatigue, headache, delirium, confusion, and hallucinations. A wide variety of cardiac problems are common and represent the most serious form of toxicity.

Treatment

Management of mild overdose may require only stopping the drug. Acute poisoning requires gastric lavage or induced vomiting, followed by the administration of activated charcoal and a cathartic as soon as possible after ingestion.

See also CARDIAC GLYCOSIDES; DIGITOXIN; DIGOXIN; FOXGLOVE.

digitoxin This cardiac glycoside is used to regulate the heart's rhythm after a congestive heart failure, increasing contractions and reducing fluid retention. While some physicians have prescribed digitoxin to treat obesity, its adverse affects can be fatal.

Symptoms

Almost immediately, overdose causes nausea, vomiting, diarrhea, blurred vision, and heart problems such as premature contractions and heart rhythm disturbances.

Treatment

Wash the stomach with tannic acid (strong tea) and keep the victim lying down. Give stimulants such as caffeine, ammonia, or atropine; if the pulse drops below 50 beats per minute, atropine is administered.

See also DIGITALIS; DIGOXIN; FOXGLOVE.

digoxin (Lanoxin) This cardiac glycoside is used to regulate the heart's rhythm after a congestive heart failure, increasing contractions and reducing fluid retention.

Symptoms

Within six hours, overdose causes nausea, vomiting, diarrhea, blurred vision, and heart problems such as premature contractions and atrial fibrillation.

Treatment

Discontinue administration; acute ingestion requires induced vomiting, gastric lavage, and the administration of activated charcoal and a cathartic as soon as possible.

See also CARDIAC GLYCOSIDES; DIGITALIS; DIGITOXIN.

digoxin-specific antibodies The antidote for poisoning by digoxin and, to some degree, digitoxin and other cardiac glycosides. Digoxin-specific antibodies are produced in immunized sheep and can reverse the signs of digitalis poisoning within 30–60 minutes of administration with complete reversal within three hours.

See also CARDIAC GLYCOSIDES; DIGITOXIN; DIGOXIN.

Dilantin See PHENYTOIN.

Dilaudid See HYDROMORPHONE.

dimercaprol This chelating agent is used to treat poisoning of arsenic, mercury, lead, antimony, bismuth, chromium, copper, nickel, tungsten, zinc, or gold. It is not effective in the treatment of iron, selenium or cadmium poisoning. Dimercaprol is toxic; about 50 percent of patients taking six milligrams per kilogram intramuscularly (2.5 mg/kg is normal) develop reactions such as hypertension, nausea, vomiting, chest pain, headache, and tachycardia.

dimethyl sulfate (sulfuric acid dimethyl ester, methyl sulfate) This colorless, odorless oily liquid is used to manufacture dyes, drugs, pesticides, and perfumes; most poisonings occur when liquid or vapors leak from industrial machines. Its very mild oniony odor is barely perceptible and not useful as a warning. Dimethyl sulfate does not dissolve readily in water but does dissolve well in organic solvents.

Symptoms

When absorbed through the skin or eyes, it is extremely irritating, although there is a latency period of up to five hours. Exposure to the vapors produces an immediate reaction of runny eyes and nose and swelling of the mouth, lips, and throat, with hoarseness and sore throat. There may also be conjunctivitis (pink eye), perforation of the nasal septum similar to the side effects of cocaine, and permanent vision problems. Liver and kidneys may also be damaged.

Upon ingestion, dimethyl sulfate hydrolyzes to sulfuric acid and methanol. Ingestion causes breathing problems and bronchitis within 12 hours, together with central nervous system side effects including drowsiness, temporary blindness, heart irregularities, and irritation, followed by convulsions and death from pulmonary edema. Dimethyl sulfate causes cancer in animals.

Treatment

Symptomatic treatment, including hydrocortisone to reduce injury.

dinoflagellate (*Gonyaulax catenella, G. tamarensis* and others) The organisms responsible for "red tide," dinoflagellates are extremely toxic one-celled aquatic animals found on the Pacific coast of North America (*G. catenella*) and the east coast of North America (*G. tamarensis*). Dinoflagellates, some of which (*Noctiluca*) also produce part of the luminescence in the sea, have the characteristics of both plants and animals; most are microscopic and marine. A person becomes poisoned with dinoflagellates when eating contaminated shellfish; primarily, dinoflagellates cause paralytic shellfish poisoning, although at least one variety causes a type of poisoning more similar to ciguatera.

Under good conditions (warm climate, warm water), dinoflagellates may reach 60 million organisms per liter of water; these rapid growths (referred to as a "bloom") cause red tides that discolor the sea and poison fish and marine life. Usually, a person becomes poisoned with dinoflagellates when eating shellfish that have been feeding on the toxic protozoa. Bivalve shellfish (mussels, clams, and oysters) are the primary shellfish at risk, and mussels are the most susceptible. Healthy bivalve shellfish filter large amounts of dinoflagellates, which form the primary ocean food from May through August. During these warm times, the dinoflagellates thrive by photosynthesis and can be so invasive that they kill birds and fish.

The first large epidemic of poisoning caused by dinoflagellate-contaminated shellfish occurred in San Francisco in 1927, when 102 people were sickened and six died. Today, largely because of the prohibition against eating certain shellfish during the summer months, such epidemics are rare.

Still, red tides and the resultant paralytic shellfish poisoning (PSP) and ciguatera are a problem in the warm months (May to November) on the Pacific coast between central California and the Aleutian Islands and on the Atlantic coast (St. Lawrence River estuary in Canada, the Bay of Fundy, and several northeastern states in the United States). Other countries have also experienced outbreaks of PSP, including England, Wales, France, Scotland, Germany, Norway, Ireland, Belgium, Denmark, Portugal, South Africa, Japan, New Guinea, and New Zealand.

Not all dinoflagellate species are toxic to humans or marine creatures, and many varieties of phytoplankton bloom to large proportions without causing harm. Harmful dinoflagellates found in North America include *G. catenella, G. acatenella,* and *G. tamarensis,* all of which cause PSP; *G. breve,* found on the Florida Gulf coast, which causes a ciguatera-like poisoning; and *G. polyedra,* found on the southern California coast, causing a paralytic poison different from PSP. In Japan, the dinoflagellate *Exuviaella mariaelebouriae* causes "oyster poisoning," damaging the liver and kidneys. Several other dinoflagellates are injurious to fish and other marine creatures but do no harm to humans.

Symptoms

Similar to curare poisoning and extremely fast acting (within 10 minutes), dinoflagellate poisoning causes a tingling and burning sensation and numbness of the lips, tongue, and face, spreading elsewhere to the body; it can also cause weakness, dizziness, joint pain, intense thirst, and difficulty in swallowing. As the illness progresses, breathing problems and muscular paralysis become more severe. Death is caused by respiratory paralysis within two to 12 hours, depending on the dose. Fatalities occur in 10 percent of poisoning cases. If the victim survives for 24 hours, prognosis is good and there do not seem to be lasting effects of poisoning.

Treatment

There is no antidote for shellfish poisoning caused by dinoflagellates. Gastric lavage and activated charcoal may be administered, since saxitoxin is readily absorbed by charcoal. It may be necessary to monitor blood pressure and the heart, and to provide respiratory support, since patients are often in critical condition.

See also CIGUATERA; PARALYTIC SHELLFISH POISONING; SHELLFISH POISONING.

dioxins A group of highly toxic substances used in a variety of industrial and other applications. The herbicide Agent Orange used during combat in Vietnam contained small quantities of one type of dioxin. However, diagnosis of dioxin poisoning is difficult, since it is hard to detect dioxin in blood or tissue and there is no established correlation with symptoms.

According to research released by the Environmental Protection Agency, dioxin is a potent carcinogen with subtle immunological, developmental, and neurological effects that may be even more of a public health threat than its carcinogenic problems. A July 2002 study found dioxins to be significantly related to an increase in breast cancer.

Dioxin has spread well beyond its main industrial sources (paper processors, herbicide manufacturers, and garbage incinerators) and can be found today in the bodies of anyone who eats fish, meat, or dairy products. Research suggests dioxin may affect the body's hormonal messenger system; it may affect sex hormones and insulin and could create permanent health problems for children exposed in the womb—lowering sperm counts, interfering with sexual development, and impairing brain development.

Symptoms

After exposure, victims experience skin, eye, and mucous membrane irritation, nausea, and vomiting. After a latency period of up to several weeks, additional symptoms appear, including chloracne, excessive hair growth, pigment abnormalities, motor weakness, and sensory impairments. In animals, death occurs a few weeks after a lethal dose as the result of a wasting syndrome in which the animal stops eating and loses weight.

Treatment

There is no specific antidote, only symptomatic treatment, with induced vomiting or gastric lavage followed by the administration of activated charcoal and a cathartic. For eye or skin contamination, flush with water and soap; irrigate eyes with tepid water or saline. Anyone helping to wash the affected clothing or skin should wear protective clothing.

diphenhydramine This antihistamine is used both as a treatment for the itchy skin rash from a wide variety of plants (such as poison ivy or sumac) and to partially prevent anaphylaxis caused by horse serum–based antivenins or antitoxins.

See also ANTIVENIN.

diphyllobothriasis A type of food poisoning caused by eating fish infested with a broad fish tapeworm *(Diphyllobothrium latum).* Now uncommon in the United States, it was formerly often found in the Great Lakes area, where it was known as "Jewish, or Scandinavian, housewife's disease" because the preparers of gefilte fish or fish balls tended to taste their food as they prepared it, before fish was fully cooked. The parasite is now supposedly absent from Great Lakes fish; recently, however, cases have been reported along the west coast.

Foods are not routinely analyzed for this parasite. In 1980, an outbreak involving four Los Angeles physicians occurred when they all ate sushi made of tuna, red snapper, and salmon. At the time of this outbreak, there was also a general increase in requests for niclosamide (the drug used to treat the infestation). Interviews of 39 patients with similar symptoms at the time showed that 32 remembered eating salmon before becoming sick.

The disease is caused by parasitic flatworms and other members of this tapeworm family; the larva are often found in the viscera of fresh and marine fishes. After eating an infected fish, an adult tapeworm between 3 and 10 feet long grows in the small intestine; about a month later, it releases more than a million eggs into the stool every day. Infection is usually limited to one worm.

It is found in freshwater fish, or fish that migrate from salt water to freshwater for breeding, including pike, salmon, trout, whitefish, and turbot.

Symptoms

Symptoms appear about 10 days after eating raw or poorly cooked fish. Many people don't have any symptoms, but others report a variety of minor complaints including distended abdomen, flatulence, nausea, headache, nervousness, weakness, cramping, and diarrhea. Some report a sensation that "something is moving inside." Those who are susceptible (usually those of Scandinavian heritage) may experience a severe anemia as a result of this tapeworm infection, caused by the tapeworm's absorption of vitamin B_{12}.

Diagnosis

The disease is identified by finding eggs in the patient's feces.

Treatment

The drug niclosamide or praziquantel will cure the infection.

dishwasher detergent See ALKALINE CORROSIVES.

disulfiram See ANTABUSE.

diuretics These are the most commonly prescribed drugs for the treatment of high blood pressure. The four types of diuretics are thiazide and thiazidelike, loop, potassium-sparing, and combination. Each type works by affecting a different part of the kidneys and may also have different uses, side effects, and precautions. Overdoses are not generally harmful; more serious are the adverse effects from chronic use or misuse. Examples of some of the drugs within each diuretic type are thiazides (chlorthalidone, hydrochlorothiazide, metolazone; loop (bumetanide, furosemide, torsemide);

potassium-sparing (amiloride, eplerenone, spirono-lactone, triamterene); and combination (amiloride and hydrochlorothiazide, spironolactone and hydrochlorothiazide, and triamterene and hydro-chlorothiazide). Because the potassium-sparing diuretics are not very effective alone, they are often combined with another diuretic.

Symptoms

Lethargy, weakness, and dehydration, which may be delayed for two to four hours until the diuretic action begins. The diuretic spironolactone may not produce symptoms until the third day; thiazide diuretics may cause hyperglycemia.

Treatment

There are no specific antidotes; treatment is symp-tomatic. Replace fluid loss and correct electrolyte abnormalities; monitor potassium levels. Induce vomiting or perform gastric lavage followed by activated charcoal and a cathartic (unless the patient is dehydrated).

DMSA (Meso-2,3-dimercaptosuccinic acid)   This chelating agent (also known as succimer) is a com-monly used drug for reducing toxicological effects of lead and methylmercury poisoning. DMSA is currently the only approved oral medication in the United States for children with high levels of lead. It works by chemically binding with lead in the patient and removing the poison from the body.

dog button plant   See NUX-VOMICA.

dog hobble *(Leucothoe)* [**Other names: dog laurel, fetterbush, pepper bush, sweet bells, switch ivy, white osier.**]   This deciduous or evergreen shrub grows from Virginia to Florida, Tennessee, Louisi-ana, and California. Its white or pink flowers grow in clusters.

Poisonous part

The leaves and nectar (in honey) are toxic and con-tain the toxin grayanotoxin (andromedotoxin).

Symptoms

Burning in the mouth, followed gradually by increased salivation, diarrhea, and prickly skin; headache, vision problems, bradycardia, severe hypotension, and possibly convulsions and coma.

Treatment

Fluid replacement, atropine for bradycardia; ephed-rine for hypotension that does not respond to fluid replacement.

drain cleaners   See ALKALINE CORROSIVES.

dyphylline (7-dihydroxypropyltheophylline)   One of the group of bronchial tube relaxers given to control asthma, bronchitis, and emphysema, dyphylline was introduced in 1946 and is available in time-release tablets or syrup.

Symptoms

Within one hour, overdose produces headache, nervousness, insomnia, nausea, vomiting, rapid heartbeat, low blood pressure, convulsions, and circulatory failure.

Treatment

Perform gastric lavage, followed by symptomatic treatment.
See also BRONCHIAL TUBE RELAXERS.

E. coli 0157:H7 The most deadly of the hundreds of strains of *Escherichia coli,* this type of *E. coli* has been recognized as a cause of foodborne illness leading to kidney failure and death since 1982. It's known popularly as "the hamburger disease" because of its links with undercooked fastfood hamburgers.

Although most strains of *E. coli* are harmless and live in the intestines of both humans and animals, the 0157:H7 strain produces a powerful toxin that can cause severe illness. An estimated 70,000 cases of infection occur in the United States each year. Most illness has been associated with eating undercooked, contaminated ground beef. Other outbreaks have been traced to many different types of food. *E. coli* has been discovered surviving in dry fermented meat and salami despite production standards that meet federal and industry food processing requirements. It has also been found in unpasteurized milk, cider, and apple juice, in lettuce, and in untreated water.

It's especially common in day care centers and among toddlers who are not yet toilet trained. Patients are infectious for about six days while bacteria are excreted in their stool. There is no solid evidence, but it appears that victims can get this infection more than once. Most states now ask doctors to report outbreaks of the disease, but none regularly tests for other strains of *E. coli* that produce the toxin.

Symptoms

The toxins cause severe cramps and watery or bloody diarrhea lasting for 6 to 8 days. Other symptoms include nausea and vomiting appearing within hours to a week after eating, but not usually any fever. Most people recover quickly and completely, but the complications are what make this a serious disease (see "Complications").

Diagnosis

Identification of the bacterium in stool. Most labs that culture stool don't test for *E. coli* 0157:H7, so it's important to request that the stool be tested for this organism. Everyone with sudden bloody diarrhea should have the stool checked for this bacterium.

Treatment

Most patients recover within 10 days without specific treatment. There is no evidence that antibiotics help and some evidence to suggest it may trigger kidney problems. Antidiarrhea medicine should also be avoided. Hemolytic uremic syndrome (see under Complications), on the other hand, is a life-threatening condition that is treated in a hospital intensive care unit, with blood transfusions and kidney dialysis.

Complications

In certain people (the very young or old), the bacteria may cause hemolytic uremic syndrome (HUS), a condition in which the red blood cells are destroyed and the kidneys fail. Between 2 and 7 percent of infections lead to this complication. In the United States, HUS is the main cause of kidney failure in children. There is no cure. Adults may develop an extremely serious bleeding disorder called thrombotic thrombocytopenic purpura in which blood stops clotting, small red spots and large bruises appear all over the body, and blood oozes through the mouth.

Patients with only a mild infection usually recover completely. Of those who develop HUS, one-third have abnormal kidney function years later, and a few need long-term dialysis. Another 8 percent suffer with other complications such as high blood pressure, seizures, blindness, and paralysis for the rest of their lives. Even with intensive care, the death rate from HUS is between 3 percent and 5 percent. In addition, the outlook is not promising for adults who develop thrombotic thrombocytopenic purpura.

ecstasy Also known as methylenedioxymethamphetamine (MDMA), ecstasy is a synthetic, psychoactive drug that is chemically similar to methamphetamine and the hallucinogen mescaline. It is taken as a capsule or tablet and was initially popular among white adolescents and young adults who took it at all-weekend parties (raves) and at dance clubs. Use has now expanded to include other ethnic groups and gay males. The attraction is the feeling of euphoria, emotional warmth, and distortions in tactile experiences and time perception that the drug causes. Acute, negative effects of ecstasy begin about 30 minutes after oral intake. Within 60 minutes, however, the jaw clenching, dry mouth, blurry vision, and sweating give way to feelings of relaxation. The effects plateau for up to 90 minutes and then diminish over three to four hours. As users come down from their high, some take additional ecstasy to prolong the effect, and this practice can lead to serious, life-threatening effects.

Ecstasy affects the brain by binding to the transporter for the brain chemical called serotonin, which plays a critical role in regulating mood, sexual activity, sleep, aggression, and sensitivity to pain. The drug is also addictive for some people. A survey of ecstasy users found that 43 percent met the diagnostic criteria for dependence, and these results are similar to those found in other countries.

Symptoms

Ecstasy can produce confusion, memory problems, increases in heart rate and blood pressure, blurry vision, nausea, chills, sweating, depression, sleep problems, drug craving, and severe anxiety. These symptoms can occur soon after taking the drug or even days or weeks later. In high doses, ecstasy can disrupt the body's ability to regulate temperature and may cause hyperthermia, which then can result in liver, kidney, and cardiovascular

system failure and death. In fact, most ecstasy-related deaths are caused by hyperthermia and heat stroke. Animal research showed that exposure to ecstasy for only four days caused damage to serotonin nerve terminals that was still evident up to seven years later. Symptoms associated with withdrawal from the drug include fatigue, loss of appetite, depressed feelings, and difficulty concentrating.

Treatment

Management of ecstasy overdose/poisoning is similar to that for amphetamines. The individual should be checked for clear airways, breathing, and circulation, as well as hypertension and ventricular dysrhythmias. Activated charcoal should be administered and symptoms should be managed, including oxygen and intravenous fluids for hypotension; benzodiazepines for agitation or seizures; dopamine or norepinephrine for hypotension that does not respond to fluid; lidocaine for ventricular dysrhythmias; correction of electrolyte abnormalities; and other measures as needed.

edrophonium chloride Antidote used in the treatment of curare poisoning reversing the neuromuscular blockade produced by curare, tubocurarine, or gallamine. It also treats the respiratory depression caused by curare overdose. It must be used with caution, however, among patients with chronic lung disease and heart problems.

See also CURARE.

elderberry, black and scarlet elders (*Sambucus canadensis* and *S. pubens*) [Other names: American elder, sweet elder.] Often cultivated for its ornamental foliage, this indigenous shrub is found throughout the United States and Canada in low, damp ground and waste places. The elderberry grows from five to 12 feet with a rough gray bark and a faintly sweet odor. It flowers in June and July with white, star-shaped clusters; its black berries mature in September and October. Sometimes, flower and fruit appear at the same time. The European elder is larger than its American cousin but is otherwise quite similar.

Poisonous part

The entire plant is toxic, although the ripe fruit is edible when cooked, and in limited amounts it may not cause symptoms even if eaten raw. According to some sources, the flowers are probably nontoxic and the berries cause nausea only if eaten raw in large numbers. The poison is cyanogenic glycosides found mostly in the roots, stems, and leaves and an unidentified cathartic mostly in the bark and roots of some species. Proper cooking destroys the toxic principle. Children have been poisoned by eating the roots or using the pithy stems as blowguns.

Symptoms

Eating leaves, bark, root, or immature berries may cause serious diarrhea. Juice from the berries of *S. mexicana* has caused nausea, vomiting, and cramps within 15 minutes, dizziness, numbness, and stupor. At least one anecdotal case of cyanide poisoning in humans from this plant has been recorded.

Treatment

Administer fluids.

See also CYANOGENIC GLYCOSIDES.

endrin [Trade names: Compound 269, Experimental Insecticide 269.] A highly toxic chlorinated hydrocarbon insecticide and rat poison, endrin has been responsible for numerous fatalities. This white crystalline solid can be inhaled, ingested, or absorbed through the skin.

Symptoms

Between 30 minutes and 10 hours after ingestion, symptoms appear including giddiness, weakness, nausea, confusion, insomnia, lethargy, repeated convulsions, and loss of consciousness followed by respiratory failure and death.

Treatment

There is no specific antidote. Perform gastric lavage but do not induce vomiting because of the risk of sudden onset of seizures; administer activated charcoal and a cathartic. Irregular heartbeat may respond to propranolol.

See also CHLORINATED HYDROCARBON PESTICIDES.

ephedrine A potent central nervous system stimulant used to treat low blood pressure following overdose with antihypertensive drugs such as beta blockers, calcium channel blockers (verapamil, nifedipine), vasodilators (minoxidil, prazosin), etc.

See also BETA ADRENERGIC BLOCKERS.

epinephrine This catecholamine produced naturally in the body is used to treat anaphylaxis or cardiac arrest. It may also be helpful in raising low blood pressure resulting from an overdose of beta adrenergic blockers and other heart-depressant drugs.

See also BETA ADRENERGIC BLOCKERS.

ergot *(Claviceps purpurea)* This parasitic fungus is found primarily in rye grain, which can also contaminate flour made from the grain. Ergot poisoning can occur after eating rye meal or bread that has been prepared from the contaminated grain. Originating in Europe, ergot is now found throughout the world.

Ergot poisoning was epidemic during the Middle Ages, when 40,000 Frenchmen died from "St. Anthony's Fire." It is no longer a danger today because of widespread screening programs used to check cereal grains for the fungus.

Ergot was used in earlier tunes as an abortifacient because of its ability to contract the uterus; however, doses necessary to expel the uterine contents also tended to be fatal. In the 17th century, midwives used ergot to help the uterus contract after childbirth, and today it is still found in hospitals, where it is used for the same purpose.

Symptoms

Drowsiness, headache, giddiness, nausea, vomiting, cramps, itching, and respiratory and cardiac arrest. In severe poisoning cases, gangrene involving the fingers, toes, ears, and nose may occur. Ingestion can also cause painful convulsions, permanent damage to the central nervous system, and psychosis.

Treatment

Gastric lavage followed by activated charcoal, together with symptomatic and supportive treatment. Amyl nitrate is sometimes used to ease spasms.

See also NITROGLYCERIN.

Escherichia coli   See *E. COLI* 0157:H7.

ethanol   The alcohol in alcoholic drinks; ethanol is administered either intravenously or orally to treat methanol or glycol poisonings.

See also ISOPROPYL ALCOHOL; METHYL ALCOHOL.

ether (diethyl ether)   The first general anesthetic, ether was first demonstrated successfully in Boston in 1846, when a tooth was extracted without pain while the patient was breathing ether. Soon after, the anesthetic properties of chloroform and nitrous oxide were added to the anesthesiologist's arsenal.

A colorless liquid, ether is administered on a gauze mask over a patient's nose and mouth and produces unconsciousness when inhaled. It is so flammable that even static electricity can cause an explosion. For this reason, ether was abandoned after the 1930s when it was replaced by other, safer anesthetic agents.

Symptoms

Overdose depresses the central nervous system and stops breathing.

Treatment

Remove the gas and force ventilation, maintain breathing and keep warm to avoid shock. If a high fever develops, pack the body in wet towels or administer dantrolene sodium and procainamide.

See also ANESTHETICS, GASEOUS/VOLATILE; CHLOROFORM; NITROUS OXIDE.

ethyl alcohol   Another name for ethanol, the alcohol in alcoholic drinks. It is used as an antidote to antifreeze poisoning.

See also ANTIFREEZE; ISOPROPYL ALCOHOL.

ethylene chlorohydrin   This colorless, odorless liquid is used as an industrial solvent and to facilitate seed germination. It evaporates quickly at room temperature. Because it has no smell and does not irritate the mouth or nose, it is possible to become exposed before danger is realized.

Symptoms

In the wake of continued exposure, ethylene chlorohydrin is a central nervous system depressant and damages the heart, lungs, liver, and kidneys. It is not yet certain whether it causes cancer or fetal damage. Symptoms appear soon after exposure, including nausea, vomiting, headache, vertigo, delirium, low blood pressure, slow breathing, cyanosis, and coma. Death occurs from respiratory and circulatory failure. In addition, there have been reports of impaired DNA and possible birth defects.

Treatment

Move the victim into fresh air and remove all contaminated clothing. Perform artificial respiration or administer oxygen as needed. For ingestion, perform gastric lavage followed by a saline cathartic. Do not administer epinephrine or other stimulants.

ethylene dibromide (EDB)   This volatile liquid is used in antiknock gasoline mixtures, especially aviation fuel, and as a pesticide and fumigant for soil, fruits, and vegetables. It can cause chemical burns or (if inhaled) respiratory tract irritation and pulmonary edema. Its use as a pesticide has been restricted since 1984 because of its suspected carcinogenic role. In cases of inhalation poisoning, rescuers must wear breathing apparatus and protective clothing to avoid exposure. Once absorbed in the body, EDB can disrupt cell metabolism and initiate multisystem failure throughout the body.

Symptoms

If inhaled, EDB can irritate the eyes and upper respiratory tract; pulmonary edema is found within six hours but may take as long as two days to develop. Ingestion causes vomiting, diarrhea, central nervous system depression, seizures, and metabolic acidosis. In fatal cases, there is acute kidney failure, liver damage, and muscle necrosis. Ingestion of 4.5 ml of liquid EDB can be fatal.

Treatment

There is no specific antidote. Treat symptoms, and provide oxygen if needed. For skin/eye contamination, remove clothes and wash with soap and water; irrigate eyes with saline or tepid water. For ingestion, do not induce vomiting because of corrosive effects and danger of rapid onset of coma or seizure. Perform gastric lavage followed by the administration of activated charcoal and a cathartic.

See also PESTICIDES.

ethylene glycol   See ANTIFREEZE.

eucalyptus *(Eucalyptus globulus Labill)*   Also known as a gum tree, this genus includes more than 600 species (both trees and shrubs) in the myrtle family. It is the essential oils of this tree that can be toxic. The eucalyptus is native to Australia, New Zealand, Tasmania, and nearby islands and is cultivated throughout the temperate regions of the world as shade trees or in forestry plantations. About 90 species are grown in California, and a few are found in Florida.

The bark of the eucalyptus tree is distinctive, peeling off in long strips exposing the inner layer. Leaves are leathery and smooth, and the flower petals (white, yellow, or red) form a cap when the flower expands and attract honeybees. The fruit is surrounded by a woody, cup-shaped receptacle and contains many tiny seeds.

Poisonous part
The leaf glands of many species contain a volatile aromatic oil known as eucalyptus oil, and is an active ingredient in expectorants and inhalants. It contains 70 percent eucalyptol; the toxic dose is 5 ml.

Symptoms
Following an acute overdose by mouth, symptoms may appear within five to 30 minutes and include burning in the mouth and throat followed by nausea and vomiting. Drowsiness, confusion, restlessness, delirium, muscle twitching, and coma may follow. Death may occur as a result of depression of the central nervous system and respiratory arrest.

Treatment
Treat seizures and coma if they occur. There is no specific antidote. Perform gastric lavage but do not induce vomiting because of the risk of inducing seizures. Administer activated charcoal.

exotoxin   Exotoxins include some of the most poisonous substances known, which are released by some types of bacteria into the bloodstream. Tetanus and diphtheria bacilli produce some of the best-known exotoxins; the former affects the nervous system and causes muscle spasms and paralysis, and the latter damages the heart and nervous system. Vaccinations for some of the potentially fatal bacterial diseases use detoxified exotoxins to prevent the disease. Once infection has occurred, however, treatment includes antibiotics and an antitoxin to neutralize the exotoxin.

See also TOXOID.

false Jerusalem cherry *(Solanum pseudocapsicum)*
This decorative pot plant has spread through cultivation from its native Gulf Coast region and Hawaii. It is a member of a very large genus with 1,700 species, most of which have not been evaluated toxicologically.

Poisonous part
Human poisoning is usually attributed to immature fruit, which contains the toxin solanine glycoalkaloid.

Symptoms
While there is little danger of fatal poisoning in adults, children may ingest a fatal amount of this plant. Symptoms appear several hours after ingestion and include gastric irritation, scratchy throat, fever, and diarrhea (solanine poisoning is often confused with bacterial gastroenteritis).

Treatment
Provide the same general supportive care that would be given in gastroenteritis cases; fluid replacement may be required.

false morel   See TURBANTOP.

fenoprofen   See NONSTEROIDAL ANTI-INFLAMMATORY DRUGS.

fentanyl   See NARCOTICS.

fer-de-lance   This extremely venomous pit viper lives in cultivated lands and tropical forests of cen-tral Mexico into South America. A member of the viper family, it is considered a pit viper because of its sensory pit between each eye and nostril.

The fer-de-lance is gray or brown with black-edged diamonds on a lighter border and is found in tropical America ranging from farms to tropical forests. Its name (French for "lancehead") is sometimes used to refer collectively to all snakes of the Central and South American genus *Bothrops* and the Asian genus *Trimeresurus,* and it is called *barba amarillo* ("yellow chin") in Spanish. Other pit viper relatives include the dangerous South American wutu *(Bothrops alternatus),* the jumping viper or tommy-goff *(B. nummifera)* of Central America, the Okinawa habu *(Trimeresurus flavoviridis)* found in the Ryukyu Islands, and Wagler's pit viper *(T. Wagleri).*

Symptoms
With a bite from this viper, blood cannot coagulate and hemorrhages into muscles and the nervous system. There is local pain, bleeding from the bite, gums, nose, mouth, and rectum. Shock and respiratory arrest are followed by death.

Treatment
Antivenin is available.
See also ANTIVENIN; PIT VIPERS; SNAKES, POISONOUS.

fertilizers   Plant foods that contain one of three ingredients necessary for plants to grow: potassium, nitrogen, or phosphorous. They are not generally considered particularly toxic even if ingested by children, *unless the fertilizer also contains herbicides or insecticides.* If a child ingests products containing only these three ingredients, usually the only symptoms that occur will be vomiting or diarrhea. However, many fertilizers also contain additives that could be toxic.

See also HERBICIDES; INSECTICIDES.

fire ant *(Solenopsis)* Several species of these small, aggressive ants, also known as thief ants, are found in North America. These red or yellow ants live in loose mounds with open ventilation craters and long tunnels, usually located in meadows of clover and Bermuda grass and in row crops; they occasionally invade homes.

Poisonous part

The release of histamine causes the painful symptoms common in fire ant stings.

Symptoms

A sting from the fire ant can cause severe pain, swelling, itching, reddening, warmth, and burning. Blisters may form and they are prone to infection if broken.

Treatment

Ice, compresses, and cleansing of the wound to prevent infection. Neither antihistamines, corticosteroids, nor antibacterial ointments significantly ease symptoms.

fireworks According to federal regulations, all fireworks must be sealed to prevent leakage of gunpowder during shipment and handling and must be constructed to prevent burnout through the sides or blowout through the bottom of the device after ignition. Still, each year fireworks injure many thousands of Americans, usually children and teenagers. These products are also toxic if ingested.

Gold sparklers may contain barium nitrate, paste, chalk, dextrin, iron, and aluminum; green sparklers contain barium nitrate, potassium perchlorate, wheat pastes, gum, dextrin, and aluminum powder. Red sparklers contain strontium carbonate, nitrate, and potassium perchlorate, plus gums, wheat pastes, dextrin, and aluminum powder.

Symptoms

If ingested, the soluble barium salts contained in these products can cause vomiting, abdominal pain, bloody diarrhea, shallow breathing, convulsions, coma, and death from respiratory or cardiac failure. Strontium may cause vomiting, abdominal pain, bloody stools, and methemoglobinemia; perchlorates may cause vomiting, abdominal pain, and methemoglobinemia.

Treatment

When a sparkler has been eaten, induce vomiting or perform gastric lavage; in the case of nitrate-induced methemoglobinemia, intravenous solution of 1 percent methylene blue is recommended.

first aid It is not always easy to know whether someone is the victim of poisoning or has the signs and symptoms of conditions that mimic poisoning, such as seizures, stroke, insulin reaction, and alcohol intoxication. Some signs and symptoms of poisoning include

- Redness or burns around lips and mouth, which may occur when certain poisons are ingested
- Burns, odors, or stains on the individual, the clothing, furniture, floor, rugs, or other objects in the surrounding area
- Breath that smells like chemicals
- Vomiting, breathing problems, confusion, excessive sleepiness, or other unexplained signs
- Empty medication bottles or scattered pills

If you suspect poisoning, check for the signs and symptoms but also contact the poison control center at 800-222-1222 before you give anything to the affected individual. You can also call 911 for emergency help or if you don't know the number for the poison control center at the time of the poisoning. Below are the recommended actions to take for different types of poisoning situations.

Inhaled Poisons

Immediately carry or drag the victim to fresh air. If you think you need protection, such as a respirator before you approach the victim, call the fire department and wait for emergency equipment to arrive.

After you find the victim and move him or her clear of the affected area, do the following:

- Check for breathing. If you are trained in CPR, try to resuscitate the individual.
- Check the eyes and skin for chemical burns.
- If there are burns on the skin, flush them thoroughly with water.
- Loosen tight clothing.
- If the person's skin is blue or if the person has stopped breathing, give artificial respiration if you know how, and call rescue services.

On the Skin

If chemicals have splashed onto the skin, get the victim away from the poisonous substance. Remove contaminated clothing and flood the skin and hair with soap and water for at least 15 minutes. Seek medical treatment. Later, throw away the contaminated clothes or thoroughly wash them separately from other laundry.

In the Eyes

Eye membranes absorb pesticides and other chemicals faster than any other external body part, and eye damage can occur in a few minutes with some types of chemicals. Therefore, it is critical to act immediately if poison has splashed into the eye(s): hold the eyelid open and wash quickly with clear running water from the tap or a gentle stream from a hose for at least 15 minutes. Do not use eye drops, chemicals, or drugs in the wash water as you cleanse the eye(s). If possible, have someone else contact poison control while you help the victim.

Stings

- Remove the stinger by scraping with a hard, flat object, like a credit card or the back of a knife.
- Apply cold towels or compresses to the sting site.
- Position the bite area lower than the heart.
- Be prepared to administer CPR.

- In case of an allergic reaction (e.g., facial swelling, shock, breathing difficulties, abdominal pain), call 911.

fish contamination   High in protein, low in calories, fat, and cholesterol—and widely suspected to fight against heart disease and cancer—this highly praised health food can also be a site of contamination and spoilage.

The problem is that fish readily soak up poisons and contaminants in water; tiny fish pick up contaminants from the plankton they feed on in polluted water, concentrating heavy metals (such as methyl mercury) in their organs. These fish are eaten by larger fish, further concentrating the toxins, and in big fish, such as swordfish and tuna, the contaminants may reach levels harmful to humans.

Fatty fish like salmon, bluefish, and herring are vulnerable to chlorinated compounds such as PCBs, dioxins, and DDT, which linger in the body for years. Very minute quantities of these substances in the water will produce very high concentrations in fish.

One of the more insidious types of mercury poisoning occurs through the contamination of fish in lakes and streams throughout the United States as a result of extensive agricultural fungicide and pesticide use and the industrial by-products of chlorine production. Estimates suggest up to 10,000 tons of mercury infiltrates the sea each year; once in the water, it enters the food chain where it is converted into organic methyl mercury, one of the most toxic substances known. The presence of sewage in the water facilitates this deadly conversion by bacteria living in the mud; once it occurs, the contaminated bacteria are then eaten by plankton, which are in turn eaten by pike, pickerel, perch, walleye, muskie, and white bass.

Unlike inorganic mercury compounds, methyl mercury is hard to detect in the blood; it does not readily break down in the body and can take months to be excreted. In addition, it can pass easily through the blood-brain barrier, irreversibly damaging brain cells; it also crosses the placenta and builds up in the fetal brain and blood. Methyl mercury seems to affect women more than men, and children and infants most of all.

The first cases of contaminated fish poisoning occurred in Japan in 1953 and 1970, when more than 121 cases—and 46 deaths—were reported. At that time, methyl mercury chloride flowed directly into a bay and river near a manufacturing plant.

According to research conducted in the 1970s, fish in the Great Lakes were also contaminated with methyl mercury (2.8 parts per million). Today, the Food and Drug Administration mandates that tuna must contain less than 0.5 mg/kg, but scientists estimate that to be safe, humans should ingest no more than 0.1 mg of mercury per day; if a fish contains 1 parts per billion of mercury, then the safe weekly limit would be about three portions of fish a week (1½ lb.). Still, no methyl mercury fish poisonings have been reported since Japan's incidences.

Low levels of mercury in fish may not be as harmful to regular fish eaters as experts once thought, according to a recently released study. Heavy consumption of mercury-tainted fish has long been considered particularly dangerous to pregnant women and their unborn babies. But in a new study conducted by the University of Rochester over a period of 15 years in the Seychelles islands, tests show no link between the children's development over their first five and a half years and the levels of mercury found in their mother's hair during pregnancy. (Concentration of mercury in the mother's hair is a measure of the amount of mercury to which fetuses were exposed.)

The journal *Neurotoxicology* published 11 articles on the study, which tracked the mental and physical development of more than 1,500 children starting at six months of age. The study is expected to sharpen the debate over mercury poisoning in the United States, where 37 states advise people to limit consumption of freshwater fish because of mercury.

There is very little known about ways to remove the methyl mercury pollutants from contaminated water, which may remain poisoned for between 10 and 100 years.

Fish spoilage

The danger of fish contamination is not just with the contaminants they ingest. Because bacteria that live on fish are adapted to withstand the cool and cold waters of lakes and oceans, they can thrive in temperatures cold enough to preserve other food. These microbes will quickly spoil the fish, unless it is kept at temperatures close to freezing. Even under the best conditions, fish lasts only seven to 12 days; but it often takes seven days for fish to get from the water to the supermarket, where it may sit for several more days.

How to protect against contamination

Seafood should look and smell fresh, with vivid skin and bright eyes and no fishy or ammonia odor. It should be displayed on ice in the store; otherwise, fish is best selected from the bottom of the refrigerator case where it is coldest. Once home, it should be kept very cold and eaten within one or two days. Cook thoroughly, but no amount of cooking will destroy contaminants. Scrape off the fatty skin before cooking. Pregnant women, nursing mothers, and young children should limit

FISH AND SHELLFISH POISONING			
Type	Onset	Fish/Shellfish	Effects
Ciguatera	one to six hrs.	Barracuda, grouper, red snapper	Gastroenteritis, hot and cold reversal, weakness, myalgia
Scombroid	Immediate to delayed	Tuna, mahimahi, mackerel, bonita	Gastroenteritis, flush, wheezing, rash
Neurotoxic shellfish	Up to three hrs.	Mussels	Gastroenteritis, ataxia, paresthesias
Paralytic shellfish	Within 30 min.	Mussels, clams, "red tide"	Gastroenteritis, ataxia, respiratory paralysis
Tetrodotoxin	30–40 min.	Pufferfish, sunfish, porcupine fish, California newt	Vomiting twitches, weakness, respiratory paralysis

consumption of fish that might have high levels of mercury and PCBs.

flea and tick killers See ORGANOPHOSPHATE INSECTICIDES.

floor polish and wax See PETROLEUM DISTILLATES.

Flumazenil This nontoxic drug is used to rapidly reverse a coma brought on by benzodiazepine overdose. After intravenous administration, the reversal takes effect within two minutes.

See also BENZODIAZEPINES.

flunitrazepam [street names: roofies, rophies, forget-me pill, circles, Mexican valium, rib, roach-2, roonies, rope, ropies, ruffies, roaches] A sleeping pill prescribed for insomnia in Mexico, Europe, Asia, and South America, flunitrazepam (Rohypnol) has not been approved for use in the United States. This benzodiazepine is effective for short-term treatment of insomnia and as a sedative hypnotic and preanesthetic drug. The effects of the drug are similar to those of diazepam (Valium), although flunitrazepam is about ten times more potent. Because the drug cannot be detected by routine benzodiazepine screens, it can be used by people who want to become intoxicated but avoid driving-under-the-influence charges.

In the United States, flunitrazepam is often used along with alcohol, which results in a synergistic effect and produces disinhibition and amnesia. This combination, along with the fact that the drug is inexpensive (typically less than five dollars per tablet) has made flunitrazepam popular as a date rape drug. Perpetrators slip a tablet into the drink of their intended victim, and the drug, which is colorless, odorless, and tasteless, dissolves quickly. When flunitrazepam is taken along with alcohol or other drugs (e.g., marijuana, cocaine), sedation can occur as soon as 20 minutes after ingestion. The drug's effects will peak within two hours and can impair judgment and motor skills and cause blackouts that can last eight hours or longer, depending on the dosage.

Cases of date rape have been reported across the United States, primarily on college campuses, in which victims—usually women—wake up in unfamiliar surroundings with no memory of what occurred in the preceding hours. Although most cases are reported by women, flunitrazepam has the same effect on men.

In March 1995, flunitrazepam was classified as a Schedule III drug by the World Health Organization. Based on an increase in abuse of the drug in the United States, however, the Drug Enforcement Agency is considering making flunitrazepam a Schedule I drug—a high potential for abuse, with no currently accepted medical use in treatment, and lacking accepted levels of safety for use under medical supervision.

Symptoms

In addition to impaired judgment and motor skills, symptoms include visual disturbances, drowsiness, confusion, decreased blood pressure, gastrointestinal disturbances, urinary retention, and memory impairment. When combined with alcohol, flunitrazepam may cause aspiration, respiratory depression, and death.

When dependence develops, withdrawal symptoms can include headache, muscle pain, extreme anxiety, tension, restlessness, confusion, and irritability, along with delirium, hallucinations, tingling of the extremities, convulsions, shock, and cardiovascular collapse.

Treatment

As is necessary with other benzodiazepines, treatment for flunitrazepam dependence must be done gradually with use tapering off. If alcohol and flunitrazepam have been used together, treatment may need to include additional medication for alcohol withdrawal. Once patients receive their initial phenobarbital doses, a benzodiazepine such as diazepam or lorazepam may be given to alleviate emerging alcohol withdrawal symptoms.

fluoride Fluoride poisoning is usually caused by the accidental ingestion of roach powder insecticides, although it can also occur in children who eat large amounts of vitamin-fluoride tablets or too much fluoride toothpaste. The recommended dose of fluoride for children under age two is 0.25 mg/day; vitamin-fluoride tablets contain 1 mg, as does the average amount of toothpaste on a toothbrush. If too much toothpaste is swallowed by a child in one day, it could result in fluoride poisoning and severe mottling of the tooth enamel. For this reason, new research suggests children under age two should brush without toothpaste; those between ages two and five should be given toothpaste no larger than a pea and required to rinse their mouths thoroughly after brushing.

In addition, the American Dental Association Council of Dental Therapeutics suggests that fluoride supplements prescribed by pediatricians should be limited to those children whose drinking water has a fluoride concentration less than 70 percent of the one-part-per-million level recommended for community water. Still, fluoride is an effective weapon against the development of dental cavities and should not be abandoned because of potential problems.

The most famous case of fluoride poisoning occurred at the Oregon State Hospital in 1943, when workers accidentally mixed 11 pounds of fluoride sodium salt with 10 gallons of scrambled eggs, killing 47 of the 263 patients who ate the tainted breakfast.

Symptoms

Following ingestion, symptoms include pain, salivation, nausea, vomiting, and diarrhea. Vomiting and diarrhea usually get rid of most of the poison in the stomach, although the gastrointestinal tract readily absorbs fluoride salts. In the event of ingesting large amounts of fluoride, death from respiratory paralysis can result within a few minutes. Death may also be caused by shock as a result of the effects of fluid loss from violent vomiting and the effects of the fluoride on the heart muscle, causing arrhythmias and heart failure.

Although the lethal dose of sodium fluoride in adults is fairly large (5 grams), a fatal dose as low as two grams has been recorded.

Treatment

Intravenous glucose in isotonic saline in order to increase the amount of water in the urine secreted from the body is the most effective way of removing fluoride from the body. Administer limewater, calcium chloride solution, or milk in order to bind as much fluoride ion as possible, followed by gastric lavage with any of the above fluids. This is followed by administration of calcium gluconate or calcium chloride to head off muscular spasms; calcium solution should also be used to wipe away corrosive materials after being vomited or excreted. For hydrofluoric skin burns, wash with cold water and administer magnesium oxide. Treat shock as it occurs.

fluoroacetate See COMPOUND 1080.

fly agaric (yellow or red) *(Amanita muscaria)* Sometimes confused with its close relative, the panther mushroom *(Amanita pantherina),* this is a member of the poisonous *Amanita* mushroom genus that has been used for at least 3,000 years as an intoxicant in the rituals of many Asian and Indian tribes. Some mycologists believe it is the source of Soma, the mystical drug of the ancients. It gets its common name from its ancient use as a fly poison, since it attracts—and kills—any fly that lands on it.

This mushroom is found in pastures and fields in summer throughout Europe and the United States in wooded areas and conifer forests, and sometimes in open pastureland. It generally appears at the beginning and end of the summer months and in many places is more abundant than common edible mushrooms.

Similar in appearance to the *Amanita phalloides,* the fly mushroom cap ranges in color from yellow, red, orange to deep brown, all with white warty patches on the caps that disappear as the mushrooms age. Because of its color variations, the panther mushroom is sometimes confused with the fly agaric. Both varieties have the unattached, white gills with white spores that are typical of the *Amanita* genus. While both varieties are poisonous, the panther mushroom is the more deadly of the two. The taste is bitter and unpleasant.

In most cases, people who have been poisoned by eating this mushroom have done so deliberately to experience hallucinations.

Poisonous part

The fly agaric and *A. pantherina* mushrooms contain the strong hallucinogen muscimol and the potent insecticide ibotenic acid. Despite its name, *A. muscaria* usually contains insignificant quantities of muscarine.

Symptoms

While poisoning is rarely fatal, severe symptoms appear quickly, between 30 minutes and three hours, and include severe gastrointestinal distress, drowsiness, lowered blood pressure, slow heartbeat, blurred vision, watery diarrhea, and intoxication featuring euphoria and hallucinations. There may be intermittent drowsiness and manic behavior. In more severe cases, psychosis, convulsions, and coma can follow.

Deaths have been reported in those whose immune systems were already compromised or in those who ate large amounts of the mushroom. Although deaths are rare in adults, they must be protected against injury during the manic phase of the intoxication. In preadolescents, however, ingestion of these mushrooms may cause convulsions and coma.

Treatment

Vomiting soon after ingestion will lessen the severity of symptoms. While some scientists have advocated the administration of atropine as a specific antidote, many others prefer to counteract delirium and coma with the use of physostigmine.

See also AMANITA MUSHROOMS; MUSHROOM POISONING; PANTHER MUSHROOM.

fly mushroom   See FLY AGARIC.

folic acid   A B-complex vitamin that is very helpful in the treatment for methanol and ethylene glycol poisoning. Folic acid is essential for the synthesis of protein in the body and is believed to help eliminate the toxic metabolite formic acid from the body.

See also METHANOL; VITAMINS.

fomepizole   A new drug approved in 1999 as a safe, effective antidote to antifreeze poisoning that offers advantages over other treatments and works extremely well.

Automobile antifreeze consists almost entirely of ethylene glycol, a chemical that is harmless on its own. If swallowed, however, antifreeze is changed by the liver into dangerous substances that can lead to renal failure and death. Fomepizole works by blocking the liver enzyme that converts ethylene glycol into toxic substances.

Antifreeze is usually ingested by mistake, as a suicide attempt or as a cheap substitute for ethanol. Experts estimate that there are about 5,000 cases of antifreeze ingestion each year in the United States.

Previous treatments for antifreeze poisoning caused problems of their own. Before this treatment was approved, most patients were treated with high doses of ethanol (alcohol), which could lead to drunkenness, a dangerous drop in blood sugar level (hypoglycemia) or liver poisoning. Moreover, this type of treatment required intensive monitoring, and most of these patients required hemodialysis.

The drug works better and has none of the complications associated with ethanol treatment, according to researchers. Still, about 17 patients in the most recent study of the new antidote needed hemodialysis. However, if the problem is caught early, treatment with this antidote should eliminate the need for hemodialysis. The new treatment may also be useful for pets who accidentally consume antifreeze.

See also ANTIFREEZE.

food poisoning   Food poisoning and foodborne infections are caused by eating food that has been contaminated by toxic substances or bacteria that contain toxins. Researchers have identified more than 250 different diseases that can be caused by contaminated food or drink; most food items that carry disease are raw or undercooked foods of animal origin, such as meat, milk, eggs, cheese, fish, or shellfish.

Any illness that appears suddenly and within 48 hours of eating questionable food and causes stomach pain, vomiting, and diarrhea should be treated as a case of food poisoning. Estimates of the number of foodborne illnesses range from a low of 6 million to a high of 81 million cases yearly, with 9,100 deaths, according to the Centers for Disease Control and Prevention (CDC). At least a third of these have been traced to poultry and meat.

According to the Food and Drug Administration, just about everyone experiences a foodborne illness at least once a year, whether they realize it or not. The CDC estimates that 76 million cases of foodborne illness occur in the United States each year, and that most of these cases are mild and cause symptoms for only one or two days. The CDC also estimates that 325,000 people are hospitalized and 5,000 people die each year because of foodborne illnesses. The most susceptible are the very young, the very old, and those that have a condition that compromises the immune system, such as HIV/AIDS, cancer, or chronic fatigue syndrome. Some foodborne diseases such as botulism or trichinosis are becoming less common, whereas others such as salmonellosis or *E. coli* infection are becoming more common.

Types of food poisons

Food can be affected by various contaminants, including bacteria, viruses, or parasites, all of which cause foodborne illness. Bacteria that may cause food poisoning include *Campylobacter, Bacillus cereus, Clostridium perfringens, Listeria monocytogenes, Salmonella, Shigella, Staphylococcus aureus, Streptococcus A* and *D, Vibrio,* and *Yersinia.*

A surprising number of parasites contaminate undercooked and raw fish and shellfish, and may pose a health threat to anyone who eats them. They include a parasitic worm *Anisakis simplex, Cryptosporidium, Cyclospora Diphyllobothrium latum, Entamoeba histolytica, Giardia, Nanophyetus salmincola* or *N. schikhobalowi, Toxoplasma gondii,* and *Trichinella spiralis.*

Seafood contaminated with toxins may look and taste normal, but standard cooking methods don't affect the toxin. State shellfish screening programs test shellfish for the presence of toxins and monitor the safety of shellfish harvest beds. However, people who catch their own shellfish from unapproved beds are at risk for various toxic infections. The toxins may be produced as fish spoil (as in scombrotoxin) or as the byproducts of toxic plankton (causing paralytic shellfish), or they may naturally be present in the fish itself (tetrodotoxin). They include ciguatoxin; paralytic, amnesic, diarrhetic, or neurotoxic shellfish poisonings; scombroid poisoning; and tetrodotoxin.

Food can also be contaminated by viruses, such as hepatitis A or the extremely common calicivirus, or Norwalk-like virus, which is rarely diagnosed because the lab test for it is not widely available. Unlike many foodborne pathogens that have animal reservoirs, it appears that the Norwalk-like viruses are spread mainly from one infected person to another, especially among food handlers, including restaurant workers and food processors. Fungi, such as aflatoxins, and metallic contaminants, such as chlorinated compounds and mercury, can also cause food poisoning.

Prevention

The single most important way to prevent foodborne illness is thorough cooking, which kills most foodborne bacteria, viruses, and parasites. In addition, proper food preparation, such as washing your hands, the cutting board, and knife with soap and water immediately after handling raw meat, poultry, seafood, or eggs, will help stop the spread of contamination. Anyone who is experiencing diarrhea or vomiting should not prepare food for others.

To prevent the spread of foodborne diseases take the following steps:

- Make sure food is thoroughly cooked or pasteurized; avoid eating raw or undercooked food from animal sources.

- Keep the juices or drippings from raw meat, poultry, shellfish, or eggs separate from other food.

- Do not leave potentially contaminated food for extended periods of time at room temperature.

- Properly refrigerate leftovers and food prepared in advance of serving.

- Keep the temperature in your refrigerator at 40°F or below and 0°F in the freezer.

- Allow air to circulate around refrigerated items, and always wrap food that is stored in a refrigerator to keep out bacteria.

- Before and after preparing food, wash your hands thoroughly with soap and water to avoid contamination by *Salmonella* and other organisms.

- After using cutting boards and utensils, wash them thoroughly with hot soapy water before you allow any other food to touch them. Acrylic cutting boards are best because they can be put into a dishwasher and they resist cuts and pits where bacteria can hide.

- Thaw meat and poultry in a microwave oven or in the refrigerator and then cook them immediately. Never thaw meat at room temperature.

- If you marinate meat or poultry, do not serve the marinade unless you cook it at a rolling boil for several minutes.

- Cook meat, poultry, and fish thoroughly and check the internal temperature using a meat thermometer. The thermometer should be placed into the thickest portion of the food and not touch bone. According to the CDC, the thermometer should register a minimum of 145°F for roasts and steaks, 165°F for poultry, and 160°F for ground meat and pork. Juices should run clear when the food is pierced.

- Keep hot foods at 140–160°F until you serve them, especially those served in chafing dishes or warmers. Food should never be kept between 40 and 140°F for more than two hours as this encourages bacterial growth.

- Serve meat, poultry, and fish on clean plates with clean utensils; do not use the plates and utensils you used to thaw or prepare the food.

- Cool poultry and meat quickly when refrigerating leftovers. Do not let stuffed poultry stand for long periods. Do not refrigerate stuffed poultry: remove the stuffing and store it separately.

- Do not partially heat food and then finish cooking it later. This is an invitation for bacterial growth that might not be killed during subsequent cooking.

- Never use cracked eggs because they may contain *Salmonella*. However, even uncracked eggs

SAFE FOOD STORAGE
Basic Guidelines by the U.S. Department of Agriculture and the Food Marketing Institute

Food	Where	How Long
Poultry		
Raw	Refrigerator	1–2 days
	Freezer	9 months
Cooked	Refrigerator	3–4 days
	Freezer	4–6 months
Seafood		
Lean fish, raw	Refrigerator	1–2 days
	Freezer	6–8 months
Fatty fish, raw	Refrigerator	1–2 days
	Freezer	4 months
Raw shrimp	Refrigerator	1–2 days
	Freezer	9 months
Cooked seafood	Refrigerator	3 days
	Freezer	2 months
Meat		
Ground meat	Refrigerator	1–2 days
	Freezer	3–4 months
Chops (all)	Refrigerator	3–5 days
Lamb chops	Freezer	6–9 months
Pork chops	Freezer	4–6 months
Roasts (all)	Refrigerator	3–5 days
Beef roasts	Freezer	6–12 months
Veal/pork roast	Freezer	4–6 months
Lamb roast	Freezer	6–9 months
Steak	Refrigerator	3–5 days
Cooked leftovers	Refrigerator	3–4 days
	Freezer	2–3 months
Luncheon meats		
Unopened	Refrigerator	2 weeks
Opened	Refrigerator	3–5 days
	Freezer	1–2 months
Dairy		
Raw eggs in shell	Refrigerator	3 weeks
Hard-boiled (in shell)	Refrigerator	1 week
Milk	Refrigerator	5 days
	Freezer	1 month
Mayonnaise (opened)	Refrigerator	2 months

can contain the bacteria, so always cook eggs thoroughly to kill the salmonella.

- Store eggs in their cartons in the coldest part of the refrigerator, never on the refrigerator door, to prevent multiplication of bacteria.
- Generally, throw out any food that has mold (except cheese, which can be consumed safely once the mold has been removed).

- Use a microwave that has a turntable because microwaves heat food unevenly.
- Do not season wooden salad bowls with oil because the oil can become rancid.
- Thoroughly clean the sink after working with meat and poultry. Clean the sink and counters with detergent that contains bleach, which kills bacteria.

SYMPTOMS OF FOOD POISONING

If you have	It could be
Ulcer pain, abdominal pain, fever, nausea, vomiting, and diarrhea one week after poisoning	Anisakiasis
Explosive watery diarrhea, abdominal cramps, dehydration from a few hours to a few days after ingesting the bacteria	Asiatic cholera
Gastroenteritis, diarrhea, nausea/vomiting appearing 1–6 hours after eating	*Bacillus cereus*
Slurred speech, double vision, muscle paralysis 4–36 hours after meal	Botulism
Cramps, fever, diarrhea, nausea/vomiting appearing 1–5 days after eating and lasting up to 10 days	Campylobacteriosis
Nausea, vomiting, and diarrhea within 6–12 hours after eating, followed by low blood pressure and heart rate; severe itching, temperature reversal, numbness/tingling of extremities (may last months)	Ciguatera
Watery diarrhea, nausea/vomiting appearing within hours to a week after eating (severe cases include blood in diarrhea; enterhemorrhagic infection includes bloody diarrhea and kidney failure)	Enteric *E. coli*
Mild abdominal pain and diarrhea, nausea/vomiting 6–16 hours after eating	Food poisoning
Explosive diarrhea, foul-smelling, greasy feces, stomach pain, gas, appetite loss, nausea/vomiting within 1–2 weeks	Giardiasis
Fever, headache, diarrhea, meningitis, conjunctivitis, miscarriage appearing within days to weeks after ingestion	Listeriosis
Burning mouth/extremities, nausea, vomiting, and diarrhea within a few hours	Neurotoxic shellfish poisoning
Burning mouth/extremities, nausea/vomiting, diarrhea, muscle weakness, paralysis, breathing problems within a few minutes	Paralytic shellfish poisoning
Diarrhea, rumbling bowels, fever, vomiting, cramps 6–72 hours after eating	Salmonellosis
Itching, flushing cramps, diarrhea, nausea/vomiting, burning throat (severe infection includes low blood pressure and breathing problems) within a few minutes to hours	Scombroid poisoning
Gastroenteritis, diarrhea, nausea/vomiting 1–7 days after eating	Shigellosis
Explosive diarrhea, cramps, vomiting not longer than a day between 30 minutes–6 hours after eating	Staphylococcal food poisoning
Diarrhea, nausea/vomiting, fever followed by muscle pain and stiffness 2–3 weeks later	Trichinosis
Gastroenteritis, explosive diarrhea, nausea/vomiting, cramps 8–30 hours after eating (*V. vulnificus* can lead to fatal blood infection)	Vibrio food poisoning (*V. parahaemolyticus, V. vulnificus*)

• Sponges used to clean the sink, dishes, and/or countertops should be decontaminated by microwaving them or putting them in the dishwasher. Both methods remove virtually 100 percent of bacteria, mold, and yeasts.

Treatment (general)

In all cases of food poisoning, symptoms should be treated much like a bout of flu, including drinking fluids (water, tea, bouillon, and ginger ale) to replace fluid loss. Mild cases may be treated at home, with a soft diet, including some salt and sugar. Most cases of food poisoning are not serious (except for botulism) and recovery usually occurs within three days. Samples of any food left from recent meals should be saved for testing if possible.

The greater danger from food poisoning is not the toxin itself but the body's natural response to poison—vomiting and diarrhea—which robs the body of vital fluids. If dehydration becomes serious, food poisoning victims need to be hospitalized and given fluids intravenously. However, poisoning from *E. coli* bacteria can lead to severe enterhemorrhagic infection, which can include bloody diarrhea, leading to kidney failure. One of the most recent *E. coli* scares occurred in September 2007, when the CDC announced that at least 28 people in eight states had become ill after consuming hamburger meat tainted with *E. coli*.

Although the time between ingestion and onset of symptoms varies according to the cause of poisoning, symptoms usually develop within one to six hours for some types of shellfish poisoning, between one and 12 hours for bacterial toxins, and between 12 and 48 hours for viral and salmonella infections. Symptoms also vary depending on how badly the food was contaminated, but there will often be nausea and vomiting, diarrhea, stomach pain, and—in severe cases—shock and collapse.

A doctor should be called if severe vomiting or diarrhea appears suddenly, if the victim collapses or if there is a suspicion of food poisoning and the victim is a *child, an elderly person, or someone with a chronic illness.*

Symptoms

Typical symptoms of food poisoning and their possible causes are provided in the table presented here.

Reporting food poisoning

According to the U.S. Department of Agriculture's Safety and Inspection Service, consumers should report possible food poisoning if the food was eaten at a large gathering: if the food was from a restaurant, deli, sidewalk vendor, or other kitchen that serves more than a few people; or if the food is a commercial product (such as canned goods or frozen food), since contaminants may have affected an entire lot or batch.

When making a report, officials need to know:

• Your name, address, telephone number

• Detailed explanation of the situation that leads you to believe this is a case of food poisoning

• When and where the suspected food was consumed

• Who ate it

• Name and address of where the food was obtained and/or consumed

• If the food is a commercial product, the manufacturer's name and address and the product's lot or batch number

• If the tainted food is meat or poultry, the USDA inspection stamp on the wrapper identifies the plant where the food was made or packaged

formaldehyde This colorless, pungent irritant gas has an unpleasant odor and is considered to be supertoxic. It is most commonly found as formalin, a solution of 40 percent formaldehyde, water, and methanol used in medicine to preserve tissue specimens. It is also found in many everyday products: the glue and resin odor in new automobiles and furniture is formaldehyde; it is also contained in antiseptics, disinfectants, fabric sizing, some explosives, and adhesives. The higher the concentration of formaldehyde in a product, the greater the danger of explosion.

Formaldehyde is the most common chemical irritant in modern buildings—found in plywood, particleboard, stain-resistant carpets, insulation, and adhesives in flooring. However, the amount of formaldehyde emitted by these products fades in time. Workers and homeowners are exposed to low levels of formaldehyde from cloth, foam insulation, and plywood (especially in mobile homes). Formaldehyde has been classified as a human carcinogen by the International Agency for Research on Cancer and as a probable human carcinogen by the U.S. Environmental Protection Agency.

Symptoms

Most dangerous when inhaled or ingested, formaldehyde is less toxic when absorbed through the skin. It attacks the respiratory system, and, if it is ingested, victims experience immediate severe abdominal pain, with vomiting, pain in the throat and diarrhea, corrosive gastritis and collapse within a few minutes, loss of consciousness and liver failure, with death from circulatory failure. Shock may cause death within a few hours up to two days. If the patient does not die, recovery may be rapid.

Inhalation of fumes irritates the eyes, nose, and respiratory tract; chronic inhalation causes pulmonary edema and death. Skin contact (especially with paper and cloth containing formaldehyde) causes discoloration and may result in sloughing and allergic dermatitis.

Treatment

Gastric lavage immediately after ingestion, followed by large amounts of water and then a saline cathartic. In the event of skin contamination, wash thoroughly. Otherwise, treatment is supportive; dialysis may be effective.

formalin   See FORMALDEHYDE.

foxglove *(Digitalis)* **[Other names: dead man's thimbles, fairy bells, fairy cap, fairy finger, fairy glove, fairy thimbles, folks gloves, foxes glofa.]** Named for the resemblance of its flowers to fingers of the fairy "folks gloves," the foxglove has been considered medically useful since the first century A.D. and was first written about as a drug in the year 1200. The name refers to any of about 30 species of plants including the common foxglove *(D. purpurea)*, which is a powerful poison and plant source of the heart drug digitalis.

Together with paintbrush, speedwell, snapdragon, and monkeyflower, foxglove is a biennial member of the figwort family (Scrophulariaceae). During its first year, the plant produces a soft rosette of full, tapering, finely toothed leaves covered with white down, and on the second year it produces a beautiful, tall flower stalk column of three to five feet, with bell-shaped hanging flowers of yellow, white, pink, and purple. The stalk has a few small leaves and a long succession of flowers that open from the bottom to the top; each flower droops over the one below it on the stalk, and the flowers bloom in midsummer.

Native to Europe, the Mediterranean region, and the Canary Islands, foxglove is grown as an ornamental in the United States and is often seen in foundation plantings of older homes. It is also naturalized on the Pacific coast from northern California to British Columbia.

Its name originates in Britain, where residents called it "folks gloves" (the gloves of the little people, or fairies) and believed that the small spots on the lower lip of the foxglove flower were tiny fairy fingerprints. It was also called "dead man's thimbles" because of its shape and toxicity, and its Latin genus—*Digitalis*—also refers to a finger, or thimble.

In fact, it was in Britain that its usefulness as a heart medication was first discovered in 1775, when the physician to Benjamin Franklin discovered that a cold infusion made from the dried, powdered leaf of the foxglove acts as a heart stimulant and also a diuretic. The strengthened heart pumps more blood through the kidneys, carrying off water that has accumulated in the tissues.

Foxglove is considered by some to be a magical plant, ruled by the planet Venus, and has, since ancient times, been considered to be an herb of protection. Welsh housewives rubbed foxglove leaves into the stone cracks in their floors and painted crossed lines on the floor with foxglove dye to prevent evil from entering their homes.

Digitalis works by slowing the heartbeat and making it stronger, thereby increasing the efficiency of the heart. It reduces congestion in the veins and causes the kidneys to produce more urine. In the past, digitalis was administered by using the entire leaf, until digitoxin was isolated in 1869. Digoxin was isolated in 1930, which allowed physicians to refine the dosage and control the drug's action on the heart. No synthetic drug has been discovered that can take the place of *Digitalis purpurea.*

Recent research also suggests digitalis may be beneficial against glaucoma and as a component in a drug program in the treatment of muscular dystrophy.

Poisonous part

All parts of this plant—particularly the leaves—are poisonous and contain several glycosides that affect the heart and kidneys as well as irritant saponins. Ingestion of the dried or fresh leaves, which are not rendered harmless by cooking, will cause a severe case of poisoning. Most cases of foxglove poisoning have resulted from therapeutic overdose or by drinking foxglove herbal teas, not from accidental ingestion. Children have been poisoned after sucking on flowers or swallowing the seeds.

Symptoms

Eating even small amounts of foxglove leaves, flowers, or other parts can dangerously disrupt heartbeat rhythm. In large amounts it can depress heart function or stop it completely. Symptoms appear within 20 to 30 minutes after ingestion and include nausea, vomiting, diarrhea, stomach pain, severe headache, blurred vision, loss of appetite, irregular heartbeat and pulse, delirium, tremors, convulsions, and death from paralysis of the heart muscle. In excess amounts, foxglove increases the force of the heart's contractions to the point where it causes irritation and stimulates the central nervous system. Some sensitive individuals experience headache, rash, and nausea from handling the plant.

Treatment

Gastric lavage followed by the administration of activated charcoal, together with potassium chloride every hour (unless urination stops). Victims must have their heart and potassium levels constantly monitored.

See also DIGITALIS; DIGITOXIN; DIGOXIN; GLYCOSIDES; SAPONIN.

fugu See PUFFERFISH; TETRODOTOXIN.

fungicide Fungicides are inorganic and organic compounds used to protect against rot and eliminate fungi. While some are fairly nontoxic to humans, others are extremely poisonous. Among the most common substances used as fungicides are mercury and copper compounds, pentachlorophenol, dithiocarbamates, tetramethylthiuram disulfide, hexachlorobenzene, and iodine.

galerina mushroom *(Cortinarius speciosissimus, C. gentilis, Galerina venenata, G. autumnalis and C. orellanus)* Members of the *Cortinarius* genus, they cause some of the same symptoms. The brown-capped galerinas are also known as deadly cort, deadly galerina, and deadly lawn galerina; all are supertoxic.

C. orellanus is found primarily in Europe; *C. gentilis, G. venenata, G. autumnalis* (deadly galerina) and *C. speciosissimus* are found throughout the United States, particularly in the Northeast.

Poisonous part

The poison orellanin found in these mushrooms is toxic to the kidneys, but experts believe the mushrooms contain other as-yet-unidentified poisons.

Symptoms

Latency period following ingestion is longer than 10 hours and may last as long as two weeks; when symptoms appear, they include acute stomach pain, headaches, back or joint pain, kidney failure, damage to the intestines, genital organs, liver, heart, and nervous system. The victim's course may seem to improve, only to worsen and improve again until death finally occurs several months later.

Treatment

There is no antidote or successful treatment known. Vomiting soon after ingestion may expel the poison, and medical treatment may save some victims.

See also CORTINARIUS MUSHROOMS; MUSHROOM POISONING; MUSHROOM TOXINS.

gasoline See PETROLEUM DISTILLATES.

gelsemine A plant alkaloid found in yellow jessamine, gelsemine depresses and eventually paralyzes motor nerve endings, with contractions or spasms and—in severe cases—convulsions and respiratory arrest.

See also ALKALOIDS; JESSAMINE, YELLOW.

gelsemium *(Gelsemium sempervirens)* [Other names: Carolina Jasmine, yellow jasmine, sariyasemin.] This flowering climbing vine belongs to the family Loganiaceae and grows in the piedmont and coastal areas of the southeastern United States. Its flowers are funnel shaped and have a strong fragrance. Historically the roots and rhizome of the gelsemium were used to treat neuralgia and migraine.

The woody stem of gelsemium contains a milky juice and bears shiny lanceolate leaves and axillary clusters of one to five flowers, which bloom in early spring. The fruit is composed of two jointed pods that contain many flat-winged seeds.

Gelsemium sempervirens contains a long list of ergot type alkaloids, including gelsemicine, which is a central nervous system depressant and convulsant; and gelsemine, which has analgesic, hypotensive, cardiodepressant, and central nervous system depressant properties. In 2006, Chinese researchers announced that they had isolated three new alkaloids and a new extract artifact, gelsebamine, from gelsemium. The gelsebamine was found to inhibit a specific human lung adenocarcinoma cell line.

Use of gelsemium for treating various ailments in cats has been reported anecdotally, while use in humans is most widespread in Mexico, where it has been given for asthma, dysmenorrhea, gonorrhea, hypertension, malaria, and rheumatism. The fresh root is used to make a homeopathic remedy.

Poisonous part

All parts of the plant are poisonous, including the nectar and the flowers. The most toxic compounds are gelsemine and gelseminine, which depress the motor nerves. The toxic and therapeutic doses of gelsemium are very close. Eating just one flower has reportedly been deadly for children. It is possible to absorb the toxins through the skin, especially if there are cuts, abrasions, or it has been otherwise compromised.

Symptoms

Symptoms typically begin within 30 minutes of ingestion but may start immediately. These include difficulty in the use of voluntary muscles, muscle rigidity and weakness, dizziness, dry mouth, visual disturbances, trembling of the extremities, profuse sweating, respiratory depression, convulsions, and loss of speech. With large doses, paralysis, feeble respiration, and death from respiratory failure can occur. Death may occur within one to seven and one-half hours from ingestion.

Treatment

Prompt evacuation of the stomach by an emetic if the patient's condition allows. Equally important is artificial respiration, aided by early subcutaneous administration of ammonia, strychnine, atropine, or digitalis.

GHB (gamma-hydroxybutyric acid) [street names: "G," goop, scoop, liquid x, liquid ecstasy, caps, grievous bodily harm] Initially used by body builders to stimulate muscle growth, GHB has become a popular recreational drug used by adolescents and young adults, especially during parties and raves, because it induces relaxation and a high that can last up to four hours. GHB can be made from ingredients such as gamma-butyrolactone, a solvent used as a paint stripper, or butanediol, which is used in the production of plastics and adhesives. The drug is available as a powder, tablet, capsule, and clear liquid.

Because GHB is odorless, colorless, and virtually tasteless (it is slightly salty), it can be slipped into drinks without detection, and so it has become a popular date rape drug, along with ecstasy. The drug was banned by the Food and Drug Administration in 1990 after 57 people sought emergency treatment at poison control centers and emergency rooms for serious to life-threatening symptoms. Since that time GHB has been associated with several deaths and has been categorized as a Schedule I drug according to the Controlled Substances Act. However, a form of GHB—sodium oxybate, Xyrem—was approved by the FDA on July 17, 2002, for treatment of a rare form of narcolepsy. It is available only by prescription and is tightly regulated. Most of the GHB used in the United States is manufactured illegally in the States.

Symptoms

The effects of GHB can be felt within five to 20 minutes of taking the drug and the high can last up to four hours. At lower doses, GHB relieves anxiety and produces relaxation. When it is combined with other drugs such as alcohol it can cause nausea, breathing difficulties, and loss of muscle control. Withdrawal effects include insomnia, tremors, sweating, and anxiety. At higher doses, users may encounter difficulty thinking, hallucinations, slurred speech, headache, amnesia, coma, or death.

Treatment

Because absorption and onset of symptoms are so rapid after ingestion, washing out the stomach typically has little impact. Thus treatment for GHB poisoning is largely supportive. Activated charcoal can be tried. There is no known antidote to GHB.

giant milkweed (Calotropis procera, C. gigantea) This tree is found in the tropical Americas and Africa; its sap is used as an arrow poison in Africa. The treelike shrubs have rubbery leaves and clusters of white or lilac flowers with a sweet scent. The seeds have silky attachments, similar to other types of milkweed seeds, which are shaken from the pods as they dry. The two species are different heights (C. procera is less than six feet; C. gigantea may grow to 15 feet).

Poisonous part

The latex sap contains a mixture of cardiac glycosides with digitalis-like action, and unidentified allergens.

Symptoms

Ingestion results in irritation, burning, and swelling of the mucous membranes, but because of the bad taste ingestion of large amounts is not normally a problem. In addition, skin contact may cause an allergic reaction. Exposure to the eyes (cornea) may cause a severe keratoconjunctivitis.

Treatment

The ingestion of a large amount of this plant may produce heart irregularities, which are managed by monitoring by electrocardiogram.

See also CARDIAC GLYCOSIDES; DIGITALIS.

giardiasis An infection of the small intestine caused by the protozoan *Giardia lamblia,* which is found in the intestinal tract and feces. Contamination occurs when sewage is used as a fertilizer or when food handlers don't wash their hands. Although giardiasis is generally found commonly in tropical countries and travelers to those areas, in recent years outbreaks have been common in the United States among people in institutions, preschool children, and in catered affairs and large public picnic areas. It is most common in this country where large numbers of young children gather. It is spread by contaminated food or water or by direct personal hand-to-mouth contact. Infection can be prevented by thoroughly washing hands before handling food.

Symptoms

Giardiasis is not fatal and will eventually pass, and about two-thirds of infected people have no symptoms. When they do occur, symptoms appear about one to three days after infection and are uncomfortable. They include explosive diarrhea, foul-smelling and greasy feces, stomach pains, gas, loss of appetite, nausea, and vomiting. In some cases, the infection can become chronic. Giardiasis is diagnosed by examining a fecal sample for the presence of the parasites.

Treatment

Acute giardiasis usually runs its course and then clears up, but antibiotic metronidazole or quinacrine will help relieve symptoms and prevent the spread of infection.

Gila monster (*Heloderma suspectum*) The Gila monster is one of only two poisonous lizards in the world; both are similar in appearance and habits. This sluggish, shy little fellow grows to about 20 inches, with a stout body, black and pink spots, and bands extending onto a blunt tail and beadlike scales. It has a black face, with large toes and strong claws, and is smaller than its poisonous relative, the Mexican beaded lizard.

Named after the Gila River basin, the Gila monster lives in the gravelly and sandy soils found in the deserts of the Southwest, particularly in Arizona, southern Utah, and New Mexico. It prefers rocks and other animals' burrows; it may also dig its own holes. Gila monsters mate during summer and lay between three and five eggs in autumn and winter, and more than 95 percent of their time is spent underground.

Poisonous part

The venom of this lizard, used principally to immobilize prey, is extremely dangerous for humans as well. It is produced in eight glands in the lower jaw; venom is secreted into the mouth and then flows through the grooves of the teeth into the bite wound as the lizard chews; it is not injected as is snake venom. The whole system is not particularly efficient, requiring the Gila monster to hang on to its prey for some time and chew its tissues, enabling the poison to flow. The bite is extremely painful but rarely fatal (no deaths have been reported in modern times), but the Gila monster is extremely tenacious; often the victim must be cut away.

Symptoms

Severe pain at the wound site, swelling, weakness, tinnitus (ringing in the ears), nausea, breathing problems, cardiac failure, and sometimes death are symptoms that occur within one to three hours after the bite; their severity depends on the amount of venom injected, where the wound is located, and the victim's health.

Treatment

There is no known antivenin. Treatment is supportive, with tetanus prophylaxis and pain relief.

See also MEXICAN BEADED LIZARD.

glue See SOLVENT ABUSE.

glycoside Also known as glucosides, the glycosides are more common in the plant kingdom than alkaloids. Glycosides are a group of compounds containing at least one type of sugar that are released when the plant is eaten. (*Glyco* comes from the root word meaning "sugar.") The amount of glycoside in a plant depends on genetics, the part of the plant, its age and, to a large degree, environmental factors such as climate, moisture supply, and fertility of the soil. While many glycosides are not poisonous, a number of them are, including cardiac glycosides, cyanogenic glycosides, and saponins.

Glycosides that yield hydrocyanic acid after hydrolysis are called cyanogenetic; one of the most common is the glycoside amygdalin, found in many members of Rosaceae plants that have cyanogenetic compounds, including hydrangea, flax, cassava, lima bean, cherry, apple, white clover, and vetch seed.

See also ALKALOIDS; CARDIAC GLYCOSIDES; CYANOGENIC GLYCOSIDES; SAPONIN.

golden dewdrop (*Duranta repens* L.) [Other names: pigeon berry, sky-flower.] This large shrub usually cultivated as a hedge is native to Key West and is also found in southern Texas, the West Indies, Hawaii, Guam, and Australia. It produces small, light blue or white flowers and masses of poisonous orange berries.

Poisonous part
The berry contains toxic saponins, but reports of poisoning with them have occurred only in Australia.

Symptoms
Sleepiness, fever, tachycardia, swelling of the lips and eyelids, convulsions, and gastrointestinal irritation.

Treatment
Gastric lavage, control of convulsions with diazepam and maintenance of fluid and electrolyte balance.

See also SAPONIN.

gout stalk (*Jatropha podagrica*) This plant is a member of a large genus of shrubs or small trees with a three-sided seed capsule, found throughout the Western Hemisphere.

Poisonous part
The seeds are poisonous and contain jatrophin (curcin), a plant lectin (toxalbumin), and cathartic oils. Ingestion of just one seed can be serious. The plant lectin inhibits protein synthesis in cells of the intestinal wall and may cause serious or fatal poisoning.

Symptoms
The onset of symptoms (nausea, vomiting, and diarrhea) occurs rapidly, unlike poisoning with other plants with toxic lectins.

Treatment
Treat symptoms; give fluids.

ground cherry (*Physalis*) There are about 17 species of this plant growing in the United States, most with an attractive fruit resembling a Chinese lantern; inside the papery pod is a berry filled with tiny seeds.

Poisonous part
The unripe berries are poisonous and contain toxic solanine glycoalkaloids.

Symptoms
While solanine rarely is toxic to adults, children can be fatally poisoned. Symptoms include stomach irritation, a harsh, scratchy feeling in the throat, diarrhea, and fever.

Treatment
Replace fluids, treat symptoms, and give supportive care.

grouper, spotted Any of a number of species of fish in the family Serranidae (including yellowfin) widely found in warm seas with large mouths and heavy bodies; they can grow to be more than six feet long. Many carry a toxic substance in the flesh that can cause a type of food poisoning called ciguatera.

Poisonous part

The toxin believed to be involved in ciguatera is fat soluble, odorless and tasteless, and is not destroyed by heat.

Symptoms

After eating, symptoms may develop quickly or slowly and involve tingling sensations in the lips and mouth followed by numbness, nausea, vomiting, abdominal cramps, weakness, paralysis, convulsions, skin rash, coma, and death in about 12 percent of cases.

Treatment

Recent research suggests that pralidoxime chloride (a cholinesterase reactivator) is an effective antidote.

See also CIGUATERA; FISH CONTAMINATION.

grouper, yellowfin   See GROUPER, SPOTTED.

Gyromitra   This genus of mushroom, also known as the false morel, contains a toxin usually removed during cooking, although a few individuals are sensitive to it even when the mushroom is cooked completely. The species has no gills, and its spores develop in microscopic sacs on the surfaces of the fruiting bodies. The appearance of the body of the fungus gives this mushroom its nickname, brain fungi. While many species of *Gyromitra* are edible, it usually takes an expert to tell the difference.

Poisonous part

While the chemical ingredient in this species is not known, many varieties contain gyromitrin, which is hydrolyzed to form the active toxin monomethylhydrazine, a substance that affects the central nervous system and is also used as rocket fuel. This toxin is volatile and dissolves readily in water; therefore, the mushroom may be made edible by air drying or extracting the toxin with boiling water.

Symptoms

Between six and 24 hours after ingestion or inhalation of the vapor while cooking, symptoms suddenly appear: The victim begins to vomit and develops dizziness, fatigue, and muscle cramps. In severe cases, this may be followed by delirium, coma, and convulsions and can sometimes be fatal. In nonfatal cases, victims recover within two to six days.

Treatment

Supportive, which may include blood transfusions and correction of acidosis. Intravenous pyridoxine is the specific antidote.

See also MONOMETHYLHYDRAZINE; MUSHROOM POISONING; MUSHROOM TOXINS.

habu, Okinawa *(Trimeresurus flavoviridis)* The most dangerous pit viper in Asia, this large, aggressive snake, known as one of the collective group called fer-de-lance, is found on the Amami and Okinawa groups in the Ryukyu Islands—often in houses. Marked with a wavy band of dark green splotches, it sometimes grows to be five feet long and can cause disability or death. Its smaller relative, the kufah *(Trimeresurus okinavesis)*, is also dangerous. Both are happy to live in trees, along with the other genus of this group, *Agkistrodon.*

Symptoms

Because the venom interferes with the coagulation of the blood, it hemorrhages into muscles and the nervous system and results in bleeding from the gums, nose, mouth, and rectum. Shock and respiratory distress is followed by death if untreated.

Treatment

Antivenin is available.

See also ANTIVENIN; FER-DE-LANCE; PIT VIPERS; SNAKES, POISONOUS.

Halcion See BENZODIAZEPINES; SLEEPING PILLS.

Haldol See ANTIPSYCHOTIC/PSYCHOMETRIC DRUGS.

hallucinogenic mushrooms A group of mushrooms, important to the sacred ceremonies of the American Indian religions (and also to drug abusers), that produce hallucinations when eaten. These mushrooms include three main groups: the psilocybes *(Psilocybe caerulescens, P. mexicana, P. pel-*

liculosa, P. cyanescens, P. baeocystis, P. cubensis), conocybes *(Conocybe cyanopus, C. smithii),* and stropharias, all of which produce visual and auditory hallucinations about 15 minutes after eating.

The *Conocybe* and *Psilocybe* mushrooms contain psilocybin and psilocin as active constituents.

Symptoms

The onset of effects for all varieties usually occurs within three hours of ingestion, and symptoms include drowsiness, loss of ability to concentrate, dizziness, and sometimes muscle weakness. The hallucinogenic effects are dose dependent and may vary according to the personality of the person; both space and time distortion are reported, together with visual and auditory imagery. The hallucinations are usually described as pleasant.

Treatment

Recovery following ingestion of such a mushroom is normally uneventful. The period of intoxication is not long, usually between three and six hours, after which all symptoms disappear. However, there is a danger that patients may become destructive during the hallucinatory period, and therefore their movements should be restricted. Phenothiazine drugs may be used to end the psychosis if extreme agitation is experienced.

See also MEXICAN HALLUCINOGENIC MUSHROOM; MUSHROOM POISONING.

harlequin snake See CORAL SNAKE, EASTERN.

Helicobacter pylori This bacterium is believed to cause most stomach ulcers and almost all duodenal ulcers, and is believed to exist in groundwater throughout the United States. In 1983, the bacterium was first found in the stomach tissue of ulcer patients. While half the world's populations are believed to be infected (including an estimated 40 million Americans), it only causes ulcers in 10 to 20 percent of its hosts. Still, one out of every 10 Americans has an ulcer, and *H. pylori* is implicated in 90 percent of those cases.

Symptoms

Nausea and stomach pain, vomiting and fever lasting between three and 14 days. Virtually everyone with the bacteria has chronic gastritis (a mild inflammation of the stomach lining), which may last for decades. Some people with the infection don't have ulcers but have nausea, gas, bloating, and burning stomach pain.

Diagnosis

Blood tests can determine the presence of antibodies to the bacteria, which can tell if you have ever had the infection but not if it's active. A biopsy can reveal *H. pylori*. Breath tests are currently being studied and may be available in the near future.

Treatment

About 90 percent of *H. pylori* infections can be cured with a combination of anti-ulcer medication and specific antibiotics. However, the treatment is not easy; it involves taking 12 to 16 pills a day for two weeks and carries the risk of some side effects, such as fatigue and dizziness. Because the treatment may not be completely successful, follow-up testing at least four weeks after completing treatment may be needed to make sure the bacteria are no longer present. If tests reveal no bacteria, the patient is not likely to be reinfected ever again. Persistent infection may require a different medication for longer period of time.

Complications

The organism has also been found in a disproportionately large number of patients with certain kinds of stomach cancer. Some scientists suggest the infection may triple the risk of this rare cancer. While there appears to be a relationship between the bacteria and stomach cancer, these cancers are becoming less common in the United States, and

therapy for *H. pylori* has not been recommended as a preventive measure.

Prevention

Chlorine in public drinking water kills the bacteria, but shallow wells may be contaminated by surface water tainted with the bacterium (deeper wells are less likely to have the bacterium). Normal water testing procedures can't identify the presence of *H. pylori*, and there is no test at present that you can use to test your well. However, private water-testing labs can test water for microscopic particulates, which will determine if the well water has been contaminated with surface water and thus, by bacteria. You can install an ultraviolet disinfection system to treat contaminated water. Charcoal-based tap filters may not be a good choice, because bacteria can form on the charcoal.

hemlock, deadly   See HEMLOCK, POISON.

hemlock, ground   See YEW.

hemlock, lesser   See HEMLOCK, POISON.

hemlock, poison *(Conium maculatum)* **[Other names: California fern, deadly hemlock, herb bonnett, kill cow, lesser hemlock, muskrat weed bunk, Nebraska fern, poison parsley, poison root, snake weed, spotted hemlock, spotted parsley, wode whistle.]**   The ancient poison drink of Socrates, poison hemlock is rapidly fatal. The plant (which resembles a carrot) has large lacy leaves as much as four feet long that produce a disagreeable garlicky odor when crushed, and a white root. It is found in South America, northern Africa and Asia, and in the United States and Canada where it has been naturalized. In Europe, it is called "fool's parsley."

Poisonous part

Leaves are most toxic when the plant is flowering, but all parts of the hemlock are deadly. Its root resembles the wild carrot, and its seeds have been mistaken for anise. Hemlock contains coniine, a muscle relaxant similar to curare, and related alkaloids. In addition, quail may eat poison hemlock seeds and pass on the poison to a human who consumes the flesh. This type of secondary hemlock poisoning can cause diarrhea, vomiting, and paralysis in humans within three hours of eating the affected quail.

Symptoms

Responsible for many human fatalities, hemlock poisoning can begin within 30 minutes after ingestion. Symptoms include gradual muscular weakness and increasing muscular pain, paralysis, blindness, respiratory problems, and death within several hours, which comes from paralysis of the lungs.

Treatment

Gastric lavage must be performed immediately after ingestion of the poison or it is ineffective; give diazepam to relieve convulsions.

See also ALKALOIDS; CONIINE.

hemlock, water *(Cicuta maculata, C. californica, C. douglasii, C. vagans, C. bolanderi, C. bulbifera, C. curtissii, C. occidentalis)* One of the most poisonous plants and the most violent poison contained in plants in the United States, the several species of water hemlock are found in waste places, pastures, and swamps of the northern temperate regions. Water hemlock is a perennial herb and member of the carrot family, growing up to eight feet tall with purple spots and small, white, heavily scented flowers. Underground, there is a bundle of roots that, when cut, smell very much like parsnips. Water hemlock *(C. maculata)* is found in eastern North America to the Great Plains; California water hemlock *(C. californica, C. bolanderi)* in midwestern California; Douglas water hemlock *(C. douglasii)* along the Pacific coast and British Columbia; tuber water hemlock or Oregon water hemlock *(C. vagans)* in the Pacific Northwest; western water hemlock *(C. occidentalis)* in the Rocky Mountain states to the Pacific coast; bulbous water hemlock *(C. bulbifera)* in the northern United States.

Poisonous part

The entire water hemlock contains the poison cicutoxin, although the root has the most. Many people have been poisoned by mistaking water hemlock for parsnips or artichokes, and children have been poisoned by using water hemlock to make peashooters and whistles. One mouthful of the root may kill an adult, and many Americans (especially children) have died after eating this plant; 30 percent of water hemlock poisonings are fatal. The powerful nerve toxin causes excruciating spasms and convulsions so powerful that people have been known to bite through their own tongue and break their teeth.

Symptoms

This is a fairly fast acting toxic plant, with symptoms beginning 15 minutes after ingestion, including restlessness, abdominal pain, nausea, vomiting, diarrhea, respiratory problems, hypersalivation, weak and rapid pulse, delirium, violent convulsions, and—within one hour—death.

Treatment

Both emetics and cathartics are used to get the poison out of the body, and morphine and barbiturates can control convulsions. Once seizures appear imminent or have already occurred, gastric lavage should not be attempted without an anesthesiologist. Prolonged problems in mental function and abnormal brain waves have been reported.

henbane *(Hyoscyamus niger)* [Other names: black henbane, devil's eye, fetid nightshade, henbell, hog's bean, insane root, Jupiter's bean, poison tobacco, stinking nightshade.] This powerful plant is the most common species of the nightshade/potato family Solanaceae, comprising 11 biennials or perennials. Naturalized in the eastern United States, it is grown commercially in North America and is found wild in garbage dumps and in isolated spots in Great Britain, central and southern Europe, and western Asia.

The annual form of the plant grows to one to two feet tall and then flowers and sets seed; the biennial produces only a tuft of basal leaves that disappear in winter leaving a root. In the spring, a branched flowering stem grows from this root that is usually much taller and more vigorous than the flowering stems of the annual plants. The whole henbane plant has a strong, unpleasant odor, and its leaves, if bruised when fresh, emit a strong narcotic smell similar to that of tobacco. Its root is a long, tapering brown tuber with a bad odor and could be mistaken for parsnips and eaten, with fatal results.

Three drugs are made from the dried leaves of the henbane plant: Atropine, hyoscyamine, and scopolamine. In addition, the leaves are smoked as a narcotic and are prepared as a beverage in India.

Poisonous part

All parts of the plant are poisonous, especially the seeds, pods, and leaves, which contain varying amounts of the belladonna alkaloids atropine, hyoscyamine, and scopolamine. The seeds have the highest amount of scopolamine, which depresses the central nervous system.

Symptoms

A fast-acting toxin (within 15 minutes), henbane produces symptoms similar to those caused by deadly nightshade or atropine poisoning. Children are poisoned by eating seeds and pods. Poisoning causes dry mouth, tachycardia, fever, blurred vision, excitement, delirium, and confusion; hallucinations are frequently reported in children.

Treatment

If poisoning is severe, a slow intravenous administration of physostigmine is given until symptoms subside.

hepatitis A   The hardy hepatitis A virus is the most common type of all the alphabet hepatitis viruses. It is spread by eating food or drinking water contaminated with the virus. It then multiplies in the body and is passed in the feces. It can then be carried on an infected person's hand and spread by direct contact or by eating food or drink handled by that person. Unlike many other viruses, it can live for more than a month at room temperature on kitchen countertops, children's toys, and other surfaces, and it can be maintained indefinitely in frozen foods and ice.

In 1992, 22,000 Americans were reported to have hepatitis A. Since 1996, however, with the introduction of a vaccine, the Centers for Disease Control and Prevention (CDC) has recommended vaccination for persons at increased risk. In 1999 it was recommended that children who lived in 11 states with the highest incidence of hepatitis A be vaccinated routinely, and that children in six additional states that had an incidence above the national average also be considered for vaccination. A study compared incidence rates in 2003 with those of the prevaccination period and found that rates declined 76 percent overall and 88 percent in the vaccinating states. Since 2001, rates in adults, especially men aged 25 to 39, have been higher than among children.

Hepatitis A may be found in shellfish (especially oysters), raw or undercooked food, fruits and vegetables, and well water contaminated by improperly treated sewage. Although there is no typical "season" for hepatitis A, it tends to occur in cycles. Mass foodborne contaminations have been found in frozen strawberries, imported lettuce, restaurant iced tea, raw oysters, and shellfish.

Symptoms

Incubation period of the virus ranges from 15 to 50 days. A quarter of all people with hepatitis A won't have any symptoms; a few young children may have a low fever and achiness, but rarely jaundice. Children over age 12 may be much sicker, with fever (100–104°F), extreme tiredness, weakness, nausea, stomach upset, pain in the upper right side of the stomach, and appetite loss. Within a few days, a yellowish tinge appears in the skin and whites of the eyes. Urine will be darker than usual, and the stool is light colored. Once the jaundice appears, patients begin to feel better.

Diagnosis

Blood tests showing antibodies to hepatitis A are the best diagnosis. Symptoms of hepatitis A are so similar to other diseases that a doctor needs test results to make the correct diagnosis.

Treatment

There is no drug treatment for hepatitis A. While symptoms appear, patients should rest and eat well; low-fat, high-carbohydrate, easily digested foods, such as crackers, noodles, rice, or soup, in small amounts are good choices. Antinausea medicine and acetaminophen can be prescribed.

Complications

Rarely, hepatitis A develops into fulminant hepatitis in which the liver cells are completely destroyed. As the liver function stops, toxic substances build up and affect the brain, causing lethargy, confusion, combativeness, stupor, and coma. This can often lead to death, although the patient may live with aggressive treatment. If the victim does not die, the liver is able to regenerate and resume function and the brain recovers.

Prognosis

Hepatitis A is less serious than other types of hepatitis viruses and causes only temporary liver damage, which is reversed as the body produces antibodies. Most people recover in a few weeks without any complications. However, it can occasionally be fatal; about 100 people die each year from this infection.

Prevention

To inactivate the virus, food must be heated at 185°F for one minute. It is difficult to test water for hepatitis A, but treated municipal or county water supplies are safe. Patients are most infectious in the two weeks before symptoms develop. Food handlers who know they are infected should not work until they are past the infectious stages, which ends one week after first becoming jaundiced. Even though federal regulations and posting of contaminated waters offer some protection, there is still a risk of contracting viruses when eating raw shellfish.

A new vaccine said to be 100 percent effective after a single dose became available in 1996. With earlier vaccines, more than 99 percent of people became immune after two doses; a booster is recommended for this vaccine between six and 12 months after the first dose.

Those who aren't vaccinated who are exposed can prevent infection by getting a shot of immune globulin (pooled human blood plasma that contains protective antibodies against the disease). People who would need this shot include

- all household members and sex partners of hepatitis A patients,
- close friends of infected schoolchildren,
- food handlers whose coworker(s) gets the disease,
- staff of prisons and institutions where at least two residents have hepatitis A.

herbicides Chemicals used to kill weeds. They can be divided into two groups: those that are poisonous to anything with which they come in contact, including animals and humans in addition to weeds; and those that are poisonous only to a selected group of weeds and will not harm humans or animals. Contact weed killers commonly used include sodium chlorate, dinitrophenol derivatives, potassium cyanate, sodium arsenite, caustic acids and alkalis, petroleum distillates, trifluralin, diquat, and paraquat.

See also PARAQUAT; PETROLEUM DISTILLATES.

herbs, unsafe Long before the beginnings of modern medicine, the earliest health care practitioners—the shamans, the medicine men, and the healers—prescribed herbs and herb extracts to treat disease. Many of these herbal medicines were beneficial (for example, digitalis heart drugs are extracted from foxglove). But many of the early remedies have been discovered to be quite dangerous—even toxic—inducing violent episodes of vomiting or seizures and causing serious liver, kidney, or other organ damage. Some cause abortions, and others are simply of no value at all.

According to the Food and Drug Administration, there are three categories of herbs: unsafe herbs, herbs of undefined safety for food use and safe herbs (GRAS—generally recognized as safe). For its own purposes, however, the FDA considers herbs as foods, not as medicine. Still, the FDA notes that even the GRAS herbs can cause problems if used to excess. "Too much of any herb is toxic," the FDA warns in one of its reports. In particular, eating too much red pepper, sorrel, or nutmeg can be decidedly toxic.

While plant ingestions are second only to drugs as the most common poisoning emergency in children, serious poisoning or death from ingesting herbs is rare because the amount of toxin is usually quite small. However, there has been an increase over the past 20 years in the public use of herbal remedies and traditional herbal healing products.

In fact, brewing or mixing some herbal remedies can be dangerous, not only because of the toxic makeup of the plants, but because the content of various toxins varies considerably with the soil and climate conditions in which the plant was grown. Beneficial and harmful components in any herb can vary tremendously from one garden to another, from one year to another, and even from one plant to another in the same garden grown at the same time.

Unfortunately, in addition to natural toxicity in some plants, "herbal" or "traditional" preparations may sometimes actually contain drugs such as phenyllbutazone, corticosteroids, salicylates, ephedrine, or toxic metal salts (mercury or lead).

Herbal mail-order suppliers and health food stores do a brisk business in health food products, and there are almost 400 different herbs available in the form of commercial teas. But some teas contain plants that can be very dangerous—nutmeg, mandrake, or jimsonweed (identified as "thorn apple," its other name). There are also almost 200 herbs blended into a variety of commercial cigarettes or smoking mixtures.

See also COMFREY; DIGITALIS; FOXGLOVE; JIMSONWEED; MANDRAKE, AMERICAN; NUTMEG.

heroin (diacetylmorphine) A narcotic drug derived from morphine, the principal alkaloid of opium, which is extracted from the pods of the opium poppy and often processed in Turkey. Currently, Afghanistan is the world's primary morphine/heroin source.

Heroin was created in an attempt to find a safer type of morphine, and the resulting product was a would-be cough medicine called Heroin, named for the drug's presumably "heroic" ability to mimic the effects of morphine without causing addiction. Developers hoped the new drug would be used to cure morphine addiction. Unfortunately, heroin is in fact four times more addictive than morphine.

Heroin is a white or brown powder (depending on where it has been processed) that can be smoked, sniffed, or dissolved in water and injected. It can be smoked when the end of a cigarette is dipped in heroin powder and lighted (this is called ack-ack); "chasing the dragon" or "playing the organ" involves mixing heroin with barbiturates. The drug is lighted and the smoke inhaled. Subcutaneous injection is called skin popping; intravenous injection is mainlining.

In addition to its painkilling properties, heroin produces sensations of warmth, calmness, drowsiness, and a loss of concern for outside events. Long-term use causes tolerance, which means the user needs more and more of the drug to maintain the same level of intoxication. It also produces both psychological and physical addiction. Sudden withdrawal of the drug causes shivering, abdominal cramps, diarrhea, vomiting, sleeplessness, and restlessness.

As yet, there is no legal medical use for heroin in the United States, although a few researchers are investigating its ability to control cancer pain. Heroin is an accepted cancer painkiller in Britain; because it is stronger than morphine, it is a better and longer-lasting pain reliever.

Symptoms
Heroin is a central nervous system depressant. An overdose frequently results in death. Following an injection, the user feels an immediate rush; if an overdose, death occurs within a few minutes unless the drug was sniffed or injected under the skin (then death may take up to four hours). Symptoms include pinpoint pupils, slow and shallow breathing, vision problems, restlessness, cramps, cyanosis, weak pulse, low blood pressure, coma, and death from respiratory paralysis.

Treatment
The antidote is naloxone; treat symptoms.

See also MORPHINE; NARCOTICS; OPIUM.

hexachlorophene See PHENOL.

holly (Ilex) There are about 400 species of red- or black-berried plants, including the popular Christmas hollies, American holly *(Ilex opaca)*, and English holly *(I. aquifolium)*. The hollies have alternate, glossy and thick-spined leaves (either single or clustered) with small, green flowers and bright red or black berries. Male and female flowers are usually on separate plants.

American holly is native from Massachusetts to Florida, west to Missouri and Texas; English holly is cultivated from Virginia to Texas, the Pacific Coast states, and British Columbia. Yaupon *(Ilex vomitoria),* also known as Carolina tea and emetic holly, is native to the Atlantic and Gulf coast states and North Carolina to Texas and Arkansas.

Poisonous part

Berries (and in some reports, leaves) of this plant are poisonous and contain alkaloids, glycosides, saponins, terpenoids, caffeine, and theobromine (a caffeinelike alkaloid). In some species, the leaves are brewed for their caffeine and other xanthines.

Symptoms

In small doses, holly may be a nervous system stimulant. In large doses, it can cause nausea, vomiting, diarrhea, inflamed and numb sensations in the mouth, drowsiness, and altered state of consciousness. The berries are particularly poisonous and can be fatal to children if enough are eaten and the symptoms are not treated. Some estimate that 20 berries are poisonous, but a fatal dose may be less in children.

Treatment

Administer fluids to prevent dehydration.

See also ALKALOIDS; GLYCOSIDE; SAPONIN.

honey Honey of any type can contain *Clostridium botulinum* spores, which are harmless to everyone *except infants under one year of age.* For this reason, infants should never be fed raw honey of any type, since botulism spores can be fatal to this group.

See also BOTULISM; BOTULISM, INFANT; *CLOSTRIDIUM BOTULINUM.*

hormone disruptors Researchers are gathering a growing amount of evidence that some persistent organic pollutants (POPs), such as DDT, dieldrin, furans, dioxins, and PCBs, among others, mimic, inhibit, and/or disrupt hormones and interfere with their natural regulatory processes, even at very low doses. These substances are called hormone disruptors (also endocrine disruptors, xenoestrogens [estrogen disruptors]), and they have well-documented negative effects on wildlife and reportedly similar effects on humans.

In animals, for example, hormone disruptors are causing feminization of male fetuses, dysfunctions in reproductive processes, behavioral changes, and development problems. Scientists are seeing examples of partially developed male and female sexual organs in alligators and polar bears and abnormally small genitals in males. In the Great Lakes, herring gull nests have twice the number of eggs but they are unfertilized and cared for by pairs of female birds, because the males have lost interest in the natural processes of mating and rearing young. Amphibian, reptile, and marine mammal populations around the world are declining, possibly due to a reduced fertility in males.

In humans, studies show that hormone disruptors may cause ovarian, breast, testicular, and prostate cancers; suppress the immune system; stimulate early puberty; impair fetal development, with the result being smaller babies; reduced intelligence; hyperactivity and violence; and reduced sperm counts. One hormone disruptor, bisphenol-A, has been shown to disrupt hormones at very low doses in animals and is suspected of causing birth defects and reproductive damage that may lead to prostate and breast cancer. Bisphenol-A has been shown to cause changes in estrogen in animal cells at the same concentrations that are found in pregnant women and their fetuses.

Xenoestrogens—substances foreign to the human body that directly or indirectly act like estrogens—are the most studied of the hormone disruptors, primarily because of their apparent impact on women's reproductive health. Although the majority of the studies have been done in animals, the results thus far strongly implicate xenoestrogens in disorders ranging from infertility to endometriosis, breast and ovarian cancer, birth defects, and premature puberty. Among the more commonly recognized xenoestrogens are bisphenol-A, DDT (banned), endosulphan (not banned), and atrazine, the most commonly used weed killer for corn in the United States.

Hormone disruptors are found in a wide range of products and in the environment: from solvents to detergents, plastics (bottles, bags, wrap, food containers), pesticides, industrial chemicals, dry-cleaning solvents, carpet, furniture, and byproducts of industry. They are also found in foods, including milk, soy beans, fish, meat, and poultry, and in drinking water.

See also BISPHENOL-A, PERSISTENT ORGANIC POLLUTANTS.

horse chestnut *(Aesculus hippocastanum)* The horse chestnut tree is a native of the Balkan Peninsula but it also grows throughout the Northern Hemisphere. Also called Spanish chestnut and buckeye (but not to be confused with the California or Ohio buckeye trees), the seed extract of the horse chestnut plant is used throughout Europe for chronic venous insufficiency, a condition characterized by swollen legs, varicose veins, skin ulcers, itching, and leg pain. It is also used to treat hemorrhoids.

Poisonous part

Unprocessed horse chestnut seeds are poisonous, as are the leaves, bark, and flowers, all of which contain the toxin esculin. Properly processed horse chestnut seeds contain little or no esculin. When purchasing horse chestnut seed extract, products should be standardized to a substance called escin.

Symptoms

If poisoning occurs, symptoms include muscle twitching, vomiting, diarrhea, headache, confusion, weakness, poor coordination, coma, paralysis, and death. Based on animal studies, horse chestnut seed extract may lower blood sugar, and so patients with diabetes or hypoglycemia should be cautious when using this supplement. Serum glucose levels may need to be monitored by a healthcare provider. Use of topical horse chestnut may cause skin irritation. People with bleeding disorders are cau-

tioned when using horse chestnut as the herb may increase the risk of bleeding.

Treatment

Symptomatic.

horse nettle See CAROLINA HORSE NETTLE.

huffing Inhalant abuse, also called huffing, sniffing, and bagging, is the intentional inhalation of chemical vapors for the purpose of achieving an altered mental and/or physical state. Most of the people who practice huffing are adolescents, and they are after a euphoric effect to enhance their experiences during clubbing and raves. Nearly 3 million teenagers are believed to practice huffing. Adult abusers typically huff to enhance their sexual experiences. Huffing is widespread across the United States, but it may be underreported because many people, including healthcare providers, law enforcement officials, and parents, are not familiar with the signs of inhalant abuse.

The chemical vapors sought after as inhalants for huffing can be found in more than 1,000 common products often available in most homes. These products fall into some general categories. *Aerosols* are sprays that contain solvents and propellants. The most popular among inhalant abusers are silver and gold spray paint, deodorant, hair products, cooking products, and fabric protector. *Gases* such as medical anesthetics and refrigerants are popular. Users turn to butane lighters, air-conditioning units, and propane tanks. Laughing gas (nitrous oxide) is abused more frequently than any other gas, and it can be found in whipped cream dispensers or products that enhance the octane levels in cars. Drug paraphernalia stores also sell sealed vials called whippets that contain the gas.

Volatile solvents are liquids that vaporize at room temperature. They include felt-tip markers, nail polish and remover, glue (rubber cement), paint thinner, gasoline, and correction fluid. *Nitrites* are used primarily to enhance sexual experiences and are a group of chemicals that include cyclohyxyl nitrite, amyl nitrite, and butyl nitrite. Cyclohexyl nitrite is found in room deodorizers; amyl nitrite and butyl nitrite are sold in small bottles referred to as poppers.

Symptoms

Initially users experience excitation, then drowsiness, lightheadedness, loss of inhibitions, and agitation. Additional effects during or shortly after use include dizziness, strong hallucinations, delusions, belligerence, apathy, and impaired judgment. Long-term users may exhibit weight loss, disorientation, lack of coordination, irritability, and depression. Withdrawal symptoms include sweating, rapid pulse, hand tremors, insomnia, nausea, vomiting, hallucinations, and in severe cases, grand mal seizures. Inhaled nitrite users experience dilated blood vessels, increased heart rate, excitement, and a sensation of heat.

Chronic huffing may result in irreversible damage to the heart, kidneys, lungs, brain, and liver. Brain damage may appear as memory impairment, slurred speech, and personality changes. Death can occur after a single use or prolonged use. Causes of death may include heart failure, asphyxiation, aspiration, or suffocation.

Treatment

If someone is in a state of crisis, stay calm, because agitation may cause the user to become violent or suffer heart dysfunction, which can result in sudden death. Make sure the user is in a well-ventilated area and call emergency medical services. Enrollment in a treatment facility is often recommended.

hyacinth *(Hyacinthus orientalis)*   A plant widely cultivated throughout the United States for its fragrant bell-shaped flowers.

Poisonous part

The bulb of this plant is poisonous.

Symptoms

Ingestion of the bulb of the hyacinth causes severe stomach problems, which, while not fatal, can be very painful.

Treatment

Perform gastric lavage or induce vomiting; treat symptoms.

hydrangea *(Hydrangea)*   The hydrangea is considered to be one of the most poisonous plants. About 80 species of this common flowering shrub are found throughout the entire Western Hemisphere; *H. macrophylla* is the most popular.

This deciduous mounded shrub can grow to be 15 feet, with large oval leaves with toothed edges up to 6 inches long, and white, pink, or blue flowers in a showy cluster. Flower color usually depends on the acidity of the soil, and the color grows brown as the flowers age.

Poisonous part

All parts of the plant (but especially the flower buds) are toxic and contain the poison hydrangin, which is believed to produce toxic cyanide compounds activated by stomach acids.

Symptoms

Several hours after ingestion, the glycosides decompose in the gastrointestinal tract and release the poison, which causes gastroenteritis and other cyanide poisoning symptoms. Cyanosis may develop, and in cases of large doses, convulsions, coma and death.

Treatment

Gastric lavage followed by a 25 percent solution of sodium thiosulfate. In unconscious victims, acidosis should be corrected and shock treated together with the administration of oxygen to aid breathing. Cyanide antidote should be administered.

hydrocarbon   An organic compound that contains primarily hydrogen and carbon atoms, usually of biological origin. Hydrocarbons include ethylene, acetic acid (vinegar), methylene chloride, formaldehyde, benzene, DDT, PCB, propylene, butylene, toluene, and xylene.

hydrochloric acid (hydrogen chloride)   Hydrochloric acid is usually marketed as a solution containing 28 to 35 percent by weight hydrogen chloride, commonly known as concentrated hydrochloric acid. It is also found in the stomach lining, forming part of the stomach juices and is important in the digestion of proteins.

A fatal dose of hydrochloric acid is almost impossible to swallow, since the highly corrosive nature of the acid would close up the throat. Skin absorption or breathing in the vapors can cause fatalities, however. The acid produces burns, ulcers, and scarring, destroying any tissue it touches.

Symptoms

Eye contact will cause blindness; skin contact will result in redness, peeling, burns, and scarring. Inhalation will inflame the throat, tongue, and lungs and cause coughing, choking, headaches, dizziness, and weakness followed some hours later by chest constriction, foaming at the mouth, and cyanosis. Blood pressure falls while pulse races, as pulmonary edema is followed by death.

When ingested, hydrochloric acid can cause burning pain, vomiting, bloody diarrhea, low blood pressure, swelling of the throat (causing suffocation), and a usually fatal peritonitis.

Treatment

Administer a mild alkali (such as milk) to neutralize acid; treat symptoms as they appear.

hydrogen peroxide This popular antiseptic found in most home medicine cabinets is used as a mouthwash, to treat infections, and to bleach hair and is usually sold in concentrations of 3 percent. Toddlers frequently ingest hydrogen peroxide, but it is considered to be of low toxicity. It generally breaks down in the gastrointestinal tract before it can be absorbed in the body; as it decomposes, however, it may release large amounts of oxygen, causing stomach distention and nausea.

hydrogen sulfide This is an irritant gas that occurs in the presence of decomposing vegetables or animals, such as in liquid manure pits, sewers, tanneries, fishing boats, or coal mines; its presence is announced by the distinctive smell of rotten eggs. Hydrogen sulfide is also an industrial byproduct of petroleum refineries and blast furnaces.

Symptoms

Poisoning with this gas resembles that of cyanide and interferes with the body's oxygen supply. In mild exposure, it causes painful and reddened eyes, blurred vision, and seeing colored halos around lights. In higher amounts, it can cause cyanosis, confusion, and pulmonary edema; at very high levels, it can cause an almost immediate fatal coma. In the case of serious poisoning, the fatality rate is 6 percent.

Treatment

Remove the victim from exposure; give oxygen and intravenous nitrite therapy. There is no antidote to hydrogen sulfide poisoning. If the victim lives for four days, recovery is likely, although there are lingering side effects for months (including lethargy, headache, fatigue, memory loss, and lack of initiative).

hydromorphone The chemical name for Dilaudid, this is a potent analgesic used for moderate to severe pain available in a wide variety of forms (tablet, injection, rectal suppositories, and oral solution). It has become a highly abused drug because of its euphoric effects. Clinical effects of this drug are quite similar to those of morphine at similar doses.

Symptoms

Chronic use may result in both physical and psychological addiction, but an overdose—even in those who have been chronic abusers—may cause breathing problems and death. Acute overdose causes depression of the central nervous system, convulsions, shock, cardiopulmonary arrest, low body temperature, pneumonia, low blood pressure, and slow heart rate.

Treatment

Induced vomiting is not recommended; however, gastric lavage may be performed even several hours after ingestion, followed by the administration of activated charcoal and a saline cathartic. Seizures may be controlled with intravenous diazepam. Naloxone may be administered.

See also MORPHINE; NARCOTICS.

hypochlorite See ALKALINE CORROSIVES.

ibuprofen (Trade names: Motrin, Nuprin, Motrin IB, etc.)   See NONSTEROIDAL ANTI-INFLAMMATORY DRUGS.

indane derivatives   These insecticides are chemicals that dissolve readily in fat and include aldrin, dieldrin, endrin, kepone, chlordane, and heptachlor, although chlordane, heptachlor, aldrin, and dieldrin have all been banned. Of these, aldrin is the most toxic; recent cancer studies in rodents have suggested that heptachlor (contained in chlordane) is a carcinogen. Food and Drug Administration studies suggest that 70 percent of all meat, fish, dairy products, and poultry in the United States contain residues of these pesticides.

Symptoms

After ingestion or skin contamination, acute poisoning causes excitability, tremors, restlessness, and convulsions. In animals, lower doses are associated with liver problems; humans with liver disease may be more sensitive to indane exposure.

Treatment

Gastric lavage followed by saline cathartics. Avoid all fats and oils (including milk), since they increase the rate of absorption. Administer phenobarbital sodium for tremors and barbiturates for convulsions, and provide oxygen if necessary. If the skin has been contaminated, wash with soap and water immediately to head off skin problems and systemic absorption. Remove contaminated clothing.

See also ALDRIN; CHLORDANE; DIELDRIN; ENDRIN; INSECTICIDES.

Indian tobacco *(Lobelia inflata)* **[Other names: asthma weed, bladderpod, eyebright, lobelia.]**   This deadly poisonous plant with its attractive red, white, and blue flowers is found in waste areas, along roadsides and in woodland throughout eastern North America, westward to Nebraska and Arkansas. Used homeopathically to treat laryngitis and asthma, it was also dried and smoked by Native Americans. It gets its name from the Flemish botanist Matthais de L'Obel.

Indian tobacco is an annual or biennial relative of the bellflowers, with its flowers appearing in July and August as loose spikes and alternate, toothed leaves. Similar in many aspects to nicotine, Indian tobacco has been advertised as a substitute for tobacco and as a weight-reducing aid.

Poisonous part

The entire plant is poisonous and contains alkaloids of lobeline and lobelamine. These toxins act by exciting, and then depressing, the central nervous system. In limited amounts Indian tobacco can open the bronchioles, but in larger amounts it can slow breathing and cause a drop in blood pressure. In addition, leaves, stems, and fruit cause a skin rash.

Symptoms

Quite similar to nicotine poisoning, ingesting Indian tobacco causes symptoms within one hour, including nausea, vomiting, weakness, tremors, convulsions, coma, and death. As little as 50 mg of the dried plant, or 1 ml of tincture of Indian tobacco, can cause these reactions.

Treatment

Gastric lavage, artificial respiration, and the administration of atropine and Valium.

See also NICOTINE.

indomethacin (Indocin)   See NONSTEROIDAL ANTI-INFLAMMATORY DRUGS.

inky cap *(Coprinus)*   The inky cap is the common name for the 100 different types of mushroom species of the genus *Coprinus*, which get their name from the fact that after the mushrooms discharge their spores, the cap disintegrates into an inklike liquid that has been used for writing. The mushrooms are found growing on dung or buried wood, and the caps of *C. atramentarius* and *C. comatus* (shaggy mane or shaggy cap) are edible if picked young, before the gills turn black.

Symptoms

While these mushrooms are edible, the coprine in the mushrooms is similar to disulfiram (Antabuse) and interferes with the metabolism of ethanol, causing intoxication when alcohol is drunk within 72 hours of eating the mushroom. The alcohol is believed to increase the solubility and absorption of the poison and causes giddiness, nausea, vomiting, sweating, breathing problems, and even tachycardia. Many victims recover within a few hours, but eating a large amount of mushrooms with alcohol can result in low blood pressure and cardiovascular collapse. The reaction persists for several hours.

Treatment

Supportive, including the administration of intravenous fluids. There is no antidote, and once they appear, the symptoms usually fade within several hours.

See also ANTABUSE; COPRINE; MUSHROOM POISONING; MUSHROOM TOXINS.

inocybe mushroom   These members of the cort family range in toxicity from mild to fairly poisonous, but none is as toxic as the *Amanita* genus of mushrooms. The most dangerous are the *Inocybe napipes* and *I. fastigiata*. They are found in pine forests throughout the United States, with gray-brown spores and small, brown caps.

Poisonous part

These mushrooms contain the parasympathetic stimulant muscarine, which is not affected by cooking and affects the autonomic nervous system and the liver.

Symptoms

Ingesting small concentrations of muscarine is associated with sweating and sometimes abdominal pain; other symptoms develop rapidly and include salivation, cyanosis, weak muscles, twitching, weak pulse, delirium, hallucinations, and convulsions, but rarely death. Heart attacks occur in only 4 percent of cases, since treatment is generally started in time to prevent this. Intoxication usually subsides within two hours.

Treatment

Induce vomiting or perform gastric lavage, since it is possible to get rid of the poison this way and recover quickly. Atropine is the antidote for muscarine poisoning and may be given to those who experience severe discomfort or anxiety.

See also AMANITA MUSHROOMS; CORTINARIUS MUSHROOMS; MUSCARINE; MUSHROOM POISONING; MUSHROOM TOXINS.

inorganic chemical insecticides   One of four major groups of insecticides, the inorganic chemical insecticides include arsenic compounds, fluorides, thallium, selenium, metaldehyde, mercury, phosphorus, sodium borate, hydrocyanic acid (cyanide), pyrethroid, and antimony.

See also ANTIMONY; ARSENIC; CYANIDE; INSECTICIDES; MERCURY; METALDEHYDE; PHOSPHORUS; SELENIUM; THALLIUM.

insecticides   There are many wide-spectrum or all-purpose products to kill insects, and in the past most were synthetic chemical compounds created in laboratories to mimic nature. These products were convenient and effective; however, gardeners came to recognize that such panaceas carry certain penalties—they poisoned more than the insects they were designed to attack.

Today, insecticides fall into two groups: those that coat the outside of a plant, and those that are absorbed by the roots, stems, or leaves into the plant itself. There are six major types: minerals, such as kerosene or borax; botanicals or natural organic compounds (nicotine, pyrethrin, and orotenone); chlorinated hydrocarbons (DDT, lindane, chlordane); organophosphates (malathion and diazinon); carbamates (carbaryl and propoxur); fumigants (such as naphthalene) and benzene (mothballs, etc.).

Newer insecticides include insect-growth regulators and natural predators (such as beetle-eating wasps, or insect-killing bacteria).

While all insecticides are toxic, most fatal poisonings occur only when large quantities are accidentally or intentionally ingested or inhaled.

See also BENZENE; BOTANIC INSECTICIDES; CARBAMATE; CHLORDANE; CHLORINATED HYDROCARBON PESTICIDES; DDT; LINDANE; MALATHION; NAPHTHALENE; ORGANOPHOSPHATE INSECTICIDES; PHOSPHATE ESTERS; PHOSPHORUS.

insect repellents   Substances that, when applied or sprayed on the skin, repel mosquitoes, gnats, and other insects. Because these products are designed for human use, they are generally considered nontoxic, although they are not recommended for use on small children. While poisoning from insect repellents is rare, there have been a few cases of toxicity with DEET (diethyltoluamide).

insulin   Insulin is a hormone produced by the pancreas. Supplements of insulin have been used to treat diabetes mellitus since 1922; today, they are used in all cases of insulin-dependent diabetes mellitus, and sometimes for noninsulin-dependent diabetes when oral hypoglycemic drugs don't work. These supplements are produced from pig or ox pancreas and by genetic engineering; there are a variety of short-, medium-, and long-acting insulins available. Insulin may either be injected by the patient before meals or introduced with an insulin pump to deliver the hormone over a 24-hour period. Oral doses of insulin are not absorbed and are not toxic.

Symptoms

An overdose can cause hypoglycemia (low sugar level) with dizziness, sweating, irritability, and weakness; severe hypoglycemia coma and permanent brain damage have occurred following injections of 800 to 3,200 units of insulin.

Treatment

Administer concentrated glucose as soon as possible after drawing blood samples; treat symptoms.

iodine   This element is one of the oldest antiseptics used in medicine, found most often in compound form as an antiseptic and cough remedy. Discovered in 1811, tincture of iodine was first used in 1839 by a French surgeon and put to work again on the battlefields of the American Civil War. It remains a popular choice for home medicine cabinets today as an inexpensive skin antiseptic. It is also used in contrast dyes for X-rays and fluoroscopy, and in making dyes, photo film, water treatment and medicinal soap.

The brownish element is not soluble in water but dissolves readily in alcohol; it is available in solid and tincture preparations. While earning a deadly reputation as a serious poison, iodine does not often cause toxic poisonings in the amounts normally found in the household. Iodoform, iodochlorhydroxyquin and sodium and potassium iodides are all powders or crystals with similar solubility.

Symptoms

Oral ingestion of iodine produces toxic symptoms similar to those of acid corrosives; absorbed through the skin, it is toxic because of its ability to be well absorbed through the skin of burn patients or neonates. Iodine is a central nervous system depressant and also interferes with cellular activity. Following ingestion, symptoms include vomiting, diarrhea, abdominal pain, thirst, shock, fever, delirium, stupor, and death. A fatal dose of iodine and iodoform is about 2 grams. However, food in the stomach inactivates iodine by converting it to harmless iodide. Fatalities from iodochlorhydroxyquin and iodide salts are rare. Accidental ingestion of the tincture is rarely fatal, since it is not rapidly absorbed.

When iodine is applied to the skin, it can cause hypersensitivity in some people, including a fever and generalized skin reaction. Because of this sensitivity in some individuals, iodophors have generally replaced the use of iodine tinctures; one of the most widely used iodophors is a complex of povidone and iodine (Betadine). These iodo-phors are compounds of iodine linked to a carrier agent.

Treatment

After acute ingestion, give milk immediately followed by a starch solution (such as 15 milligrams of cornstarch or flour to 500 milliliters of water). Vomiting is not advisable if there is any esophageal injury, and milk should be repeatedly given every 15 minutes to ease stomach irritation. Antidote is sodium thiosulfate, which reduces iodine to iodide. In the event of an allergic reaction, administer epinephrine and intravenous hydrocortisone.

ipecac syrup A substance that makes people vomit (an emetic), ipecac syrup (also called ipecacuanha) comes from the dried roots of a poisonous shrub *(Cephaelis ipecacuanha)* found in Europe and Central and South America. The commercially available syrup is used in the treatment of accidental poisoning to remove the toxic substance from the stomach before it is absorbed into the blood.

It is a thick, amber liquid that will stay fresh for several years in a tightly closed container stored at room temperature. It is available over the counter in syrup form but should be kept out of the hands of youngsters, as ipecac is poisonous.

Ipecac syrup should never be given to a suspected poisoning victim unless instructed to do so by a health care specialist. Not all poisons require the removal of the poison, and sometimes vomiting can be dangerous—especially if the toxic substance is caustic or petroleum based. Syrup of ipecac should not be given to anyone not fully conscious or to a child under age one without careful supervision. While ipecac syrup saves lives, it is itself poisonous and should never be given in more than two doses. More may be toxic.

In a recent study (the first ever done in an emergency room on pediatric poisonings), researchers at Children's Hospital of Buffalo tested whether giving ipecac in addition to charcoal would help remove poison from the body even better. In that study, 32 of 70 children less than six years old at the hospital took syrup of ipecac before taking activated charcoal; the rest of the group received charcoal alone. The children treated with both took an average of 39 minutes *longer* to recover than the group treated with charcoal alone. Doctors had to wait from 30 minutes to two hours until the ipecac's work was done and the children stopped vomiting so they could administer the charcoal. Even then, the queasy feeling caused by the ipecac made it more difficult for the children to keep from vomiting the gritty charcoal solution, while most of the children who took the charcoal alone had no problems.

Because time is so important in the treatment of poisoning cases, many scientists now believe that activated charcoal alone may be the better emergency room treatment. Ipecac only empties the stomach of its toxic contents, but by the time a child sees a physician in the emergency room, it has usually been at least an hour since the poison was ingested and chances are the poison has already traveled into the small intestine.

Ipecac taken within five minutes of ingestion will remove about 50 or 60 percent of the poison, which can reduce a substance like aspirin to a safe level. But after an hour, only 20 percent of the poison will come back up. At that point, activated charcoal does a better job, since it can pass through the intestine, bind with the poison, and move it out of the body through the stool.

Charcoal, then, may well replace ipecac in hospitals. At home, however, charcoal is more difficult to administer because children don't like the tasteless, gritty solution. According to Allan Kornberg, M.D., head of the emergency medicine department at the Children's Hospital of Buffalo and author of the above study, ipecac should continue to be used at home for emergencies—but always with the guidance of a poison control center.

While the correct dosage should be prescribed by a physician or poison control center, a normal dose for a person over age one is two tablespoons followed by at least two to three glasses of water, *not milk.* If the victim hasn't vomited within 20 minutes, the dose may be repeated. If the victim doesn't vomit after the second dose, call the poison control center for further instructions. If possible, the victim should vomit into a container so the material can be identified by medical experts at the hospital. Vomiting is effective only if it occurs within four hours of ingestion of a solid substance, or within two hours after ingestion of a liquid.

See also CHARCOAL, ACTIVATED; IPECACUANHA.

ipecacuanha *(Cephaelis ipecacuanha)* Ipecacuanha is a poisonous plant found throughout Europe and South and Central America and is the plant source for ipecac syrup, which is used, ironically, as an emetic to rid the stomach of poisons. (When used incorrectly, however, this syrup can be fatal.) *The fluid extract from the plant is 14 times more toxic than the commercially available ipecac syrup and should never be used as a substitute.*

Poisonous part

The berries and juice are most toxic and contain the alkaloid emetine, which weakens the heart.

Symptoms

Vomiting occurs immediately after ingestion but may not be fatal until 24 hours to a week later. Recovery can take up to a year.

Treatment

Gastric lavage, morphine, and bed rest.

See also IPECAC SYRUP.

iron in drugs and supplements Dietary supplements that contain iron (ferrous sulfate, ferrous gluconate, ferrous fumarate) are common—but overlooked—potential poisons in children. An acute overdose of iron can damage the stomach and small intestine, affect blood circulation and damage the liver and other organs, causing shock and even death. Young children have been seriously injured by swallowing doses of 200–400 mg of iron, equivalent to 14 to 27 children's vitamin-and-mineral supplements with iron or four to seven tablets of a typical adult iron supplement. More than 2,000 people are poisoned each year with iron, and a large number of these poisonings are fatal; mortality may be as great as 50 percent. The Food and Drug Administration ruled in 1997 that packages of all preparations that contain iron (such as iron supplements and vitamins) must now display a warning that accidental overdose of iron-containing products is a leading cause of fatal poisoning in children under the age of six. In addition, products containing 30 mg or more iron per unit must be packaged as individual doses that will limit the number of pills or capsules a small child could swallow.

Despite child-resistant packaging, accidental overdose of iron remains a common cause of poisoning in children under six. According to the U.S. Consumer Product Safety Commission, pediatric iron-related injuries increased 150 percent in 1986, from an annual average of 1,200 from 1980 through 1985 to 3,000 from 1986 through 1996. The number of accidental overdoses and deaths declined dramatically, however, after the U.S. Food and Drug Administration (FDA) proclaimed a regulation for unit-dose packaging of iron supplements in 1997. In a study that compared the 10 years prior to the regulation with the five years after its implementation, the average number of iron ingestion calls to Poison Control Centers regarding children younger than six years decreased from 2.99 per 1,000 to 1.91 per 1,000, and the number of deaths decreased from 29 to one.

Iron is used by the body to produce the red blood cells that transport oxygen, and it helps the cells in the muscles and other parts of the body turn oxygen into energy. But recent research by a team of Finnish researchers links excess iron stored in the body to heart disease. Men who ate iron-rich food (such as red meat) faced a higher likelihood of heart attack. The findings could help force public health experts to rethink dietary recommendations for iron ingestion, since even normal levels of stored iron may prove damaging. Over-the-counter vitamin supplements often contain iron, as do some enriched foods such as cereals.

Up until the late 1800s, iron therapy was used to treat anemia, but it later fell out of favor. Recently, however, ferrous sulfate has been widely prescribed to treat iron deficiency anemia, and its popularity has greatly increased the risk of poisoning. There are about 120 iron products currently marketed in the United States.

The exact mechanism behind iron poisoning is not known, nor is it understood how death results—whether from shock, from systemic effects due to the passage of large amounts of iron into the blood or from the metabolic effects of absorbed iron, which cause respiratory collapse.

Symptoms

Within 30 minutes of overdose, the first symptoms appear: lethargy, vomiting, fast and weak pulse, low blood pressure, shock, pallor, cyanosis, acidosis, clotting problems, and coma. Then, symptoms may disappear, and the victim may seemingly begin to improve. One or two days later, the victim goes into shock, with pulmonary edema, vasomotor collapse, coma, and death within 12 to 48 hours.

Treatment

Control shock; perform gastric lavage with sodium bicarbonate and administer a chelating agent. Peritoneal dialysis or hemodialysis, or early exchange transfusion, may be needed. Give supportive and symptomatic therapy as required, including multiple vitamins and antibiotics.

See also VITAMINS.

irritant oils   Some glycosidal oils in high concentrations can irritate the digestive tract. While in small quantities they are harmless (such as the oils in plants of the mustard family, horseradish, and radishes), in large amounts they are more upsetting and cause the irritations found with some plants of the buttercup family and anemone species.

See also VOLATILE OILS.

isopropanol   See ISOPROPYL ALCOHOL.

isopropyl alcohol   Widely used as a solvent, antiseptic, and disinfectant, isopropyl alcohol (also known as isopropanol) is found in products such as shaving lotions and window cleaner and is twice as toxic as its relative ethyl alcohol. It is also found in the home as a 70 percent solution (rubbing alcohol), which is commonly drunk by alcoholics as a substitute for liquor. But unlike other common alcohol substitutes (methanol and ethylene glycol), isopropyl alcohol is not metabolized to highly toxic organic acids.

While the effects of isopropyl poisoning resemble drunkenness, they may last up to four times longer than those induced by alcoholic drinks. Rubbing alcohol can be swallowed, inhaled (as a vapor), or absorbed. In fact, alcohol sponge baths were once prescribed as a way to reduce fever, until it was discovered that the alcohol sometimes produced a nonfatal coma.

Isopropyl alcohol is a potent central nervous system depressant, and ingestion or inhalation of it can cause coma and respiratory arrest. It is metabolized to acetone, which may contribute to and prolong the central nervous system depression.

Symptoms

Within 10 to 30 minutes after ingestion (depending on how much food is in the stomach), overdose symptoms appear: nausea, vomiting, stomach pain, depressed respiration, vomiting blood, excessive sweating, hemorrhage in the trachea and bronchial tubes, pneumonia, swelling, and coma.

Treatment

There is no specific antidote. Ethanol is not given as an antidote, and if the victim has only drunk a few swallows or more than 30 minutes has passed, there is no point to emptying the stomach, since the alcohol is rapidly absorbed after ingestion.

However, for large ingestions, perform gastric lavage (do NOT induce vomiting) and administer activated charcoal and a cathartic, although charcoal will not absorb isopropyl alcohol very well. Hemodialysis removes isopropyl alcohol and acetone, but it is usually not necessary because the majority of victims can be managed with supportive care alone. Dialysis is indicated when levels are very high, or if low blood pressure does not respond to fluids.

See also ETHANOL; ETHYL ALCOHOL; METHANOL.

isoproterenol   This drug, similar to catecholamines, is useful in the treatment of excessively slow heartbeat following an overdose of beta blockers.

See also BETA ADRENERGIC BLOCKERS.

ivy (Hedera)   Of the five species in the genus *Hedera, H. helix* (English ivy) is the most common.

This form is poisonous if eaten because of the presence of saponins; in small amounts it can cause stomach upset and a tingling sensation around the mouth, but large amounts can lead to labored breathing, convulsions, and coma. While no fatal cases have been reported in the United States, European children have been poisoned with this plant.

English ivy is a climbing evergreen plant with three- or five-lobed leaves and a woody stem and prefers shade and damp, moist ground. Occasionally, it produces black berries. There are more than 200 cultivars, and ivy has been a known toxicant since early Greek times.

Poisonous part

All parts of the ivy plant contain the saponin hederin and are poisonous if eaten.

Symptoms

Burning sensation in the throat, nausea, vomiting, diarrhea, excitement, difficulty in breathing, abdominal pain, excess salivation, and skin irritation; rarely, it causes coma.

Treatment

Traditional treatment of gastroenteritis and fluid replacement, especially in young children.

See also SAPONIN.

jack-o'-lantern fungus *(Clitocybe illudens)* This cousin of the *Inocybe* mushroom also contains muscarine and induces sweating. An orange fungus found growing on wood, it can induce severe vomiting but is not fatal.

Symptoms

This fungus can cause gastrointestinal upset. Ingestions of small amounts of the parasympathetic stimulant muscarine contained in these mushrooms also cause vomiting and blurred vision.

Treatment

Intoxication usually subsides after two hours; when the victim experiences severe discomfort or anxiety, atropine may be given. Other treatment is symptomatic.

See also INOCYBE MUSHROOM; MUSHROOM POISONING; MUSHROOM TOXINS.

jellyfish Although the term is used to refer to any marine member of a group of invertebrates, the true jellyfish family includes about 200 species, all of which are disk-shaped animals found drifting along the shoreline. Jellyfish, together with corals, sea anemones, and Portuguese men-of-war all belong to the group of marine animals called coelenterates, which have four, eight, or more dangling tentacles with capsules that sting when touched.

Most common in tropical waters, jellyfish float on the surface of the water, trailing tentacles that can penetrate human skin and inject venom. Most live for only a few weeks, but some live as long as a year, and the deep-sea species may live longer. Jellyfish are by far the most common of the coelenterates and cause a significant number of injuries in the United States coastal areas.

Produced in a wide variety of sizes, colors, and shapes, jellyfish often are almost transparent with brilliant tentacles, ranging from a few millimeters to more than two meters across the top. Because some varieties have such long tentacles, it is possible to be stung without ever seeing the top of the jellyfish floating on the surface. Jellyfish are also dangerous after storms have broken them up and sprinkled them across the sandy beaches, where they can still sting—even when dry.

One of the most poisonous of the jellyfish is the sea wasp *(Chironex fleckeri)* which swims from Queensland north to the central Atlantic coast of the United States; a moderate sting from a sea wasp can cause death within a few minutes. While most stings from poisonous fish and jellyfish may not cause much harm, some jellyfish and Portuguese men-of-war can inflict severe stings, and the victim may panic and drown. The lion's mane jellyfish *(Cyanea capillata)* is the giant of all jellyfish, with a sac that reportedly measures 8 feet or more across. Its tangle of poisonous tentacles arranged in groups of eight (each group with 150 tentacles) may reach over 100 feet long. The lion's mane ranges in the Atlantic and Pacific Oceans, and although it is not believed to be fatal to humans, its sting is very painful. The most common jellyfish is the moon jellyfish *(Aurelia aurita)*, which is only slightly venomous and is found in all warm and temperate waters.

Symptoms

Stings from a jellyfish cause severe burning pain and a red welt—or a row of lesions—at the site of the sting. Some victims also suffer from headache, nausea, vomiting, muscle cramps, diarrhea, convulsions, and breathing problems. In the water, the initial shock of the sting may cause a swimmer to jerk away, which stimulates the tentacles to release more poison. On shore, more poison is released if the victim tries to rip off the sticky threads. On those who have been stung by jellyfish but survive, the wounds from the jellyfish stings become red blisters that can leave permanent scars. One or two weeks after the sting, the victim may experience a recurrence of the lesions at the site, which can be treated with antihistamines.

In the United States, it is not particularly important to identify the type of coelenterate, but in Australia (where many lethal varieties exist) it is crucial.

Treatment

Alcohol, ammonia, or vinegar and salt water *(do not use freshwater)* poured over the site of the sting will deactivate the tentacles, which should then be scraped off with a towel or with sand held by a bath towel—*not the hand.* Pull off—do not rub—the tentacles. The tentacles will continue to discharge their stinging cells (nematocysts) as long as they remain on the skin. Watch carefully for signs of shock or breathing problems.

Baking soda in a paste with water should be applied to the sting to relieve pain; after an hour, moisten again and scrape off the baking soda with an object to remove any remaining nematocysts. Calamine lotion also will help ease the burning sensation, and painkillers may help with the stinging pain. (Other local remedies for pain include meat tenderizer, sugar, ammonia, and lemon juice.)

Jellyfish often cause allergic reactions, which can be eased by the administration of Benadryl or a steroid. A severe reaction to the sting requires hospitalization and perhaps CPR. Antivenin, effective against more dangerous species, may be available but must be administered immediately together with a tourniquet. Another type of jellyfish, the Portuguese man-of-war, is rarely fatal but causes hives, numbness, and severe chest, abdominal, and extremity pain. If given early, the calcium blocker verapamil may be effective.

See also PORTUGUESE MAN-OF-WAR.

Jerusalem cherry *(Solanum pseudocapsicum)*   One of the nightshade family, this popular houseplant has luscious orange or red berries that are deadly poison. It is a decorative pot plant and has escaped from cultivation in Hawaii and the Gulf coast states.

Poisonous part

Human poisoning is usually attributed to immature fruit, which contains the toxin solanine glycoalkaloid, the poison of the true nightshades.

Symptoms

While there is little danger of fatal poisoning in adults, children may ingest a fatal amount of this plant. Symptoms appear several hours after ingestion and include gastric irritation, scratchy throat, fever, and diarrhea (solanine poisoning is often confused with bacterial gastroenteritis).

Treatment

Provide the same general supportive care that would be given in gastroenteritis cases; fluid replacement may be required.

See also NIGHTSHADE, DEADLY.

jessamine, yellow *(Gelsemium sempervirens)*   Also known as Carolina jessamine, this plant is a highly toxic member of the olive family which has about 300 tropical and subtropical species of fragrant, flowering shrubs. The plants are found in woodlands and are native to all continents except North America. Still, it is found today from eastern Virginia to Tennessee, and Arkansas south to Florida and west to Texas; it is also grown in parts of California.

A perennial evergreen with lance-shaped leaves and fragrant, bright yellow flower clusters, the plant has a small fruit capsule with winged seeds. It is not a member of the jasmine species *(Jasminum),* which causes only a mild skin rash.

Poisonous part

All parts of this plant contain the poisons gelsemine, gelsemicine and other related alkaloids, which cause strychninelike effects. There are cases of children who were poisoned after sucking on the flowers; honey made from the nectar of this plant has been implicated in three deaths.

Symptoms

At high doses, poisoning can be fatal in 10 minutes, but it may take several hours in lower doses. Symptoms include frontal headache, dizziness, drooping eyelids, sweating, weakness, convulsions, anxiety, difficulty in breathing, depression, and death through respiratory failure.

Treatment

Immediate gastric lavage with instillation of a slurry of activated charcoal, intravenous fluids, and respiratory support.

See also GELSEMINE.

jimsonweed (Datura stramonium) [Other names: apple of Peru, devil's trumpet, Jamestown weed, mad apple, stinkweed, thornapple.] Responsible for more poisonings than any other plant, jimsonweed is an extremely deadly member of the potato family. Originally called "Jamestown weed," it got its name in 1666 following a mass poisoning in the town when starving soldiers ate the berries of the plant. Jimsonweed is found throughout much of the Northern Hemisphere in roadside and waste places but never in mountains or woods.

An annual, jimsonweed grows to about six feet with ovate, unevenly toothed, strong-scented leaves; large, white or violet trumpet-shaped flowers; and a large, spiny fruit (often called a thornapple). Seeds are small and dark brown or black when ripe and yield what is called "datura." Jimsonweed is the source for the alkaloidal drug hyoscyamine. There are about 15 species of *Datura*, and while all are poisonous, their fragrance can be sweet or unpleasant depending on the season.

Poisonous part

All parts of this plant are poisonous and harbor belladonna alkaloids (the poisons hyoscyamine, hyoscine, and atropine). The juices, seeds, and wilted leaves are especially deadly. Four to five grams of crude leaf or seed will be a fatal dose for a child. Poisonings have occurred from sucking nectar from the flower tube or eating fruits containing the poisonous seeds.

Symptoms

Within several hours after ingestion, the first symptoms appear: excessive thirst and dry mouth, dilated pupils, dry, hot and flushed skin, headache, vertigo, weak pulse, visual difficulty, fever, hallucinations, disorientation, urinary retention, decreased bowel activity, high blood pressure, delirium, convulsions, coma, and death. Handling the leaves and rubbing the eyes can dilate the pupils.

Treatment

Sedatives are effective for convulsions, and a purgative may also be used. If intoxication is severe, slow intravenous administration of physostigmine is usually advised until symptoms diminish.

kepone   See MIREX.

kerosene   See PETROLEUM DISTILLATES.

ketamine   "Special K," or ketamine hydrochloride, is a powerful hallucinogen that was developed for veterinary use but which has become a drug of abuse. Ketamine causes powerful hallucinations that are accompanied by visual distortions and a lost sense of time, identity, and sense. The high can last from 30 minutes to two hours, but the drug can still affect the body up to 24 hours later. It is available as a powder that is usually snorted, but it can be sprinkled on marijuana or tobacco and smoked. Some users combine it with other drugs, including heroin, cocaine, or ecstasy.

Liquid ketamine was developed in the early 1960s, and it was used as an anesthetic during the Vietnam War. The powdered version of the drug became popular as a recreational drug in the 1970s, and it has stayed on the drug scene ever since. Because it is odorless and tasteless, it can be added to beverages without being detected, and so it is sometimes used as a date rape drug. It is similar molecularly to phencyclidine (PCP) and thus produces similar effects. Because ketamine is an anesthetic, users do not feel pain, and this feature can lead users to inadvertently injure themselves.

Symptoms

Beyond the acute effects of the drug, use can result in serious physical and mental problems including delirium, amnesia, impaired motor function, depression, high blood pressure, muscle rigidity, aggressive/violent behavior, slurred speech, numbness, and potentially fatal respiratory disturbances.

Low doses (25–100 mg) produce psychedelic effects rapidly; larger doses can produce vomiting and convulsions. One gram can cause death. Some people experience flashbacks up to one year after use.

Treatment

Symptomatic; there is no antidote.

kokoi frog   One of the "arrow poison" frogs, this frog has a venom in its skin that has been used for centuries as an arrow poison by the Cholo Indians of Colombia. Ten times more deadly than the toxin found in the Japanese pufferfish, it is the most active venom known. The molecular structure of the toxin found in the kokoi frog is related to that of steroid hormones secreted by the adrenal gland.

Symptoms

The toxin in the kokoi frog blocks the transmission of nerve impulses to the musculoskeletal system, causing death within minutes.

Treatment

There is no known antidote.

See also ARROW POISON FROGS.

krait, blue (Bunguras coeruleus)   This is one of the nonhooded members of the cobra family; it has powerful venom but seldom bites humans. Still, of those who *are* bitten, nearly half die if untreated. The krait is generally passive and has shiny scales and bands of yellow and black, or white and black.

Similar to the blue krait is the banded krait, or pama *(B. fasciatus)*, also a member of the cobra family. This variety is almost harmless, although larger than its blue krait cousin. While the venom is lethal, bites are very rarely reported.

The kraits are fairly small and are mainly nocturnal; when disturbed, they tend to roll up into a loose ball and only bite under great provocation. They are found throughout most of southern Asia and range from 4 to 7 feet long with light and dark bands and short fangs.

Symptoms

The venom of snakes in the cobra family contains a neurotoxin chemically different from that of other snakes. While there is little local reaction, within 15 to 30 minutes more generalized symptoms appear: pain, swelling, a drop in blood pressure and confusion followed by death if the poison spreads to the respiratory muscles. The venom from this snake family is twice as toxic as strychnine and nearly five times more toxic than that of a black widow spider.

Treatment

Immediate administration of specific antivenin—only the specific antiserum for the type of cobra involved should be used. Many types of antivenins are available for the krait bite in southern Asia; other antivenins are produced in Bangkok for both the blue krait and the pama.

See also ANTIVENIN; COBRA; SNAKES, POISONOUS.

labetalol This drug is used in the treatment of high blood pressure and racing heartbeat associated with stimulant drug overdose (such as cocaine or amphetamines).

laudanoisine See MORPHINE.

laudanum A solution of opium once used as a sedative and painkiller and to treat diarrhea. It was created in the 16th century by the Swiss physician Paracelsus, and it was a popular medication during Victorian times, when physicians would prescribe it for women suffering from "the vapors." Elizabeth Barrett Browning, Charles Baudelaire, Theophile Gautier, Alexandre Dumas, Edgar Allan Poe, and Samuel Taylor Coleridge were all users of laudanum; in fact, Coleridge wrote his poem "Kubla Khan" while in an opium reverie. Unfortunately, the pleasurable effects that laudanum brought came at a cost: long, dry spells in their creativity and occasional loss of ambition. In order to achieve the euphoric effects, they had to risk overdose and addiction.

See also HEROIN; MORPHINE; NARCOTICS; OPIUM.

laughing gas See NITROUS OXIDE.

laurel, mountain *(Kalmia latifolia)* **[Other names: Alpine laurel, calfkill, calico bush, hook heller, ivy bush, lambkill, mountain ivy, narrow-leaved laurel, pale laurel, poison laurel, sheep laurel, spoonwood, swamp laurel.]** Like its cousin the rhododendron, the evergreen mountain laurel is a deadly narcotic poison found in moist areas and rocky hills throughout North America. Ancient Greek legends reported that these two plants poisoned Xenophon's army when they consumed honey made from the flowers' nectar. Closer to home, the Delaware Indians used wild laurel for suicide.

The ornamental bush grows to heights from four to eight feet, with three-inch-long leaves and white, pink, or purple flowers appearing in June and July. The leaves may also be poisonous to animals, which in turn can poison any other human or animal who eats the meat. Native to North America, the plant is not a true laurel but a member of the heath family.

K. latifolia grows in the northeastern United States but not in Canada; *K. angustifolia* grows in eastern North America from Ontario to Labrador east to Nova Scotia, and south to Michigan, Virginia, and Georgia; *K. microphylla* is found from Alaska to central California.

Poisonous part

All parts of the plant are poisonous, especially the leaves and nectar (in honey), and contain carbohydrate andromedotoxin, the same poison as rhododendron. A tea made from two ounces of the leaves of the laurel has caused poisoning.

Symptoms

Usually beginning within six hours, they include severe gastrointestinal distress, watery eyes and mouth, respiratory problems, and bradycardia followed by depression, convulsions, paralysis, coma, and death. Death from mountain laurel poisoning may occur anywhere from several hours to days after ingestion. Children can be poisoned by eating leaves.

Treatment

Gastric lavage, fluid replacement, and respiratory support; atropine for bradycardia and ephedrine for hypotension that does not respond to fluid replacement.

See also RHODODENDRON.

laxatives A group of drugs used to treat constipation. There are a variety of types of laxatives, each causing different symptoms in overdoses. They include bulk forming, stimulant, lubricant, and saline. In addition, chronic overuse can produce bowel function dependency.

Symptoms

Stimulant laxatives may cause abdominal cramps and flatulence; prolonged use of saline laxatives is likely to cause a chemical imbalance in the blood. Lubricant laxatives may coat the intestine and prevent vitamin absorption. Resulting diarrhea from laxative overdose causes fluid and electrolyte imbalance.

Treatment

Since systemic absorption is not really a problem, laxative overdose is simply treated by reestablishing the fluid and electrolyte imbalance caused by diarrhea. In cases where the patient is at risk for dehydration, perform gastric lavage or induce vomiting followed by the administration of activated charcoal.

lead poisoning Lead poisoning in adults is rare, but unfortunately it is one of the most common and preventable childhood health problems today. It can be a problem for those who lick or eat flakes of old paint containing lead. Lead can also contaminate water flowing through old lead pipes, slowly poisoning those who drink it. Lead poisoning causes the most damage to the brain, nerves, red blood cells, and digestive system and is considered to be a cumulative poison, since it remains in the bones for as long as 32 years and in the kidneys for seven. Several recent studies have also shown that high levels of lead in the blood can hinder a child's growth, and this may occur early in the chemical chain of events regulating bone growth—perhaps in the brain.

Symptoms

Lead is excreted very slowly from the body, so it builds up in tissues and bones and may not even produce detectable physical effects, although it can still cause mental impairment. If they do appear, early symptoms include listlessness, irritability, loss of appetite and weight, constipation, and a bluish line in the gums followed by clumsiness, vomiting, stomach cramps, and a general "wasting." Acute poisoning symptoms include a metallic taste in the mouth, abdominal pain, vomiting, diarrhea, collapse, and coma. Large amounts directly affect the nervous system and cause headache, convulsions, coma, and, sometimes, death.

Treatment

Individuals with suspected lead poisoning should be given a simple blood test, which can determine the level of lead in the blood. A person with enough absorbed lead in the body to show symptoms will probably require hospitalization. Treatment usually includes the administration of medicines (called chelating agents) to help the body rid itself of lead. In mild cases, the chelating agent penicillamine may be used alone; otherwise, it may be used in combination with edetate calcium disodium and dimercaprol. In acute cases, perform gastric lavage.

Prevention

There are many steps you can take to ensure lead is not a problem for you and your family.

- To temporarily reduce lead paint and dust, clean floors, windowsills, and window wells at least twice a week with a trisodium phosphate detergent available at hardware stores. Sponges used for this purpose should not be used for anything else.
- Move cribs and playpens away from chipped or peeling paint, mantels, windowsills, and doors. Replace or strip baby furniture that may be decorated with lead paint.
- Wash the child's hands, face, bottle nipples, and toys often
- Children and pregnant women should not be in the area while lead paint is being removed.

LEAD POISONING GUIDE
Recommendations by the U.S. Centers for Disease Control and Prevention.

Lead levels	Complications	Treatment
0–9 mcg/dl*	None	Annual checks until age six
10–14 mcg/dl	Borderline (possible test inaccuracy); risk for mild developmental delays even without symptoms	Nutrition; housecleaning changes will bring level down
15–19 mcg/dl	Risk for IQ decrease; no symptoms usually noticed	Test for iron deficiency; nutrition; housekeeping changes will lower level
20–44 mcg/dl	Risk of IQ impairment increases; usually no symptoms	Complete medical evaluation; eliminate lead; drug treatment possible
45–69 mcg/dl	Colic; anemia; learning disabilities	Remove from home until lead is removed; drug treatment
70 mcg/dl	Vomiting; anemia; critical illness	Immediate hospitalization; lead removal

* mcg/dl = micrograms per deciliter of blood

- Avoid imported canned foods; the seams of the cans may be soldered with lead, which can seep into the contents.

- Feed your child plenty of calcium, iron, and protein, with plenty of milk, breads, low-fat foods, and green leafy vegetables (they diminish lead's effects in the body).

- Limit the amount of dirt tracked into the house. Leave your shoes at the door or make sure everyone wipes their shoes on a heavy-duty mat in front of the door before they enter the house.

- If you are pregnant, do not drink out of ceramic mugs.

- Test your water's lead levels: it should not exceed 15 parts per billion.

- Avoid storing acidic food (such as orange juice and tomatoes) in ceramic or crystal containers, which may contain lead glaze.

- Never boil water to eliminate lead; boiling only concentrates lead.

- Allow water to run on cold for a few minutes before using; never cook with hot water from the tap, especially when making baby food, since lead leaches more quickly into hot water.

- If your soil tests high in lead, cover with clean soil and seed or sod.

- Consider a water-treatment device to remove lead from tap water.

lepiota mushrooms *(Lepiota josserandii, L. brunneoincarnata, L. helveola, L. subincarnata)* The poisonous mushroom *L. josserandii* contains the deadly poison amatoxin, and the others in the *Lepiota* genus are assumed to contain amatoxins as well. Amatoxins prevent protein synthesis and cause cell death, sometimes affecting the kidneys as well. These mushrooms are not made less toxic by drying, cooking, or boiling in water.

Symptoms

Initial symptoms are caused by amatoxin on the intestine. After about 12 hours following ingestion, the victim experiences persistent nausea and vomiting, intestinal pain, and watery diarrhea. This is followed by a period of remission of up to five days, followed by liver problems similar to those caused by acute viral hepatitis. Without treatment, liver and kidney damage cause coma and death.

Treatment

Give fluids and monitor electrolytes; maintain urine flow, since amatoxins are partially excreted by the kidneys. Give repeat doses of activated charcoal with water. If the patient was diagnosed promptly, massive doses of penicillin may help prevent liver damage. In more severe cases, liver transplant may be necessary. For most patients, full recovery is unlikely.

See also AMATOXINS; MUSHROOM POISONING; MUSHROOM TOXINS.

Librium   See BENZODIAZEPINES.

lidocaine   A local anesthetic related to cocaine, this is a synthetic version of the coca bush alkaloids. It is used to control possible irregular heartbeat following poisoning by a variety of heart drugs and toxins (such as digoxin, cyclic antidepressants, stimulants, and theophylline). It is also used to relieve pain and irritation caused by sunburn or hemorrhoids, to numb tissues before minor surgery and as a nerve block. It is used topically to relieve pain when inserting needles, and it is given intravenously as an antiarrhythmic agent following a heart attack to reduce the danger of ventricular arrhythmias (irregular heartbeat).

Although lidocaine is used to treat poisoning by other drugs, it is also toxic itself if used excessively.

Symptoms
Immediately upon ingestion, lidocaine causes giddiness followed by dizziness, blue color, low blood pressure, tremors, irregular and weak breathing, collapse, coma, convulsions, and respiratory arrest.

Treatment
Efforts to remove the drug after 30 minutes are useless. The ingested drug must be removed, and absorption from the injection site limited by tourniquet and wet cloths. Give oxygen and artificial respiration until the nervous system depression lifts. If the victim survives for one hour, recovery outlook is good.

See also ANTIDEPRESSANTS; DIGOXIN; THEOPHYLLINE.

lighter fluid   See PETROLEUM DISTILLATES.

lily of the valley *(Convallaria majalis)*   Often mistaken for wild garlic, the beautiful white-flowered plant is deadly—*even the water in which the flowers are kept is toxic.* Found throughout western North America through the Midwest and into Canada and Britain, the plant also occasionally bears orange-red berries. It is a hardy perennial, with hanging, bell-shaped white flowers and smooth, dark green leaves, and spreads by underground roots to form thick beds.

Poisonous part
All parts of this plant are poisonous, especially the leaves. The poison, which is similar to digitalis, is a glycoside called convallatoxin; the plant also contains irritant saponins.

Symptoms
Immediately after ingestion, the following symptoms appear: nausea, rash, headache, and hallucinations. If large amounts are eaten, dizziness and vomiting may occur one or two hours later; slow heartbeat can lead to coma and death from heart failure.

Treatment
Gastric lavage together with cardiac depressants to control cardiac rhythm. Activated charcoal may be given and repeated later, and saline cathartics may also be used.

See also GLYCOSIDE; SAPONIN.

lindane   The common name for cyclohexane hexachloride, this is a synthetic organic insecticide used to control insects resistant to DDT and those that attack cotton. A cancer-causing agent, lindane was formerly used as a general-purpose insecticide against indoor pests. The Environmental Protection Agency canceled the registration of all indoor fumigating devices containing lindane in 1986.

Symptoms
Less serious poisoning incidents will result in nausea, dizziness, headache, tremor, and weakness. Acute cases of ingestion or skin contamination cause vomiting and diarrhea, excitability, loss of

balance, and convulsions. If the insecticide also contains an organic solvent, symptoms may also include breathing problems and cyanosis followed rapidly by circulatory failure. Exposure to the fumes from a thermal insecticide vaporizer can cause eye, ear, nose, or throat irritation in addition to the above symptoms. While symptoms will fade after exposure ends, there have been reports of the development of anemia.

Treatment

Gastric lavage followed by saline cathartics. Avoid all fats and oils (including milk), since they increase the rate of absorption. Administer phenobarbital sodium for tremors and barbiturates for convulsions, and provide oxygen if necessary. If the skin has come in contact with these insecticides, wash with soap and water immediately to head off skin problems and systemic absorption. Remove contaminated clothing.

See also DDT; INSECTICIDES; PESTICIDES; SYNTHETIC ORGANIC INSECTICIDES.

lionfish *(Pterois)* **[Other names: butterfly cod, fire-fish, rock perch, turkeyfish.]** The lionfish includes any of several species of the scorpion fish family often found off the beaches in Barbados, where it hides in coral and stings unwary swimmers. Lionfish are famous for their poisonous fin spines, which can produce a painful sting that is not usually fatal but extremely uncomfortable. The fish have 18 spines along their back, which sometimes break off in the wound, leading to secondary infections and sometimes gangrene. Unaggressive fish, they drift peacefully along the coral reefs in which they live.

Symptoms

Perspiration, rapid heartbeat, vomiting, diarrhea, and intense abdominal pain. The wound site is swollen, inflamed, and painful, with the pain radiating outward.

Treatment

Supportive; local anesthetic can ease pain around the wound site.

See also SCORPION FISH.

listeriosis A rare but potentially fatal illness caused by eating food contaminated by the toxic *Listeria monocytogenes* bacterium. It is one of the most dangerous foodborne illnesses a pregnant woman can contract, causing conditions that lead to miscarriage or illness in newborns. The government estimates that there are about 2,500 cases of listeriosis each year, and 500 deaths. Some studies have suggested that as many as 10 percent of all Americans carry the bacteria in their intestines.

While pregnant women are most at risk, others at high risk include people with a compromised immune system, cancer patients (especially leukemia patients), the elderly, or people with diabetes, cirrhosis of the liver, asthma, or ulcerative colitis.

There have been outbreaks in Mexican-style cheese in California that led to numerous stillbirths and a cluster of cases in Philadelphia. The bacteria may be found in unpasteurized milk, imported soft cheese, hot dogs, lunch meats and spreads, raw vegetables, fermented raw-meat sausage, raw and cooked poultry, raw meats, and raw or smoked fish. One recent study found that 20 percent of hot dogs tested contained the bacterium. When listeria is found in processed products, the contamination probably occurred after processing (rather than due to poor heating or pasteurizing).

Symptoms

Illness occurs within three weeks after consuming tainted products; most healthy people probably won't show any symptoms. If they do appear, symptoms resemble those of the flu, including a persistent fever. Nausea, vomiting, and diarrhea may precede more serious forms of listeriosis or may be the only symptoms. In high-risk individuals, the infection may spread to the nervous system, causing a type of meningitis including intense headache, fever, stiff neck, confusion, loss of balance, or convulsions. Listeria meningitis carries a fatality rate that may reach 70 percent.

Diagnosis

Listeriosis can be diagnosed from a blood test, cerebrospinal fluid, or stool. There is no routine screening test for susceptibility during pregnancy.

Treatment

Antibiotics are most helpful in pregnant women to prevent disease in the fetus. Babies with listeriosis receive the same antibiotics as adults, although a combination of antibiotics may be used until diagnosis is certain. Even with prompt treatment, some infections result in death, especially in those with other serious medical problems.

Complications

Internal abscesses, meningitis, blood poisoning. In pregnant women, the infection can lead to stillbirth or miscarriage.

Prevention

Pregnant or high-risk patients should avoid foods linked to contamination in the past and should practice good food preparation practices and wash all vegetables and salads well.

lithium   Available either as a pill (lithium carbonate) or liquid (lithium citrate), this is the treatment of choice for manic-depression (bipolar disorder), for which it is given orally. It is also used to treat alcohol poisoning and schizoid personality disorders, and sometimes to boost the white blood cell count in persons with leukopenia.

However, toxic levels can be quickly reached, causing fatal acidosis or alkalosis, particularly in chronic overmedication for long-term treatment. For this reason, patients given lithium treatment should have frequent blood checks to make sure a toxic level has not been reached. Lithium is not recommended for those who have kidney or heart disease or for women in early or late pregnancy.

It should not be taken with alcohol (combination can result in lithium poisoning); combination with caffeine reduces lithium's effect, and combination with cocaine can cause psychosis. In addition, lithium in combination with a wide range of drugs can cause a variety of problems, including increased toxicity, hypothermia, major seizures, and sedation.

Poisonous part

It is not clear how lithium produces toxic effects, but the drug seems to focus primarily on the kidneys. Lithium is thought to stabilize cell metabolism; in large amounts it depresses neural function, but entry into the brain is slow. This explains the delay between peak blood levels and central nervous system effects after acute overdose.

Symptoms

Within 15 minutes to an hour after ingestion of an excessive dose, tremors appear, followed by twitching, apathy, speech problems, appetite loss, hair loss, dry mouth, seizures, blurred vision, confusion, coma, and death. After acute ingestion, victims experience mild nausea and vomiting, but these are delayed for several hours. Patients with long-term intoxication have more serious symptoms; toxicity may be severe with levels only slightly above recommended doses.

Treatment

There is no specific antidote. Stop administering lithium and give sodium chloride intravenously. In cases of ingestion of acute large doses, perform gastric lavage and administer activated charcoal followed by a saline cathartic. Drink plenty of fluids; dialysis may be required. Potassium may be given as well.

loquat *(Eriobotrya japonica)* [**Other names: Japanese medlar, Japanese plum.**] This small evergreen tree is cultivated in California, Florida, the Gulf coast states, Hawaii, and the West Indies. It has large, stiff leaves and fragrant white flower clusters; the fruit is yellow and shaped like a pear.

Poisonous part

While the unbroken seed is harmless, the pit kernel is toxic and contains cyanogenic glycosides that release hydrocyanic acid upon interaction with water in the gastrointestinal tract.

Symptoms

Since the glycosides must be broken down before the hydrocyanic acid is released, some hours may pass before symptoms appear. When they do, they include abdominal pain, vomiting, sweating, and lethargy. In severe poisoning cases, there may be convulsions and coma.

Treatment

If conscious, victims may be given gastric lavage followed by a 25 percent solution of sodium thiosulfate distilled into the stomach; activated charcoal absorbs cyanide but releases it slowly during passage through the intestine. In those who are losing consciousness, treat shock, correct acidosis, and give respiratory assistance with oxygen, together with the administration of a cyanide antidote.

See also CYANOGENIC GLYCOSIDES.

lorchel   See TURBANTOP.

LSD *(lysergic acid diethylamide)* **[Other names: acid, blotter acid, haze, microdots, purple haze, sunshine, window panes.]**   LSD is a synthetic hallucinogenic drug that was the drug of choice during the 1960s. A synthetic derivative of ergot, it is usually in the form of a clear liquid, and it can be either injected or ingested (often in a soaked sugar cube). Its distribution and manufacture are governed by the Controlled Substances Act because of its potential for abuse.

Symptoms

Although its mechanism is not yet clear, LSD affects the brain and produces hallucinations, hyperexcitability, tremors, prolonged mental dissociation, psychopathic personality disorders, convulsions, and coma, with a possible risk of suicide. There have been reports of numerous "flashbacks" many years after the final dose has been taken. Symptoms can appear within 20 minutes of ingestion, but there is no set toxic dose, since effects vary widely from one person to another depending on the situation and the person's current emotional state. However, hallucinations and visual illusions are dose related; the toxic dose may be only slightly greater than the dose required to produce hallucinations.

Treatment

There is no specific antidote, although Valium can control the hyperactivity or convulsions; coma is treated in the same way as barbiturate poisoning. Do not induce vomiting, since it is not effective and can worsen psychological distress; gastric lavage should be performed only if a massive dose has been ingested within 30 to 60 minutes. Administer activated charcoal.

See also BARBITURATES; ERGOT.

lye   The common name for sodium hydroxide and one of a wide variety of caustic alkalies found in drain cleaners, oven cleaners, and other household products, this is one of the most dangerous household poisons. Toddlers in particular are vulnerable to accidents, including burns to the eye, skin, and esophagus. Because of the dangers of ingestion of lye in particular, federal legislation has required safety caps on containers of more than 2 percent concentrations of lye and banned use of more than 10 percent sodium hydroxide in household liquid drain cleaners.

Symptoms

In small doses, lye causes nausea, vomiting, coughing, and the spitting of blood. Larger amounts can result in weakness, dizziness, slow, shallow breathing, and unconsciousness followed by convulsions and, sometimes, mild heart attack. Death is almost always a result of pulmonary problems. Inhalation causes lung damage.

Treatment

Gastric lavage only when preceded by endotracheal tube in comatose victims. *Do not induce vomiting.* Magnesium or sodium sulfate or citrate may be used as a cathartic. Oxygen and supportive therapy may also be needed.

See also ALKALINE CORROSIVES.

lysergic acid diethylamide   See LSD.

malathion   This is an insecticide generally considered to be safe for use around people and animals to eliminate pests such as fruit flies, mosquitoes, and boll weevils, in addition to household flies and lice on farm animals. Malathion is a colorless liquid with a definite smell, slightly soluble in water and sold as wettable powders, emulsifiable concentrates, dusts, or aerosols. While it is possible to become sick after skin contamination or inhalation, fatal cases have been reported usually only after ingestion. If heated, malathion becomes extremely dangerous, emitting toxic phosphorous oxide fumes; the addition of water transforms this into phosphoric acid.

In addition, recent research has discovered that low doses of malathion *can* cause a response in mice similar to an allergic reaction. These studies were begun following reports of rashes and allergy symptoms in humans after aerial spraying of malathion, particularly following medfly spraying in the San Fernando Valley in southern California. Although scientists at the University of Southern California at Los Angeles say the effects of the pesticide are probably not life threatening, they are unsure how the chemical would affect those with impaired immune systems.

Symptoms
Almost immediately to within several hours, symptoms begin: dermatitis, headache, nosebleeds, nausea, vomiting, diarrhea, blurred vision, excess salivation, bronchitis, shock, heart rhythm disturbances, or skin irritation; death is caused by the muscle weakness that affects the lungs, interfering with breathing.

Treatment
Respiratory support must be maintained to guard against respiratory failure.

See also INSECTICIDES; ORGANOPHOSPHATE INSECTICIDES.

mambas   The black mamba *(Dendroaspis polylepis)* is one of the most dangerous of all snakes; a large black mamba can produce enough venom to kill 10 adults. Growing up to 14 feet, its color ranges from dull gray to greenish brown or black, depending on its age. This highly aggressive snake is found in savannas, rocky outcrops, thickets, and remnant forests in Ethiopia, Somalia, and Southwest Africa. Extremely agile and speedy, it is the most territorial of all the mambas; when cornered, it rears up to strike, biting a person's head or trunk. Its potent venom is neurotoxic and cardiotoxic; the fatality rate is nearly 100 percent without antivenin.

The green mamba *(D. angusticeps)* is smaller and less aggressive and prefers to live in trees. Highly agile, this snake is found in forests and thickets and is highly dangerous when restrained.

The mambas have no upper jaw teeth behind their two fangs and are not aggressive unless provoked or restrained. Their color often conceals them until an unwary intruder gets too close.

Symptoms
Local pain, swelling, paralysis of vocal cords, sweating, vomiting, restlessness, drowsiness, collapse, coma, and death.

Treatment
Antivenin is available.

See also ANTIVENIN; SNAKES, POISONOUS.

mandrake, American [Other names: devil's apple, hog apple, Indian apple, raccoon berry, umbrella leaf, wild jalap, wild lemon.]   Also known as the mayapple *(Podophyllum pelatum)*, this plant produces fruit that, when ripe, can be eaten safely in moderation even by children. Eating the plant is fatal within 30 minutes.

The Middle Eastern variety was a famous love potion during the Middle Ages, when it was also considered to have magical properties. Some believed it would protect against evil spirits, and others believed that elves could not tolerate its smell. The ancient Greeks associated the mandrake with Circe, the witch. Because it was believed that touching the root would be fatal, dogs were trained to pull the dark brown root out of the ground, whereupon, according to legend, the root would shriek and the dog would die. Others believed that, pulled from the ground while muttering the correct incantation, the plant could bring forth the devil. In fact, the simple possession of mandrake could mark the owner as a witch, and three German women were executed in 1630 for just such a crime.

The American mandrake grows in moist woods and pastures. Found from Quebec to Florida, west to Ontario, Minnesota, and Texas, it grows about 1-foot tall, with a jointed dark root about half the size of a finger, branching in a fork that resembles a pair of legs; in fact, it resembles a tiny human being. Leaves are deeply lobed with one white flower that appears in the spring, resembling a strawberry blossom; this is followed by a yellow fruit that is edible when ripe (and is sometimes used for preserves).

Poisonous part

Rootstock, stem, flower, leaves, and unripe fruit contain several hallucinogenic alkaloids, including hyoscyamine (atropine) and mandragorin; toxins also include podophylloresin and its glucoside, and alpha- and beta-peltatin. When green, the rhizome, foliage, seeds, and green fruit are poisonous. Herbalists believe the best time for collecting the root is the latter part of October or early November, after the fruit is ripe.

Symptoms

Within a few minutes to a half hour after ingestion of large amounts of the plant or topical application of the resin, mandrake poisoning causes severe diarrhea and vomiting, sedation, slowed heart rate, pupil dilation, coma, and death. The mandrake's close relative, the mayapple, causes gastroenteritis, headache, and collapse and, when combined with alcohol, can be fatal within 14 hours.

Treatment

There is no specific antidote; give fluid replacement and blood transfusions if necessary.

manganese Workers in mining, metalworking, foundry, and welding occupations are generally the only people exposed to manganese toxicity from chronic rather than acute exposure.

Poisonous part

While the exact mechanism of manganese toxicity is not known, inhalation affects the central nervous system; manganese is not well absorbed from the gastrointestinal tract.

Symptoms

Although an acute intoxication is possible, causing pneumonitis, it is more likely that workers would be poisoned as a result of chronic exposure to low levels of manganese over a period of months or years. In the case of chronic exposure, manganese causes an affective psychiatric disorder (often misdiagnosed as schizophrenia or psychosis). This is followed by further signs of brain disease, such as parkinsonism or similar movement disorders.

Treatment

For cases of acute inhalation toxicity, administer oxygen and treat symptoms. Long-term exposure should be treated with the typical drugs for psychiatric and movement disorders. Chelating agents have not been proven effective once chronic brain damage has occurred.

massasauga *(Sistrurus catenatus)* One of three rattlesnakes from the family Viperidae, this pygmy rattler ranges from the Great Lakes southwest to southeastern Arizona and Mexico. Its name, which is from the Chippewa language, means "great river mouth" and is thought to indicate the snake's habitat in the land of the Chippewa—swamps around rivers.

The massasauga has a stocky tail with a small rattle, and rounded dark blotches on its back and sides. A light-bordered dark bar runs from the eye to the rear of its jaw. The snake may grow to

40 inches. This "swamp rattler" is found in bogs, swamps, marshes, floodplains, and dry woods in the East; grassy wetlands, rocky hillsides, and the sagebrush and desert grasslands of the West. Unlike many snakes, massasaugas do not hibernate communally in an upland den but sleep alone in a mammal or crayfish burrow. They emerge in spring in response to the rains and rising water.

While fairly poisonous snakes, they are not aggressive and normally bite only when disturbed.

Symptoms

Symptoms appear within 15 minutes and include excessive thirst, nausea, vomiting, shock, paralysis, respiratory problems, anemia, kidney problems, and sometimes death. The bite of a rattlesnake is painful. Indications of a serious bite include swelling above the elbows or knees within two hours, hemorrhages, numbness at the puncture site, tingling around the mouth, yellow vision, vomiting, and violent spasms.

Treatment

Antivenin is available.

See also PIT VIPER; RATTLESNAKE, CANEBRAKE; RATTLESNAKE, CASCABEL; RATTLESNAKE, EASTERN DIAMONDBACK; RATTLESNAKE, MEXICAN WEST COAST; RATTLESNAKE, RED DIAMONDBACK; RATTLESNAKES; RATTLESNAKE, TIMBER; RATTLESNAKE, WESTERN DIAMONDBACK; SIDEWINDER; VIPER, GABOON; VIPER, JUMPING; VIPER, MALAYAN PIT; VIPER, RUSSELL'S; VIPERS; VIPER, SAWSCALE; VIPER WAGLER'S PIT; WATER MOCCASIN; WUTU.

matches   Serious cases of poisoning from ingesting matches are quite rare since the principal component of white or yellow phosphorus was replaced by red or by phosphorus sesquisulfide. The "strike anywhere" type of match is made of a nonpoisonous paste containing 6 percent phosphorus sesquisulfide and 24 percent potassium chlorate, plus zinc oxide, red ochre powdered glass, glue, and water. "Safety" (or strike-on-box) matches are nonpoisonous; their chief ingredient is potassium chlorate. Book matches are similar to the safety type of match.

Accidental ingestion of matches by children often occurs, but it produces relatively insignificant side effects. Even if a child ate an entire book of 20 match heads, the total amount of potassium chlorate is still only 1/20 of the toxic dose.

meadow saffron (Colchicum autumnale, C. speciosum, C. vernum) [Other names: autumn crocus, fall crocus, naked ladies.]   This crocus look-alike and ancient abortifacient is a member of the lily family and is often mistaken for an onion. It has long, tubular purple or white flowers that emerge from an underground bulb. Highly toxic, it is found in damp and woodsy areas in England, Wales, and Scotland. Goats, which are immune to the poison, can eat the plant and pass on the poison in their milk, which will sicken anyone who drinks it.

Poisonous part

All parts (especially the bulbs) are toxic; tincture of colchicine is made from the seeds of *C. autumnale*, and the drug colchicine is used as a rheumatic.

Symptoms

Within two to six hours after ingestion, the victim begins to exhibit some symptoms similar to those of arsenic poisoning: burning throat, intense thirst, vomiting, difficulty in swallowing, bloody diarrhea, stomach pain, sensory disturbances, muscle weakness, delirium, and heart and breathing failure. Meadow saffron poisoning is fatal in half of all cases, although it may not occur until three days after ingestion.

It is also possible to suffer chronic colchicine poisoning, with symptoms of hair loss and blood and protein in the urine and colchicine in the feces.

Treatment

Because colchicine is only slowly excreted, the victim is often ill for a long time. Painkillers and atropine may be given to alleviate stomach pain and diarrhea; fluids are required.

meclofenamate   See NONSTEROIDAL ANTI-INFLAMMATORY DRUGS.

meperidine (Demerol) Introduced in 1939 as a means of reducing the pain associated with muscle spasms, this drug was later found to have many other painkilling abilities. It soon became almost as popular a drug as morphine, but it is only about one-tenth as potent. Still, meperidine is a fairly strong analgesic and is used for treatment of moderate to severe pain, to supplement anesthesia before an operation and to relieve the pain of labor during childbirth.

Symptoms

Large doses of meperidine can cause twitches, tremors and convulsions, and the drug is especially dangerous when mixed with monoamine oxidase (MAO) inhibitors (a class of antidepressants). In fact, if it is taken within two weeks of an MAO inhibitor, it can cause symptoms similar to those in acute narcotic overdose (including convulsions, high blood pressure, coma, and death).

Treatment

Medical help should be sought immediately. Stimulants such as strong tea and coffee will help to keep the victim awake. If the victim is discovered soon after ingestion and is conscious, induce vomiting.

mercury Every known form of this highly toxic, silvery liquid metal is poisonous, and since there are more than 115 known mercury compounds, there are many opportunities for mercuric poisoning to occur. It is widely used in skin and hair bleach, dusting or wettable powders and fumigants, cathartics, antiseptics and diuretics, and in explosives, tooth fillings, electrical lamps, batteries, paints, and felt. In the past, many milliners used mercury to help shape hats; it has been suggested that Lewis Carroll's Mad Hatter may really have been suffering from mercury poisoning, as did many hatters of the 1800s.

Its toxicity depends on the chemical form in which it appears, and in its most common form, as a free metal in fever thermometers, mercury is not a serious threat if ingested, since it is not well absorbed by the body. However, breathing mercury vapor is more hazardous. Employees in dental offices may also be exposed to excess levels of mercury, via recirculation ventilation systems or sloppy conditions. Mercury chloride found in antiseptics is the most toxic of all mercury compounds. Organic mercurials that are used to treat seeds are highly toxic, and acute cases of poisoning have been reported from fish contamination or water pollution.

There is a large number of professions whose workers are exposed to mercury, including those who make barometers, batteries, boilers, calibration instruments, caustic soda, carbon brushes, ceramics, chlorine, dental amalgam, electrical apparatus, neon lights, pressure gauges, disinfectants, dyes, explosives, fireworks, inks, drugs, insecticides and pesticides, and wood preservatives.

Symptoms

Acute poisoning from inhaling mercury vapor occurs almost immediately, causing stomach problems, coughing, fever, nausea, vomiting, and diarrhea. The vapor affects the brain and lungs, attacking the respiratory system and causing pneumonia, pulmonary edema, and ventricular fibrillation followed by death. Chronic poisoning results in damage to the central nervous system and can cause psychosis. Ingestion of mercuric chloride and other soluble mercuric salts can cause thirst, abdominal pain, vomiting and diarrhea, followed by kidney damage, and death. Skin contamination with mercury compounds causes a variety of symptoms, including depression, sleeplessness, weight loss and anorexia, headaches, anxiety, hallucinations, loose teeth, and tremors.

Treatment

Dimercaprol and treatment of symptoms.

See also FISH CONTAMINATION; MERCURY AND DENTAL FILLINGS.

mercury and dental fillings For decades, experts in the field of toxicology were sharply divided over whether mercury contained in dental fillings posed a hazard to human health. In a study published in 2006, for example, 465 patients with chronic mercury toxicity reported severe fatigue (32.3 percent), memory loss (88.8 percent), and depression (27.5 percent). When amalgam mercury fillings were removed and appropriate treatment was administered, patients experienced a significant reduction in symptoms to a level reported by healthy subjects. Yet other experts, including those at the Food and Drug Administration (FDA) and the National Institutes of Health, for many years insisted that amalgams were at least as safe as the available alternatives.

Then in June 2008, the FDA announced that "dental amalgams contain mercury, which may have neurotoxic effects on the nervous systems of developing children and fetuses." It also added that when amalgam fillings are "placed in teeth or removed they release mercury vapor," and that this effect also occurs when people chew. The FDA has decided to review its rules about amalgams and may alter its position on the use of mercury in fillings.

See also MERCURY; FISH CONTAMINATION.

metal cleaner   See ALKALINE CORROSIVES.

metaldehyde   This is a type of inorganic chemical insecticide often used in combination with calcium arsenate and used to control slugs and snails. It is also sold as fuel for small heaters that can cause toxic vapors if not properly ventilated. Poison control centers report incidences of children being poisoned after mistakenly eating slug or snail bait or heater fuel tablets.

Ingestion of 100 to 150 milligrams per kilogram may cause convulsions, and ingestion of more than 400 mg/kg is potentially lethal.

Symptoms

Metaldehyde is a stomach irritant; between one and three hours after ingestion it causes nausea, vomiting, stomach pain, flushed face, fever, muscular rigidity, and twitching. In severe poisonings, convulsions and coma are followed by death from respiratory failure. Liver and kidney damage have been reported.

Treatment

There is no specific antidote. Perform gastric lavage immediately after ingestion, followed by activated charcoal and cathartics, with supportive therapy including plenty of fluids. Do NOT induce vomiting. Demulcents (such as milk) may relieve gastric distress; sedation may also be required.

See also INORGANIC CHEMICAL INSECTICIDES.

methanol   See METHYL ALCOHOL.

methocarbamol   This centrally acting muscle relaxant is used in the control of painful muscle spasms following the bite of the black widow spider and strychnine poisoning. Onset of action almost immediately follows intravenous administration.

See also BLACK WIDOW SPIDER; STRYCHNINE.

methyl alcohol (wood alcohol)   Also known as methanol, this common household solvent is related to ethyl alcohol and is found in solvents, perfumes, windshield washing liquids, duplicating fluid, antifreeze, shellac, and paint removers.

It is far more poisonous than the ethyl alcohol found in cocktails, because it metabolizes into formaldehyde upon ingestion; it also takes far longer to eliminate methyl alcohol from the body. While it can produce intoxication, its metabolic products may cause metabolic acidosis, blindness, and death.

Methyl alcohol is a liquid at room temperature, evaporates quickly and can be swallowed, inhaled as a vapor or absorbed through the skin. In the past, moonshine makers (who distill ethyl alcohol from fermented grain) sometimes mistakenly mixed wood shavings in with the brew, resulting in a toxic brand of moonshine. (Methyl alcohol is made from fermented wood.)

Symptoms

The fatal oral dose of methyl alcohol is estimated to be 30 to 240 milliliters. Because methyl alcohol metabolizes slowly in the body, there is a latency period ranging from 12 to 48 hours between ingestion/inhalation and symptoms. In the first hours after ingestion, the primary symptom is intoxication because the body has not yet begun to break down the substance into more toxic products. Once methyl alcohol is transformed into formaldehyde in the body, it causes fatigue, headache, nausea and vomiting, vertigo, back pain, severe abdominal pain, vision problems, dizziness, and blindness. (These symptoms will appear even later if ethanol has been drunk at the same time.) In large doses, symptoms progress to rapid, shallow breathing, cyanosis, coma, precipitous drop in blood pressure, and death from respiratory arrest. An autopsy would show massive organ damage, especially in the eyes. Breathing fumes can cause headache, eye irritation, dizziness, visual disturbances, and nausea. In extreme cases, inhaling these fumes can be fatal; it damages the liver, heart, kidneys, and the lungs, predisposing them to pneumonia.

Treatment

Ethanol (100 proof) is administered to interfere with the metabolism of methyl alcohol; within two hours of ingestion, gastric lavage is preferred, but syrup of ipecac may be given at home to induce vomiting before medical help arrives. Ethanol is then administered orally or intravenously for the next four days until the methyl alcohol is excreted; kidney dialysis may also remove the alcohol from the blood. Folic acid may also be administered; and 4-methylpyrazole (fomepizole) can inhibit alcohol dehydrogenase and prevent methyl alcohol metabolism. Activated charcoal has not been shown to absorb methyl alcohol efficiently, and it may also delay the absorption of orally administered ethanol.

methyl bromide This odorless, colorless gas is used in insecticidal fumigants and fire extinguishers and in the production of chemicals and dyes. It is considered to be a potential industrial carcinogen by the National Institute of Occupational Safety and Health (NIOSH). It can be inhaled or absorbed easily through the skin; methyl bromide also easily penetrates protective clothing and can be retained in boots and clothing for some time.

Symptoms

Methyl bromide affects the central nervous system, the respiratory tract, the skin and the cardiovascular system. There is a wide variance in onset of symptoms, ranging from a few minutes to two days after ingestion. Methyl bromide irritates the eyes, skin, and upper respiratory tract, which may lead to pulmonary edema; skin contamination can cause a rash or chemical burns. With acute exposure, there may be malaise, vision disturbances, headache, nausea, vomiting, vertigo, tremor, seizures, and coma followed by death from pulmonary or circulatory failure. In addition, chronic exposure may lead to dementia or psychosis.

Treatment

Some scientists recommend the use of dimercaprol or acetylcysteine, although their use has not been tested in controlled studies. Remove all contaminated clothing and wash the skin with soap and water; irrigate eyes with saline or tepid water.

See also ETHYL ALCOHOL.

methyl chloroform See TRICHLOROETHANE.

methylene chloride One of a group of chlorinated hydrocarbons, this chemical solvent is listed as a human carcinogen by the National Toxicology Program of the U.S. Department of Health and Human Services. It is encountered by millions of Americans every day in products ranging from paint strippers and thinners to paint, hair spray, antiperspirants, room deodorants, and Christmas tree light sets. Upon combustion, it can produce phosgene, chlorine or hydrogen chloride; it was considered to be one of the least toxic of the chlorinated hydrocarbons, but now it is a suspected carcinogen.

Methylene chloride irritates mucous membranes and depresses the central nervous system. Carbon monoxide is generated within the body during metabolism of methylene chloride.

Symptoms

Inhalation is the most common route of intoxication and causes skin irritation, nausea, vomiting, and headache. Severe exposure may lead to pulmonary edema, heart problems, and central nervous system depression with respiratory arrest. Ingestion can lead to corrosive injury and system intoxication. Chronic exposure is toxic to bone marrow, the kidneys, and the liver.

Treatment

Administer 100 percent oxygen by tight-fitting mask or endotracheal tube; if skin or eyes are contaminated, wash thoroughly. In case of ingestion, do NOT induce vomiting, perform gastric lavage if the victim has ingested within the past 30 to 60 minutes or has ingested a large amount. Administer activated charcoal and a cathartic, although the effectiveness of the former is not known.

See also CHLORINATED HYDROCARBON PESTICIDES.

methylenedioxymethamphetamine (MDMA)   See ECSTASY.

methyl phenidate   See RITALIN.

methyl mercury   See   FISH   CONTAMINATION; MERCURY.

metoclopramide   This antinausea drug is used to control persistent nausea and vomiting often found in poisoning cases, especially when activated charcoal may not be given.

Mexican beaded lizard (Heloderma horridum) One of only two poisonous lizards in the world out of more than 3,000 lizard species, the Mexican beaded lizard is found only in Mexico and is a relative of the Gila monster, also a member of the *Heloderma* genus. Slightly larger than the Gila monster, the Mexican beaded lizard is still not a very large animal—between 19 and 29 inches long; it is a mixture of black, yellow, and pink and has knobby scales. Both lizards are sluggish but have a strong bite. Fatalities from the bite of a Mexican beaded lizard are rare.

Beaded lizards are nocturnal and mate during summer, laying between three and five eggs in autumn and winter. Although these lizards are relatively slow moving, they can bite quickly and hang on stubbornly. While biting, they chew so that the grooved teeth can allow the venom to flow from the glands at the base of the mouth. In general, the bite of the beaded lizard is not fatal, but it is quite painful. There have been only eight recorded deaths from bites of both these lizards.

Beaded lizards live underground, either in abandoned holes or ones they dig themselves, they locate their food by scent rather than sight, following a trail in much the same way as a bloodhound does.

See also GILA MONSTER.

Mexican hallucinogenic mushroom (Psilocybe mexicana) Also known as "magic mushrooms," these are a species of mushrooms that contain the hallucinogenic substance psilocin-psilocybin, which American Indians have used for thousands of years in their religious ceremonies.

The *Psilocybe* genus includes more than 100 different species of the little brown mushrooms, which are found growing in grass and manure heaps—especially after spring rains. Though found primarily in the South, they grow almost everywhere in the United States. One of the easiest ways to identify the *Psilocybe* mushroom is by its blue-green discoloration in areas where it has been handled or damaged.

Symptoms

Within an hour of ingestion, its effects—which are usually considered pleasant—appear: euphoria, loss of sense of distance and size, and hallucinations. Symptoms will last between four and six hours depending on the quantity of toxin ingested, the mood and personality of the person and the setting of the experience. Effects lasting longer than 24 hours are not due to a natural toxin but to the consumption of a mushroom with another hallucinogen added (usually phencyclidine or PCP). The mushrooms can cause high fever, convulsions, and death in children who have eaten them.

Treatment

For those who seek medical assistance, treatment usually involves reassurance, although sedation (with diazepam) is sometimes necessary. In children, treatment includes external cooling and respiratory support; it may be necessary to administer diazepam to control convulsions.

See also HALLUCINOGENIC MUSHROOMS; MUSHROOM POISONING.

Mexican moccasin   See CANTIL SNAKE.

midazolam   This ultrashort-acting benzodiazepine is used to help manage anxiety, agitation, and psychosis following overdose of hallucinogenic or stimulant drugs such as LSD or amphetamines. It is also used to induce sedation and amnesia during placement of an endotracheal tube.

See also AMPHETAMINES; BENZODIAZEPINES; LSD.

Minipress (prazosin hydrochloride)   One of a group of antihypertensives, this toxic medicine is available as a white crystalline water-soluble capsule.

Symptoms

Within 30 to 90 minutes after ingestion, Minipress overdose causes headache, drowsiness, hair loss, weakness, nausea, vomiting, diarrhea, shortness of breath, nervousness, rapid heartbeat, depression, rash, itching, blurred vision, loss of consciousness, and death.

Treatment

Atropine is administered while monitoring the cardiorespiratory systems and the kidney function.

See also ANTIHYPERTENSIVE DRUGS.

mirex   This type of synthetic organic insecticide is a chlorinated hydrocarbon that is almost impossible to dissolve in water and is generally no longer used as an insecticide. Emergency exceptions for specific uses are allowed, however.

Mirex was used throughout the southeastern United States to control fire ants, other ant species, and yellow jackets. It breaks down in the soil and forms kepone, a chlorinated organic insecticide banned from use in 1978.

Symptoms

Inhalation, ingestion, or skin contamination can cause chest pain, weight loss, rash, and a range of neurological problems including tremors, mental alterations, weakness, and slurred speech. Both mirex and its derivative, kepone, cause cancer in experimental animals.

Treatment

Gastric lavage followed by saline cathartics. Avoid all fats and oils (including milk), since they increase the rate of absorption. Administer phenobarbital sodium for tremors and barbiturates for convulsions, and provide oxygen if necessary. If the skin has come in contact with these insecticides, wash with soap and water immediately to head off skin problems and systemic absorption. Remove contaminated clothing.

See also CHLORINATED HYDROCARBON PESTICIDE.

mistletoe (American: *Phoradendron rubrum, P. serotinum, P. tomentosum*; European: *Viscum album*)   This popular winter holiday plant is a parasite of deciduous trees in the southeastern United States, and the whole mistletoe plant—especially the berries—is poisonous, although seldom fatal.

Mistletoe has thick, leathery leaves, with white translucent berries in the *P. serotinum* and *P. tomentosum* varieties and pink berries in the *P. rubrum* variety. *P. serotinum* is the variety typically sold as a decorative holiday plant at Christmas; it grows from New Jersey to Florida and west to southern Illinois and Texas. *P. tomentosum* is found from Kansas to Louisiana and west to Texas and Mexico.

V. album is a parasite found principally on apple trees and, although a European plant, has been introduced into Sonoma County, California. Its thick, leathery leaves are up to three inches long and yellow-green in color; the fruit is a sticky white berry.

Mistletoe is a plant steeped in legend and mystery. It is said that mistletoe was once a tree, the wood of which had been used to make Christ's cross, and was relegated to exist only as a parasite ever after. Similarly, it was an herb of the underworld in both Greek and Roman legends, while in Britain the Druid priests were said to use mistletoe in many important religious ceremonies. Tradition says that the mistletoe was the "golden bough" that the Trojan hero Aeneas, forefather of the Romans, carried with him on his descent into Hades. The bough opened the gates of hell for the hero and brought him safely back.

Its reputation as an herb of love, in which two people standing under it at Christmas must kiss, originated in Scandinavia, when Balder (the god of peace) was killed with an arrow dipped in mistletoe. When his fellow gods asked that his life be spared, mistletoe was given to the god of love, who announced that anyone who passed beneath it must be given a kiss as a symbol of love. It subsequently became a part of the Christmas celebrations when the Druids used the greens as a way of welcoming the New Year.

Poisonous part
Stems, leaves, and berries of this plant contain toxic amines and proteins called phoratoxins, toxic lectins that inhibit synthesization of proteins in the intestinal wall. They can cause hallucinations, slow heartbeat, high blood pressure, heart attacks, and cardiovascular collapse. While poisoning is rarely fatal, there have been cases in which children have died after eating mistletoe berries. Tea brewed from the berries has also been fatal.

In the European variety *(V. album)* only the leaves and stems are toxic, containing a toxic lectin (toxalbumin) called viscumin, which interferes with protein synthesis. In addition, related lectins called viscotoxins are also found.

In addition to its own toxic properties, mistletoe may also take up poisonous substances from the tree on which it lives.

Symptoms
Similar to those of poisoning by digitalis, symptoms appear after a delay of a few hours and include severe nausea, vomiting, diarrhea, stomach cramps, difficulty in breathing, slow pulse, delirium, hallucinations, and coma.

In the European variety, poisoning symptoms are similar to, but less toxic than, those caused by the lectins in rosary pea *(Abrus prevatorius)* and castor bean *(Ricinus communis)*. Symptoms in this variety appear some time after ingestion and include abdominal pain and diarrhea together with lesions of the intestinal tract. Severe poisoning with this variety of mistletoe is rare.

Treatment
Treat as for severe gastroenteritis, with replacement of fluids and electrolytes.

mold   The exact number of species of mold is unknown, but it is estimated to be as many as 300,000 or more. Molds are fungi that can grow and develop indoors and outdoors and can be found in virtually every environment, year round. Although they grow best in damp, warm, humid conditions, they spread and reproduce spores, which can survive harsh environments and become active again when conditions are favorable. Indoors, those environments are generally basements, showers, or damp attics, where humidity levels are high; outdoors, they can be found in damp, shady areas or places were vegetation is decomposing. Some molds are cryophytes (which can adapt to low temperatures), some are thermo tolerant (they can adapt to a wide range of temperatures), and some are thermophiles (they adapt to high temperatures). Depending on the species, these molds will grow in nearly any environment. Temperatures in excess of 500 degrees Fahrenheit have not been able to destroy some molds, including the toxic *Stachybotrys* (see below).

Some people are sensitive to molds, and their reactions can range from mild nasal stuffiness and wheezing to severe reactions such as fever and shortness of breath. Individuals who have chronic lung conditions may develop mold infections in their lungs. The term "toxic mold" is somewhat misleading: while the molds themselves are not toxic, certain types produce secondary metabolites that produce mycotoxins. When susceptible individuals breathe in mold spores and mycotoxins they can become ill. Mold and mycotoxins are implicated in some cases of sick building syndrome.

The molds most commonly found both indoors and outdoors throughout the United States are *Alternaria* and *Cladosporium;* others that are often seen are *Aspergillus, Penicillium, Helminthosporium, Epicoccum, Fusarium, Mucor, Rhizopus,* and *Aureobasidium.* One of the mycotoxins, aflatoxin, is produced by *Penicillium, Aspergillus flavor,* and *Aspergillus parasiticus.* Four different aflatoxins have been identified (B1, B2, G1, and G2), with B1 being the most toxic, carcinogenic, and prevalent.

Much less common but significantly dangerous are the molds *Stachybotrys chartarum* and *Chaetomium,* which have been proven to produce mycotoxins that can lead to autoimmune disease. *Strachybotrys* grows on cellulose products (e.g., wood, paper, insulation, fiberboard, hay, straw) that has gotten wet. This mold can be found in homes and other buildings that have been in floods, basements or attics that have been exposed to water, and barns and other outbuildings.

Symptoms

Nasal and throat irritation, cough, shortness of breath, chronic bronchitis, learning disabilities, mental deficiencies, heart problems, cancer, multiple chemical sensitivity, rash, and diarrhea are all possible symptoms associated with exposure to mold. Animal studies suggest that *Chaetomium* species may cause autoimmune disorders (e.g., rheumatoid arthritis, chronic fatigue syndrome, lupus) but no scientific studies in humans have been done. Exposure to the mycotoxins of the more dangerous molds may include nasal infections, peritonitis, and cutaneous lesions.

Treatment

Symptomatic for the signs and symptoms of mold exposure. The best "treatment" is to remove the mold and its source. If the affected area is large, professional mold removal service may be required. For smaller areas, a nonammonia soap or detergent in hot water should be used to scrub the affected area with a stiff brush or cleaning pad. Rinse the area with water and then disinfect the area with a solution of household bleach (one-half cup of bleach per gallon of water). Allow the area to dry naturally, which allows the bleach to kill all the mold.

See also SICK BUILDING SYNDROME.

monkshood *(Aconitum)* **[Other names: aconite, bear's foot, friar's cap, helmet flower, soldier's cap, western monkshood** *(A. columbianum),* **wild monkshood** *(A. uncinatum),* **wolfsbane, yellow monkshood** *(A. lutescens).*] Dubbed "queen mother of poisons" before the birth of Christ, this extremely poisonous plant may reach 6 feet in height with small blue, pink, or white flowers and a unique hood-shaped upper petal appearing from June to September. According to legend, it is ruled by Hecate, goddess of the underworld, who supposedly poisoned her father with it.

Monkshood is a strikingly beautiful plant rich in myth and medicine, history and magic. Often grown as an ornamental perennial in shady borders around older homes, this plant has flowers that resemble delphiniums; the flowers are arranged on stems of equal height and distance from each other and blossom in an orderly fashion from stem base to tip. Although the plant is a perennial, the spongy root is an annual and sprouts tiny side roots, each capable of producing another monkshood plant. Together with larkspur and columbine, monkshood belongs to the buttercup family and includes about 100 species in the genus *Aconitum.*

The name may come from the Greek *akonitos,* "without struggle" or "without dust," or from the Greek city Acona, where a naturalist in the third century once identified the plant. Other sources suggest the name comes from the hill of Aconitus, where Hercules fought with Cerberus, the three-headed dog who guards the entrance to Hades. Saliva from this dreaded dog's mouth dripped onto monkshood, making it a deadly poison.

In mythology, monkshood formed the cup that Medea prepared for Theseus. In Rome, Nero ascended to the throne after poisoning Claudius by tickling his throat with a feather dipped in monkshood. While it is named for the shape of its flower, it was also associated with political intrigue among the ranks of the Roman Catholic clergy. Traditions holds that Romeo (of Shakespeare's *Romeo and Juliet*) committed suicide with monkshood.

Witches also made wide use of this plant in herbal preparations to induce supernatural experiences, combining it with belladonna in ointments the witches rubbed on their bodies to help them "fly." In fact, these two plants produce an irregular heart action and delirium, which is believed to have caused the sensation of flying. During the Middle Ages, the plant was widely feared because it was thought witches used it to summon the devil. In Shakespeare's *Macbeth,* the witches' brew calling for "tooth of wolf" refers to monkshood, which is also known as wolfsbane because arrows dipped in the poison kill wolves. (For this same reason, medieval folks believed monkshood would protect them against werewolves).

Monkshood thrives naturally and is also cultivated as a decorative plant in Canada and the northern United States, including Alaska. Until the 1930s, monkshood was used as a painkiller, diuretic, and diaphoretic. Ointments containing monkshood have been used externally to treat rheumatism, neuralgia, and lumbago, and a tincture was used to lower pulse rate and fevers and treat cardiac failure. Because of its toxicity, monkshood is rarely used today in medicine, although it is still valued in homeopathy as an ointment for muscle and joint pain.

Poisonous part

The entire plant is poisonous. However, the roots and leaves contain the greatest concentration of the toxin aconitine and similar alkaloids, including picratonitine, aconine, benzoylamine, and neopelline. The alkaloids first stimulate and then depress the central and peripheral nerves. One teaspoonful of the root is lethal to an adult, and even handling the plant is dangerous to highly sensitive people. Because of the root's similarity to Jerusalem artichoke or horseradish, monkshood should never be planted near a vegetable garden. Even touching the plant's juices to an open wound can cause pain, fainting sensations, and suffocation.

But like many botanical toxins, the one in monkshood can be beneficial if administered in very small doses. In fact, 18th- and 19th-century physicians used monkshood as a cardiac sedative, although modern drugs have since replaced it.

Symptoms

If monkshood is eaten, symptoms start rapidly with a burning or tingling sensation of the lips, tongue, mouth, and throat. Delayed-onset symptoms include excessive salivation, nausea, vomiting, tightness and numbness in the throat, impaired swallowing, and possibly speech impairment. Intermittent visual disturbances can include blurred vision or color patches in the visual field and pronounced and prolonged pupil dilation. Dizziness, prickling skin sensation, muscle weakness, and uncoordinated movements can also occur.

In critical cases there are heart rate and rhythm disturbances followed by convulsions and death. Death may occur as early as a few minutes after ingestion or as late as four days.

Those who survive report odd hallucinations during the poisoning episode and sensory disturbances for a long time afterward. If the victim does not die, recovery occurs within 24 hours.

Treatment

There is no specific antidote, although gastric lavage and oxygen to help breathing, as well as drugs to stimulate the heart, may be used. Arrhythmias should be managed by electrocardiogram monitoring.

See also ACONITINE.

monoamine oxidase (MAO) inhibitors A class of psychiatric drugs used to treat severe depression that also stimulate the central nervous system and affect the liver. MAO inhibitors may cause serious poisoning either by overdose or through interactions with other drugs or food.

For example, eating cheese or drinking alcohol (especially red wine) can cause hypertension, stroke, and even death. Some MAO inhibitor drugs have been taken off the U.S. market because of extreme toxicity in combination with other drugs.

MAO inhibitors include furazolidone (Furoxone), isocarboxazid (Marplan), nialamide (Niamid), pargyline (Eutonyl), phenelzine (Nardil), procarbazine (Matulane) and tranylcypromine (Parnate).

Symptoms

In an acute overdose, symptoms may not appear for six to 24 hours, but they should be apparent quite soon after eating certain foods or taking certain other drugs. Symptoms include anxiety, flushing, headache, tremor, sweating, tachycardia, and hypertension; severe poisoning causes severe high blood pressure, brain hemorrhage, delirium, high fever, cardiovascular collapse, and multisystem failure.

Treatment

There is no specific antidote. Treat symptoms; monitor temperature and vital signs, with an ECG

DRUGS AND FOODS THAT DON'T MIX WITH MAO INHIBITORS

Drug	Food
Amphetamine	Beef liver/Beer
Buspirone	Beans
Dextromethorphan	Cheese
Ephedrine	Chicken livers
Fluoxetine	Game meats/Pickled herring
Guanethidine	Saver Kraut/Snails
L-Dopa	Red wine
LSD (lysergic acid diethylamide)	Yeast
Meperidine (Demerol)	
Metaraminol	
Methyldopa	
Phenylephrine	
Phenylpropanolamine	
Reserpine	
Trazodone	
Tryptophan	

for victims without symptoms. Do not induce vomiting because of the risk of seizures and worsening the high blood pressure; perform gastric lavage followed by activated charcoal and a cathartic.

See also ANTIDEPRESSANTS.

monomethylhydrazine A propellant used in rocket fuel, this is also a decomposition product of the mushroom toxin gyromitrin and the primary toxic component of the gyromitra mushroom.

Symptoms
A strong convulsant, this substance can cause central nervous system depression, pulmonary edema and cardiovascular collapse, with some kidney damage and severe liver damage.

Treatment
The antidote is pyridoxine, which may help in the control of hyperexcitability and even coma but will not protect the liver from damage.

See also *GYROMITRA;* MUSHROOM POISONING; MUSHROOM TOXINS.

monosodium glutamate (MSG) This natural salt is found in low amounts in seaweed, soybeans, and sugar beets; refined, it is used to enhance the flavor of certain foods (especially red meat, poultry, and fish). MSG is commonly used by the processed food industry and Asian restaurants as a flavor enhancer. The most common processed foods that use MSG include meat products, bouillons, precooked soups, and gravies in packages, condiments, pickles, candy, and baked goods.

Almost anyone who eats processed food, fast food or dines at an Asian restaurant will encounter MSG; most of the health complaints have come from people eating at Chinese restaurants. Soups and foods coated with a liquid sauce often contain the highest concentration of MSG, and rice used in Japanese sushi also contains high concentrations.

Labels must indicate which packaged foods contain MSG, but avoiding the additive is much more difficult in restaurants, since menus usually do not mention that the food contains this flavor enhancer. Unless it is explicitly stated otherwise, it should be assumed that Asian food contains MSG.

MSG contains the amino acid glutamate, which may be responsible for brain damage under certain conditions of oxygen deprivation in the brain (such as during a stroke), or when ingested in large quantities. While the glutamate in MSG is considered safe for adults, research at Washington University in St. Louis finding that large doses of glutamate may damage brain cells prompted the Food and Drug Administration to ban MSG from baby food in the mid-1970s.

According to a recent animal study (February 2008) and several earlier studies, MSG can lead to the development of inflammation, obesity, and type 2 diabetes. The 2008 study focused on the impact of MSG on the liver and found that the substance induces obesity and diabetes with steatosis (fatty liver) and steatohepatitis (liver inflammation caused by fat buildup). These findings caused the investigators to suggest that the safety profile for MSG be reviewed and that the substance be considered for withdrawal from the food supply.

Symptoms
Among certain individuals in a subgroup of the population, MSG causes "Chinese restaurant syn-

drome": tightness in the head and face, headache, chest pain, dizziness, sweating, and numbness. According to the Food and Drug Administration, about 4 percent of the population will have an occasional reaction to MSG; about 2 percent are highly sensitive to it.

Treatment
Symptomatic.

moonseed *(Menispermum canadense)* [Other names: Canadian moonseed, Texas sarsaparilla, vine-maple, yellow sarsaparilla.] Sometimes mistaken for wild grapes, moonseed is a woody twining vine growing on stream banks and fences in eastern North America. Its Hawaiian relative, also called moonseed (*Cocculus ferrandianus*), is used as a fish poison. A perennial, moonseed grows in the eastern part of the United States in moist woods, hedges, and streams. Its woody root is very long and yellow, and its stem is a climbing vine with round, smooth leaves and yellow flowers appearing in July, followed by one seeded fruit.

Poisonous part
Both leaves and fruit contain poisonous alkaloids.

Symptoms
Within several hours after ingestion, moonseed grapes and leaves cause bloody diarrhea, convulsions, shock, and death.

Treatment
Gastric lavage.

morning glory *(Ipomoea)* [Other names: flying saucer, heavenly blue, pearly gates.] This is the common name for plants of the Convolvulaceae family, which are popular for their hallucinogenic properties. These viny plants have large, heart-shaped leaves and flaring, brightly colored flowers; the hallucinogenic part of the plant is the black or brown seeds. The seeds' hallucinogenic properties have been known since ancient times, when Aztecs and North American Indians used them as part of

their religious ceremonies and in healing and divination. Not all species are toxic, however.

In recent times, the seeds of the morning glory have been advertised for sale in alternative publications as "hallucinogens" but also labeled "not for human consumption."

Poisonous part
The seeds of this plant are poisonous and contain an active principle similar to that of LSD, but only one-tenth as toxic.

Symptoms
Between 50 and 200 powdered seeds can produce symptoms similar to those caused by LSD, with feelings of depersonalization and visual hallucinations, in addition to psychoses and flashbacks later on.

Treatment
Supportive and symptomatic. Do not induce vomiting; gastric lavage should be performed within 30 minutes only in case of massive overdose.

morphine [Other names: lanthopine, laudanoisine, laudanum, meconidine, narcotine, protopine.] Considered to be supertoxic, this opiate is the principal alkaloid of opium and is the best-known narcotic painkiller. It is extracted from the unripe seed pods of the opium poppy. It has been used as a painkiller since 1886 and was often found in Chinese opium dens popular during the Victorian era.

A white crystalline alkaloid, it is available in liquid or tablet form and can be ingested or injected. Liquid morphine is a bluish syrup given to cancer patients to treat pain, sometimes mixed with a blue liqueur to strengthen the effects.

Morphine increases the effects of sedatives, painkillers, sleep-inducing drugs, tranquilizers, antidepressants, and other narcotic drugs. It works faster if mixed with alcohol or other solvents. It works by blocking the transmission of pain signals at specific sites in the brain and spinal cord, preventing the perception of pain. Short-term use is not likely to cause dependence, but the euphoric effects of the drug have contributed to its long history as a street drug. Long-term abuse leads to a craving for the drug and a need to have ever-greater amounts. Sudden withdrawal of the drug can cause flu-like symptoms (sweating, shaking, and cramping).

In addition, morphine cannot be used together with a wide range of drugs, including aminophylline, phenytoin, phenobarbital, and sodium bicarbonate.

Symptoms

Symptoms include sleepiness, physical ease, floating sensations, giddiness, unbalanced gait, dizziness, nausea, breathing problems, unconsciousness, and coma. Depressant effects may last longer in those persons with liver or kidney problems. Death from morphine overdose occurs between six and 12 hours after ingestion and is almost always due to respiratory failure. If the victim survives for two days, the prognosis is good.

Treatment

Naloxone is the antidote; recovery can be expected within one to four hours if administered soon after ingestion.

See also HEROIN; NALOXONE; NARCOTICS; OPIUM.

mothballs   See CAMPHOR; NAPHTHALENE.

mother-in-law plant *(Caladium)*   This popular plant is cultivated both outdoors and as an indoor plant and can grow to about 16 inches. It is a deciduous plant with large, oval arrow-shaped leaves that can grow to be 14 inches long and come in a range of colors, including pink, red, white, and green. The plants can be cultivated all year in subtropical gardens and during the summer in temperate zones.

Poisonous part

All parts of the plant are toxic and contain raphides of calcium oxalate.

Symptoms

Ingestion causes pain, swelling, and irritation of the mouth, lips, throat, and the digestive tract, which leads to nausea, vomiting, and diarrhea. Ingestion of a large amount can result in swelling of the tongue and throat, which can obstruct the airway.

Treatment

Pain and swelling subside on their own, but cool liquids and demulcents (such as milk) held in the mouth may help the pain. Painkillers are sometimes given, but the oxalates in this plant are insoluble and therefore do not cause systemic poisoning.

mountain laurel   See LAUREL, MOUNTAIN.

MSG   See MONOSODIUM GLUTAMATE.

multiple chemical sensitivity (MCS)   A physical illness clinical ecologists believe is caused by minute levels of toxic chemicals in the air, water, and food. According to this theory, people with MCS suffer from fatigue, achy muscles, headaches, mental fogginess, and other vague symptoms because of sensitivity to tiny amounts of toxic chemicals in the environment.

While many traditional physicians believe these ills are primarily psychosomatic, others believe there is evidence of a real chemical illness and that it may affect 15 percent of Americans. According to these clinical ecologists, the disease develops in one of two ways: through a slow buildup of chemicals over the years, or from one massive exposure such as an industrial chemical spill.

People are more vulnerable if they have nutritional deficiencies, a family history of allergies, a chronic disease or an infection that has weakened the immune system. Still, experts recommend that health problems must be ruled out before concluding that the environment is to be blamed for illness.

Even physicians who doubt the existence of MCS concede that it can't hurt to pay attention to chemicals and try to avoid overexposure. They recommend the following:

• Store insecticides, paint thinner, and other toxic chemicals in an outside shed or garage; never keep them under the sink where the fumes can leak into the house.

- Choose electric appliances, 100 percent cotton or wool carpets, and furniture made of glass, chrome, or solid wood instead of particleboard. Avoid "no chip" wood finishes that emit formaldehyde.
- Keep gas appliances repaired; replace filters regularly.
- Be cautious with chemicals used often: artists' oils, marking pens, and typewriter correction fluid can be highly toxic.
- Air out the house often, especially when using appliances than burn gas, propane, wood, or kerosene.
- Use your own nontoxic products: use fresh herbs and flowers as air fresheners; dust with pure mineral oil sweetened with drops of lemon; soften fabrics by adding baking soda to rinse water.
- Air dry-cleaned clothes, bedspreads, and drapes outside before bringing them into the house. If dry-cleaned goods have a chemical odor, refuse to accept them until they are properly dried; change cleaners if the problem persists.
- Read and follow labels; wear gloves and open windows when using mildew removers, rug shampoos, or other household chemicals.
- Wash permanent-press clothes and sheets before using, or buy all-natural fibers (wool, cotton, and silk).
- Avoid pesticides.
- Don't smoke. (Cigarette smoke contains 4,700 chemicals, according to the Environmental Protection Agency.)

muscarine   This alkaloid was isolated in 1869 as a minor toxic constituent in the mushroom *Amanita muscaria* (in fresh fungi, it is found in only a concentration of 0.0003 percent). It is found in much larger amounts in many species of *Inocybe* and some species of *Clitocybe* mushrooms. Eating mushrooms that contain muscarine is only rarely fatal; even without treatment, most symptoms fade within a few hours.

Symptoms

Muscarine, like pilocarpine, excites receptors of the parasympathetic and sympathetic nervous systems. Within 15 to 24 hours after ingestion, muscarine poisoning produces profuse sweating and salivation, visual disturbances, nausea, vomiting, abdominal pain, diarrhea, headache, and bronchospasm. Very high doses cause incontinence, slow heartbeat, low blood pressure, and shock.

Treatment

Symptoms will disappear even without treatment in most cases. However, vomiting and gastric lavage may help together with the administration of atropine to suppress toxin symptoms.

See also AMANITA MUSHROOMS; FLY AGARIC; INOCYBE MUSHROOMS; MUSHROOM POISONING; MUSHROOM TOXINS.

muscimol   This water-soluble toxin was first isolated in the early 1960s from the toxic mushrooms *Amanita muscaria* (or fly agaric) and *Amanita pantherina* (panther mushroom). Both muscimol and its metabolic precursor ibotenic acid are believed to be the primary cause for the toxicity of these two mushrooms and a few related species.

Symptoms

Within 20 to 90 minutes after ingestion, muscimol begins to affect the central nervous system, causing drowsiness, stupor, elation, hyperactivity, delirium, confusion, hallucinations, rapid heartbeat, gastroenteritis, and urinary retention.

Treatment

Induce vomiting and perform gastric lavage; administration of physostigmine and diazepam (Valium) may help control symptoms and convulsions. Stimulants are not advised.

See also AMANITA MUSHROOMS; FLY AGARIC; MUSHROOM POISONING; MUSHROOM TOXINS; PANTHER MUSHROOM.

mushroom poisoning   There is a reason for the saying "There are old mushroom hunters, and bold mushroom hunters, but no old bold mushroom hunters." In recent years, cases of mushroom poisoning have been on the increase, attributable to the rise of interest in "natural" foods and to better reporting of cases. At the same time, scientists have been learning more and more about the toxic properties of mushrooms, or "fungus fruit."

Out of the more than 5,000 varieties of mushrooms found in the United States, about 100 are toxic—but most of these cause only mild stomach problems. A few, however, can cause fatal reactions. Most of the toxic symptoms are caused by the gastrointestinal irritants that lead to the vomiting and diarrhea common in mushroom poisoning. In most cases, onset of stomach distress is rapid, but if the onset is delayed past six to 12 hours, the more serious amatoxin or monomethylhydrazine poisoning may be suspected. The stalk and cap of the mushroom that pops up after a spring rain are really the fruit of a vast underground network of microscopic filaments; therefore, picking a mushroom no more harms the plant than plucking an apple from a tree.

But despite the fact that scientists for the past hundred years have been trying to isolate the toxic principles in mushrooms, the exact chemistry behind the deadly poisons in these fungi is still unknown. While most of the species of mushroom are not poisonous, the few toxic ones that do exist are deadly and have been known since ancient times.

Since the first report of mushroom poisoning in 1871, much of the information about poisonous mushrooms is inaccurate—including the persistent belief that there are some ironclad "rules" that can be used to tell the difference between edible and toxic varieties. In fact, there is no rule that applies to all species of mushrooms.

For example, it's not true that a silver spoon or coin put in a pan with cooking mushrooms will turn black if the mushrooms are poisonous. *All* mushrooms will discolor silver in boiling water, if they are rotten, but *no* mushroom (toxic or edible) ever does as long as it is fresh. Toxic mushrooms won't get darker if soaked in water, nor will they get milky if soaked in vinegar.

A mycologist (mushroom expert) is the only one who can reliably detect poisonous mushrooms, and even mycologists make mistakes because the toxicity of mushrooms is complicated. Some are always deadly; others are poisonous at some times

MUSHROOMS GROUPED ACCORDING TO PRIMARY TOXIN

Amatoxins and Phallotoxins (cyclopeptides)

Amanita phalloides	A. tenuifolia
A. verna	Galerina autumnalis
A. virosa	G. marginata
A. bisporigera	G. venenata
A. ocreata	Lepiota helveola
A. suballiacea	Conocybe filaris

Muscimol and Ibotenic Acid

Amanita muscaria	A. cokeri
A. pantherina	A. cothurnata
A. gemmata	A. Strobiliformis

Monomethylhydrazine (gyromitrins)

Gyromitra esculenta	G. brunnea
G. gigas	G. fastigiata
G. ambigua	Paxina
G. infula	Sarcosphaera coronaria
G. caroliniana	

Muscarine

Boletus calopus	I. geophylla
B. luridus	I. lilacina
B. pulcherrimus	I. patouillardii
B. satanas	I. purica
Clitocybe cerrusata	I. rimosus
C. dealbata	Amanita muscaria
C. illudens	A. pantherina
C. riuulosa	
Inocybe fastigiata	

Coprine (and Cyclopropanone)

Coprinus atramentarius
Clitocybe clavipes

Indoles (psilocybin and psilocin)

Psilocybe cubensis	P. silvatica	P. semilanceata
P. caerulescens	Conocybe cyanopus	Stropharis coronilla
P. cyanescens	Gymnopilus aeruginosa	
P. baeocystis	G. spectabilis	
P. fimentaria	G. validipes	
P. mexicana	Panaeolus foenisecii	
P. pelluculosa	P. subbalteatus	

but not others, depending on the stage of growth. And other poisonous mushrooms have never been regarded as toxic simply because no one has ever eaten them yet.

The most common poisonous mushrooms in the United States are those in the genus *Amanita* (including the world's deadliest mushroom, *A. phalloides*); up to 90 percent of those who eat this mushroom will die if untreated.

Unlike most incidents of plant poisonings, which occur primarily in curious children, poisoning from mushrooms is generally found among adults who ingest them as a source of food or for their hallucinogenic effects. While it may be easier to obtain a history of the ingestion, it is usually almost impossible to identify the kind of mushroom eaten. It is possible, however, to identify the type of mushroom by evaluating the kinds of symptoms, since mushrooms produce only a small number of distinct toxic syndromes.

Identification

It's possible to identify the kind of mushroom ingested based on the following questions:

1. When was the mushroom eaten, and how long afterward did the symptoms appear? (When symptoms develop within two hours of ingestion, they are not often severe. Poisonings with a latency period of more than six hours may be severe or life threatening.)
2. What symptoms appeared first? If symptoms appeared quickly, are they primarily

  • nausea and stomach pain with vomiting/ diarrhea?

  • sweating?

  • intoxication or hallucinations but no drowsiness?

  • delirium and sleepiness or coma?

If symptoms were delayed, did they produce

  • a feeling of fullness and severe headache six hours later?

  • vomiting and watery diarrhea about 12 hours after eating?

  • extreme thirst and copious urination three days after eating?

If someone who did not eat mushrooms shows similar symptoms, it's possible the problem is bacterial food poisoning and not mushroom poisoning at all.

Symptoms

In general, symptoms that appear within two hours of eating poisonous mushrooms are rarely severe and require little intervention; symptoms that do not appear until six or more hours later are usually much more severe and can be life threatening. If more than one type of mushroom was eaten, several types of toxicity may occur. However, symptoms that appear after eating mushrooms may not be the result of systemic poisoning from a toxic mushroom. Some people are allergic to mushrooms, and others have a genetic deficiency of enzymes needed to metabolize the unusual sugars found in mushrooms; this

MUSHROOM TOXICITY		
Mushroom	**Toxin**	**Symptoms**
Amanita muscaria, A. pantherina and others	Ibotenic acid, muscimol	Muscle jerks, hallucinations
Amanita phalloides, A. ocreata, A. verna, A. virosa, Lepiota and *Galerina* species	Amatoxins	Vomiting, diarrhea, cramps, liver failure
Clitocybe dealbata, Inocybe species, *C. cerrusata, Omphalotus olearius*	Muscarine	Salivation, sweats, vomiting, diarrhea, miosis
Coprinus, Clitocybe clavipes	Coprine	Reaction with alcohol
Gyromitra (Helvella) esculenta and others	Monomethylhydrazine	Vomiting, diarrhea, weakness, seizures, hepatitis, hemolysis
Psilocybe cubensis and others	Psilocybin	Hallucinations

deficiency causes gas and diarrhea. If alcoholic beverages were drunk within 72 hours of eating mushrooms, extreme nausea, vomiting, and headache could occur as a result of the interference of edible mushrooms with the metabolism of alcohol.

Treatment

If someone becomes sickened and mushroom poisoning is suspected, first find out how many types of mushrooms were eaten, when they were eaten, the symptoms and if anyone else ate them. When determining symptoms, find out which ones appeared first. Gastrointestinal symptoms that appear more than six hours after ingestion are usually caused by a group of mushrooms including the deadly amanitas, or mushrooms containing monomethylhydrazine (including *Gyromitra* mushrooms, or false morels). If the victim has not already vomited, administer syrup of ipecac followed by activated charcoal and a cathartic. If possible, send vomited material, together with any remaining mushrooms, to a mycologist for identification. If ingested mushroom is of the *Amanita* species (except for *A. muscaria* or *A. pantherina*), the victim should be admitted to the hospital to monitor kidney and liver function.

See also AMATOXINS; COPRINE; GYROMITRA; MONO-METHYLHYDRAZINE; MUSCARINE; MUSCIMOL; MUSH-ROOM TOXINS.

mushroom toxins   Any illness due to the ingestion of a toxic mushroom (or toadstool) is known as mycetismus. Many species of wild mushrooms in many genera are poisonous; several of the toxins have been isolated and identified. It is important to remember that mushroom toxins differ among themselves and in the type of intoxication and symptoms they produce.

Poisoning by a mushroom toxin might range from mild symptoms of stomach upset to fatal disturbances of the body's major systems, including brain, heart, liver, and kidneys.

Of the approximately 5,000 different types of mushrooms in the United States, about 100 are poisonous and less than a dozen can be deadly. Amanita mushrooms account for 90 percent of deaths related to mushrooms.

See also AMANITA MUSHROOMS; AMATOXIN; COPRINE; FLY AGARIC; GALERINA MUSHROOMS; GYROMITRA; HALLUCINOGENIC MUSHROOMS; INKY CAP; INOCYBE MUSHROOM; LEPIOTA MUSHROOMS; MONO-METHYLHYDRAZINE; MUSCARINE; MUSCIMOL; MUSH-ROOM POISONING; TURBANTOP.

naloxone   This opioid drug blocks the action of narcotic drugs and reverses breathing difficulty caused by a narcotics overdose. It is also given to newborn babies who are affected by narcotics during childbirth, and to patients who have received high doses of a narcotic drug during surgery. In addition, some reports suggest that naloxone may at least partially reverse the central nervous system and respiratory depression following clonidine and ethanol overdoses.

See also HEROIN; MORPHINE; NARCOTICS; OPIUM.

nanophyetiasis   This type of infestation is caused by eating seafood tainted with worms (*Nanophyetus salmincola* or *N. schikhobalowi*) that are transmitted as a larvae that embeds itself in the flesh of freshwater fish. There have been no reports of massive outbreaks; the only scientific report has been an account of 20 people in Oregon who came down with the disease. However, the condition is endemic in Russia, where the infection rate is reported to be more than 90 percent and growing. North American cases were all associated with raw, smoked, and underprocessed salmon and steelhead.

Symptoms
Diarrhea, usually accompanied by stomach discomfort and nausea; a few people reported weight loss and fatigue.

Diagnosis
The disease is diagnosed by finding the eggs in feces. However, it's hard to tell the difference between these eggs and those of another parasite (*Diphyllobothrium latum*).

Treatment
Treatment with niclosamide or bithionol appears to cure the infection.

naphthalene   More commonly known as mothballs or mothball flakes and contained in toilet bowl cleaners, naphthalene is a white crystalline solid and a constituent of coal tar, which can be poisonous when eaten. In the past, naphthalene has also been used as an antiseptic; however, naphthalene is no longer commonly used because it has been replaced by the far less toxic paradichlorobenzene.

Too often, parents do not realize how toxic mothballs are and leave them out where toddlers can eat them. In addition, naphthalene does not easily dissolve in water and so many remain in clothes or blankets even after washing. It's even more dangerous to store baby clothes in mothballs, since naphthalene is very soluble in oil; the baby oil rubbed on an infant's skin acts as a solvent for the toxic substances in the clothes, which can then be absorbed in the baby's skin. Naphthalene products should never be used with children's clothes and diapers.

Symptoms
Symptoms appear quickly, within five to 20 minutes depending on whether naphthalene was inhaled or eaten. First symptoms are nausea, vomiting, headache, diarrhea, fever, jaundice, and pain while urinating. More serious poisoning causes excitement, coma, and convulsions. Naphthalene causes kidney damage and destroys red blood cells, clumping them together and forcing the hemoglobins out. People with a hereditary deficiency of glucose-6-phosphate dehydrogenase (most often people of Mediterranean descent) are more susceptible to naphthalene poisoning. This same deficiency makes them sensitive to aspirin.

Treatment
There is no specific antidote. If ingested, perform immediate gastric lavage followed by a saline

cathartic; alcohol, milk, oil, or fats should be avoided. Drink plenty of fluids to encourage the production of urine, and administer sodium bicarbonate orally and fluids with furosemide to stop kidney damage. With severe cases of poisoning with central nervous system problems, blood transfusions are given.

See also PARADICHLOROBENZENE.

naproxen (Naprosyn) See NONSTEROIDAL ANTI-INFLAMMATORY DRUGS.

narcissus *(Narcissus)* This extremely toxic plant genus includes about 26 varieties of common flowering plants with hundreds of cultivars; they include popular plants such as the jonquil (*N. jonquilla*) and the daffodil (*N. pseudonarcissus*)—all of which are poisonous. While native to central Europe and North Africa, they are found throughout the United States.

Poisonous part
All parts of these plants—especially the bulbs—are poisonous and contain lycorine and other alkaloids.

Symptoms
Even small amounts of the bulbs can cause poisoning in adults within several hours to a few days, including symptoms of nausea, severe vomiting, diarrhea, and colic. If eaten in large quantities, narcissus can cause convulsions, collapse, paralysis, and death. Mortality is about 30 percent.

Treatment
Gastric lavage and fluid replacement.

narcotics A group of depressants including codeine, opium, morphine, paregoric, and heroin, which are used medicinally to relieve pain, coughing, and vomiting. They require a doctor's prescription, since continued use can lead to dependence or addiction.

Depressants in addition to the above include fentanyl or Sublimaze; the eye drop DFP or diisopropylphosphate; Numorphan (oxymorphone); the painkiller Dilaudid (hydromorphone); the cough suppressant Hycodan or Dicodid; Lorfan (levallorphan); Levo-Dromoran (levorphanol); the painkiller Darvon (propoxyphene); the painkiller Talwin (pentazocine); the muscle relaxant Flexeril (cyclobenzaprine); Demerol (meperidine); and Dolantin (pethidine).

Symptoms
Soon after ingestion, the victim will become mentally stimulated and then quickly drowsy. As the body continues to absorb the narcotic, the victim will experience headache, slow, shallow breathing, and finally unconsciousness and coma.

Treatment
Medical help should be sought immediately. Stimulants, such as strong tea and coffee, will help to keep the victim awake. If the victim is discovered soon after ingestion and is conscious, induce vomiting.

See also CODEINE; HEROIN; HYDROMORPHONE; MORPHINE; OPIUM; OXYMORPHONE.

Nembutal See BARBITURATES.

neostigmine See PARASYMPATHOMIMETIC DRUGS.

neuromuscular blocking agents A group of drugs that paralyze skeletal muscles, used to counteract excessive muscular activity, rigidity, or seizures following overdoses involving stimulants (amphetamines, cocaine, phencyclidine) or strychnine. The drugs include succinylcholine, pancuronium, and vecuronium. They are also used to help paralyze muscles prior to placement of an ototracheal tube.

See also AMPHETAMINES; COCAINE; STRYCHNINE.

neurotoxic shellfish poisoning This type of toxic poisoning is associated with shellfish harvested along the coasts of Florida, North Carolina, and the Gulf of Mexico. The toxin attacks the nervous system and triggers both stomach and neurological problems. Recovery is complete with very few after-effects; no fatalities have been reported.

Symptoms

Symptoms occur within a few minutes to a few hours after eating contaminated shellfish and include tingling and numb lips, tongue and throat, muscular aches, dizziness, reversal of sensations, diarrhea, and vomiting. Symptoms last between a few hours and a few days.

Prevention

Monitoring programs can prevent human intoxication. Consumers should eat shellfish from reportable sources and approved beds only.

neutralizers Rarely used in modern hospitals, neutralizing agents at one time were sometimes employed instead of activated charcoal in certain poisoning cases: mercury and iron poisoning, iodine ingestion, and strychnine, nicotine, and quinine poisoning (see below).

Mercury

Sodium formaldehyde sulfoxylate neutralizes mercuric chloride and other mercury salts to metallic mercury, which cannot be absorbed by the body.

Iron

Gastric lavage with sodium bicarbonate converts the ferrous ion to ferrous carbonate, which is not well absorbed by the body.

Strychnine, nicotine, and quinine

Administer potassium permanganate.

Iodine

Gastric lavage with a solution of starch and water, which is continued until the stomach contents are no longer blue.

See also CHARCOAL, ACTIVATED; IODINE; IRON SUPPLEMENTS; MERCURY; NICOTINE; POTASSIUM PERMANGANATE; QUININE; SODIUM BICARBONATE; STRYCHNINE.

nicotinamide One of the B vitamins used to prevent toxic effects in the brain and endocrine system following the ingestion of the rat poison Vacor.

See also VACOR.

nicotine A plant alkaloid found in several species of tobacco and an extremely fast-acting poison that, when eaten, can cause blood vessels to collapse and the muscles of respiration to fail in much the same way as does curare. While there is no medicinal use for nicotine, some of its derivatives are used as botanic insecticides; in fact, nicotine is the oldest insecticide known.

In those who ingest nicotine by smoking cigarettes or chewing the leaves, repeated small doses soon build up tolerance to the toxins. The primary danger of poisoning lies in the manufacture and use of insecticides containing nicotine.

Toxic doses vary and range from four milligrams to two grams; generally 40 milligrams is considered fatal. Nicotine content in regular cigarettes averages about 15 to 20 milligrams per cigarette; cigars range from 15 to 40 milligrams. Eating tobacco is not generally a serious toxic risk, since the stomach does not absorb nicotine well from cigarettes.

Children may become poisoned with nicotine if they ingest tobacco or drink saliva spit out by a tobacco chewer (often collected in a spittoon or can). Adults may attempt suicide by ingesting nicotine-containing pesticides, or may be poisoned after coming in contact with tobacco while harvesting the plants.

Nicotine chewing gum (Nicorette) has been marketed as an aid for people to stop smoking, but its slow absorption makes nicotine intoxication from this product unlikely.

Symptoms

Nicotine's effects are extremely complex and vary from person to person, depending on the length of time following exposure, the amount of dosage and chronic use. Cigarette tobacco and moist snuff each contain about 1.5 percent nicotine; chewing tobacco contains 2.5 to 8 percent nicotine; nicotine gum contains two milligrams per piece in the United States (although bioavailability is only about 20 to 40 percent of that amount).

Rapid absorption of between two and five milligrams can cause nausea and vomiting, especially in a person unused to nicotine. Absorption of 40 to 60 milligrams in an adult may be lethal, although most smokers get this dose spread throughout the day. In a child, ingestion of one cigarette or three butts may be toxic, although serious poisoning from cigarette ingestion is rare.

Immediately after ingestion, nicotine causes a burning sensation in the mouth, throat, esophagus, and stomach. Once in the bloodstream, whether after inhalation from tobacco smoke or through the mouth from chewing tobacco (or, more recently, in nicotine gum or the nicotine skin patch), the substance acts on the central nervous system until it is eventually broken down by the liver and excreted. It first stimulates, and then depresses, both the brain and spinal cord. It primarily affects the autonomic nervous system, which controls involuntary body activities (such as heart rate). While effects vary from person to person, it can slow the heart rate and cause nausea and vomiting.

In habitual users, however, nicotine increases the heart rate, narrows the blood vessels (thereby raising blood pressure), and stimulates the central nervous system, reducing tiredness and improving concentration. It is uncertain whether the nicotine contained in tobacco products is responsible for coronary heart disease, peripheral vascular disease, and other heart problems.

Extremely large amounts of nicotine can affect breathing in ways similar to that of curare, paralyzing the breathing muscles and causing vomiting, seizures, and death from respiratory arrest only minutes after ingestion.

Treatment

In severe poisonings, artificial respiration and oxygen must be administered, since death occurs from respiratory paralysis. Nicotine is completely eliminated from the body within 16 hours, so victims who can be kept alive for that period may live. Mecamylamine (Inversine) is a specific antagonist of nicotine but is available only in tablets, which are not suitable for a victim who is vomiting, has low blood pressure or is having convulsions. Signs of parasympathetic stimulation (that is, slow heartbeat, salivation, wheezing, etc.) may respond to atropine.

For ingestion: gastric lavage followed by the administration of activated charcoal to absorb excess nicotine; pentobarbital, diazepam, or inhalation anesthesia to control convulsions. For skin contamination: scrub skin with plenty of soap and water and remove contaminated clothing.

See also ALKALOIDS; BOTANIC INSECTICIDES; NICOTINE GUM; NICOTINE PATCH; TOBACCO.

nicotine gum (nicotine polacrilex) Popularly known by its trade name Nicorette, this is a nicotine resin that is used to help people stop smoking. It gradually releases nicotine when chewed. However, chewing too much of the gum will release too much nicotine and cause nausea. For this reason, heart patients, pregnant women, and those with peptic ulcers should not chew the gum.

The gum was designed to be "parked" between cheek and gum, in order to maximize the nicotine's absorption. As the smoker begins to feel comfortable with the smoke-free behaviors, the amount of nicotine is decreased over a six-month period. Lower-strength versions are available without a prescription. A doctor can decide which strength is needed. Drinks will wash the nicotine to the stomach, so it needs to be absorbed by the mouth. Ten to 15 pieces a day is a normal dose.

Symptoms

The same as nicotine overdose.

Treatment

For severe overdose, see Treatment section under NICOTINE.

See also NICOTINE; TOBACCO.

nicotine patch Another innovation in the stop-smoking arsenal, the nicotine patch became available in the United States in 1994. In this form, nicotine is gradually absorbed through the skin as a means to help a smoker stop using cigarettes.

Since the introduction of nicotine gum and the transdermal patch, estimates based on FDA and pharmaceutical industry data indicate that more than 1 million individuals have been successfully treated for nicotine addiction. However, recent research reports indicate that several patients wearing a patch have died from heart attacks because they have continued to smoke.

In 1996, a nicotine nasal spray, and in 1998, a nicotine inhaler, became available by prescription. Various comparisons of the effectiveness of the many nicotine-replacement products show a wide range of results. One study found that 11 percent of people who used a nicotine patch quit smoking, compared to 4.2 percent for those who used a placebo patch. A nonnicotinic medication called bupropion led to an abstinence rate of 30.3 percent after one year compared to a 16.4 percent rate for those using only the patch. A 2008 study found that after six months, 42 percent of those using bupropion alone stopped smoking, compared to a 35 percent rate for those who used both a patch and the drug. Other studies show the nasal spray and nicotine inhalers to be more effective than the patch.

Symptoms

Nicotine acts on the central nervous system until it is eventually broken down by the liver and excreted. It first stimulates, and then depresses, both the brain and spinal cord. It primarily affects the autonomic nervous system, which controls involuntary body activities (such as heart rate). In habitual users nicotine increases the heart rate and narrows the blood vessels (thereby raising blood pressure); it can also cause a heart attack.

Treatment

The best treatment is preventive: *Never smoke cigarettes while wearing a nicotine patch.* In severe cases, artificial respiration and oxygen may need to be administered. Nicotine is completely eliminated from the body within 16 hours, so victims who can be kept alive for that period may live. Mecamylamine (Inversine) is a specific antagonist of nicotine but is available only in tablets, which are not suitable for a victim who is vomiting, has low blood pressure or is having convulsions. Signs of parasympathetic stimulation (that is, slow heartbeat, salivation, wheezing, etc.) may respond to atropine.

See also NICOTINE; NICOTINE GUM; TOBACCO.

nifedipine This substance dilates the arteries and is used to combat severe high blood pressure following overdose of artery-constricting drugs such as phenylpropanolamine, cocaine, amphetamines,

phencyclidine, (PCP) or other stimulants. It is also helpful to counteract peripheral or coronary artery spasms following poisoning by ergot or cocaine.

See also AMPHETAMINES; COCAINE; ERGOT; PHENCYCLIDINE.

nightshade, bittersweet A member of the wide-ranging nightshade family (but a less deadly relative than deadly nightshade), bittersweet nightshade can also have poisonous effects.

Poisonous part

The entire plant contains the toxin atropine and other belladonna alkaloids, including scopolamine, hyoscyamine, hyoscine, and belladonna—but these are concentrated in the roots, leaves, and berries. These alkaloids paralyze the parasympathetic nervous system (which controls the involuntary activities of the organs, glands, blood vessels, and other body tissues). Atropine can directly stimulate the central nervous system and is eliminated almost entirely by the kidneys. Taken internally, as little as 0.1 gram of atropine (one of the alkaloids extracted from nightshade) can cause poisoning.

Symptoms

Symptoms appear between 15 minutes and a few hours after ingestion and include a scratchy or burning sensation in the throat with a loss of voice, rapid pulse, fever, nausea, vomiting, blurred vision, pupil dilation, inability to urinate, difficulty in swallowing, mental confusion, aggressive behavior, reduced secretion of saliva, convulsions, coma, and death. The poison acts by paralyzing the nerve endings of the involuntary muscles. Mild poisoning acts as a euphoric, imparting a feeling of timelessness or giddiness to its victims. Severe poisoning causes blindness, rage, and paralysis of the central nervous system. Coma is followed by death from respiratory failure.

Treatment

Gastric lavage with 4 percent tannic acid solution and vomiting. Pilocarpine or physostigmine may be given for dry mouth and visual disturbances. There is no known antidote. There is risk of heart, kidney, and urinary tract damage if symptoms are prolonged or severe. If treatment is initiated, prognosis is good.

See also ATROPINE; NIGHTSHADE, DEADLY.

nightshade, deadly (*Atropa belladonna* L.) [Other names: anuncena de Mejico, banewort, Barbados lily, belladonna lily, cape belladonna, dwale, English nightshade, lirio, naked lady lily, sleeping nightshade.] Also known as belladonna, deadly nightshade is a powerful drug plant (source of the drug atropine) with a history rich in magic, witchcraft, and murder. It is a member of the Solanaceae family and is one of a group of nightshades.

However, the "true" nightshades contain the poison solanine, and they are closely related—the Jerusalem cherry, the woody nightshade or European bittersweet, and the American, or black, nightshade. Deadly nightshade (the belladonna plant) belongs to another branch of the Solanaceae, and its chief poison is atropine.

Atropine and solanine have different effects on the body, so that reporting a poisoning with "nightshade" is not specific enough to determine correct treatment.

Native to Eurasia and North Africa, this five-foot, shrublike perennial herb is found in meadows, near old buildings, and in shady, marshy places in North America and is cultivated commercially in Europe for medicinal purposes. While its fresh leaves have an unpleasant smell when crushed, the dried leaves are odorless; both have a bitter taste. Its alternate ovate leaves grow on multibranched stems, with glossy black, round berries and bellshaped flowers that have an intensely sweet smell from July to September. A horizontal, underground, thickened plant stem produces shoots above and roots below and bears buds, nodes, and scalelike leaves.

The name "belladonna" comes from the Italian, meaning "beautiful woman," a reference to its use during the Renaissance, when women used an extract to make their complexions luminous and to dilate their pupils for a wide-eyed, beautiful look. Rouge was also made from the berries. Its generic name *Atropa* comes from the Greeks, whose myth holds that when the thread of life was played out by the three Fates, Atropos cut it.

According to astrologists, deadly nightshade is ruled by Hecate and is popular in witchcraft as a shape changer, a flying ointment, and a major hallucinogen. (Of 16 recipes for flying ointments, eight call for deadly nightshade.) It is also said that deadly nightshade can change into a beautiful enchantress on Walpurgis Night, the witches' sabbath.

There is also a place for nightshade in literature; it is believed Shakespeare intended it as the poison that Juliet takes in *Romeo and Juliet* so she will seem dead but is really just sleeping.

Poisonous part

A single berry can be fatal, and the entire plant contains the toxin atropine and other belladonna alkaloids, including scopolamine, hyoscyamine, hyoscine, and belladonna—but these are concentrated in the roots, leaves, and berries. These alkaloids paralyze the parasympathetic nervous system (which controls the involuntary activities of the organs, glands, blood vessels, and other body tissues). Atropine can directly stimulate the central nervous system and is eliminated almost entirely by the kidneys.

Taken internally, as little as 0.1 gram of atropine (one of the alkaloids extracted from nightshade) can cause poisoning. The root is the most poisonous part, but the entire plant is deadly. A careful dose of deadly nightshade is antispasmodic, is a sedative and a diuretic and induces sweating; it also inhibits mucus and glandular secretions. At certain doses, the drug relieves pain and stimulates the central nervous system; it is classified as a narcotic. Its derivative atropine is considered an important drug today as an antidote for some types of nerve gas, and also as an antidote for depressant poisons such as muscarine, opium, and chloral hydrate. Atropine is also an antispasmodic to treat gastritis, pancreatitis, and chronic urethritis. Nightshade's leaves provide isolated compounds including hyoscyamine and scopolamine, and it was once used in ophthalmology for pupil dilation, although it has generally been replaced today by other chemicals.

The plant is often eaten by rabbits, which can then pass the poison on to anyone who eats the affected meat.

Symptoms

Symptoms appear between 15 minutes and a few hours after ingestion and include a scratchy or burning sensation in the throat with a loss of voice, rapid pulse, fever, nausea, vomiting, blurred vision, pupil dilation, inability to urinate, difficulty in swallowing, mental confusion, aggressive behavior, reduced secretion of saliva, convulsions, coma, and death. The poison acts by paralyzing the nerve endings of the involuntary muscles. Mild poisoning acts as a euphoric, imparting a feeling of timelessness or giddiness to its victims. Severe poisoning causes blindness, rage, and paralysis of the central nervous system. Coma is followed by death from respiratory failure.

Treatment

Gastric lavage with 4 percent tannic acid solution and vomiting. Pilocarpine or physostigmine may be given for dry mouth and visual disturbances. There is no known antidote for belladonna poisoning, and because the poison breaks down very slowly in the body, it is often impossible to save the victim. There is risk of heart, kidney, and urinary tract damage if symptoms are prolonged or severe, and poisoning can be quickly fatal if treatment is not initiated. If treatment is initiated, prognosis is good.

See also ATROPINE; NIGHTSHADE, BITTERSWEET; SOLANINE.

nightshade, yellow *(Urechites lutea)* This woody vine is found in Florida, the Bahamas, and the Greater and Lesser Antilles south to St. Vincent. It has a milky sap and long, narrow leaves with yellow flower clusters. The fruit is contained in woody pods that can grow to 8 inches, containing winged seeds.

Poisonous part

The leaves of the yellow nightshade are poisonous, containing urechitoxin, a cardiac glycoside.

Symptoms

Symptoms appear some time after ingestion, depending on the amount of material eaten. They include pain in the mouth; nausea and vomiting; abdominal pain; cramps and diarrhea; and heart problems (conduction defects and slow heartbeat).

Treatment

Gastric lavage followed by activated charcoal and saline cathartics. For heart problems, atropine, and phenytoin.

See also CARDIAC GLYCOSIDES; NIGHTSHADE, BITTERSWEET; NIGHTSHADE, DEADLY.

nitrogen oxides Nitric oxide and nitrogen dioxide are dangerous chemical gases released during a variety of chemical and industrial processes, including electric arc welding, electroplating, and engraving. The oxides are found in engine exhaust, and they are produced when stored grain with a high nitrite content ferments in storage bins. Nitrogen dioxide is a colorless gas, arising from unvented gas stoves, that causes respiratory problems in children.

Slow accumulation and hydration to nitric acid in the alveoli cause delayed onset of chemical pneumonitis. Because nitrogen oxides do not dissolve well in water, there is very little upper respiratory irritation at low levels of exposure, and prolonged contact may occur with only a mild cough or nausea. However, with more concentrated exposures, upper respiratory symptoms such as burning eyes, sore throat, and painful cough may be noted.

Symptoms

After exposure, there may be a delay of up to 24 hours before chemical pneumonia may occur, with cough and pulmonary edema; following recovery there may be permanent restrictive and obstructive lung disease because of bronchiolar damage.

Treatment

Administration of corticosteroids is the treatment of choice by many toxicologists, but there is no convincing evidence that this will improve the chances of avoiding chemical pneumonia or lung damage. Remove the victim from exposure and give oxygen; observe closely for signs of upper airway obstruction for at least 24 hours after exposure. Remove contaminated clothing and flush exposed skin with water; irrigate exposed eyes with saline.

nitroglycerin (glyceryl trinitrate) A drug used to lower blood pressure and dilate coronary vessels; when taken with alcohol, it can cause a sharp drop in blood pressure. It is available in spray or tablet form and can be ingested, injected, inhaled, or absorbed. Nitroglycerin is also given to treat coronary spasm in adults suffering from ergot poisoning.

Symptoms
Immediately after ingestion the drug begins to dilate blood vessels throughout the body; overdose causes headache, flushing of skin, vomiting, dizziness, collapse, low blood pressure, coma, and respiratory paralysis.

Treatment
Induce vomiting with syrup of ipecac followed by activated charcoal.

See also ERGOT.

nitroprusside Sodium nitroprusside is a drug that dilates blood vessels typically given to treat high blood pressure and heart failure and to induce low blood pressure for certain operations. Poisoning may occur with one single large overdose or with prolonged use. It is also used in the treatment of stimulant or monoamine oxidase (MAO) inhibitor overdose.

Poisonous part
Nitroprusside releases free cyanide; acute cyanide poisoning may be produced with a high-dose infusion of nitroprusside.

Symptoms
The most common symptom is a rapid fall in blood pressure. Cyanide poisoning includes symptoms of headache, hyperventilation, muscle spasms, anxiety, agitation, seizures, and metabolic acidosis.

Treatment
In the case of cyanide poisoning, administer sodium thiosulfate; sodium nitrite may worsen low blood pressure and is not indicated. Continue to treat symptoms; hemodialysis may help victims with kidney problems.

See also CYANIDE; MONOAMINE OXIDASE (MAO) INHIBITORS.

nitrous oxide Also known as "laughing gas" widely used by dentists and available on college campuses, nitrous oxide is a general anesthetic and is used in a wide variety of commercial products, including whipped cream and cooking oil sprays.

Discovered in 1776, it was not used as an anesthetic until 23 years later; it was not widely used until 1860. It was, however, popular at parties; Sir Humphry Davy, the first person to synthesize the gas, enjoyed nitrous oxide parties as did the poets Samuel Coleridge and Robert Southey, and Peter Roget, author of *Roget's Thesaurus.* Reportedly, students in the early 19th century used nitrous oxide for recreational purposes, and one student actually quit medical school and began selling the stuff for 25¢ per dose.

However, this nonflammable, nearly odorless gas does not produce a complete anesthesia at safe levels and is therefore used as a painkiller or together with stronger anesthetic agents. It is often abused for the euphoria it produces and is easily available on the street.

Poisonous part
Nitrous oxide depresses the central nervous system and, when used without enough oxygen, can be fatal.

Symptoms
If used improperly (that is, without sufficient oxygen), nitrous oxide can cause irregular heart patterns, brain damage, death, headache, cerebral edema, and permanent mental deficiency. Symptoms appear within a few seconds to several minutes.

Treatment
There is no specific antidote. Administer oxygen; give symptomatic treatment. Chronic symptoms should disappear between two and three months after exposure has ended.

See also ANESTHETICS, GASEOUS/VOLATILE.

nonsteroidal anti-inflammatory drugs (NSAIDs) This is a group of chemically diverse drugs widely used for the treatment of pain and inflammation. On their own, anti-inflammatory drugs are not very toxic, but victims with gastrointestinal tract disease, peptic ulcers, or poor heart function and those on anticoagulant drugs should avoid them. Inflammation results in an increased blood flow, which in turn produces swelling, redness, pain, and heat. Inflammation is one of the body's defense mechanisms in response to infection and certain chronic diseases such as rheumatoid arthritis.

NSAIDs include ibuprofen (Motrin, Rufen, Advil, Haltrain, Medipren, Nuprin), fenoprofen (Nalfon), meclofenamate (Meclomen), naproxen (Anaprox, Naprosyn), sulindac (Clinoril), indomethacin (Indocin), tolmetin (Tolectin), mefanamic acid, piroxicam (Feldene), oxyphenbutazone, and phenylbutazone.

None of these should be taken with other nonsteroid analgesics or with warfarin or other oral anticoagulants, because bleeding time may be prolonged while on anti-inflammatory pain relievers. Antacids, however, may sometimes reduce the effects of an anti-inflammatory drug.

Symptoms

While an overdose of most of the NSAIDs causes little toxicity beyond stomach pain, there are a few that do produce severe toxicity: oxyphenbutazone, phenylbutazone, mefenamic acid, piroxicam, and diflunisal. In general, symptoms appear after ingesting more than five to 10 times the therapeutic dose.

If a person is allergic to aspirin or other nonsteroid analgesic drugs, using another anti-inflammatory medicine could be fatal. Anti-inflammatory drugs become toxic when given to those with kidney problems, since the kidneys can't cleanse the blood. Overdose causes kidney failure and severe liver reactions, including fatal jaundice.

Normally NSAID overdose produces mild stomach upset, with nausea and vomiting plus abdominal pain. Occasionally, other symptoms might include sleepiness, lethargy, nystagmus (an involuntary oscillation of the eyeball), tinnitus (ringing in the ears), and disorientation. However, with the more toxic drugs listed above and significant overdose of ibuprofen (in excess of 3,200 mg per day), symptoms may include seizures, coma, metabolic acidosis, kidney and liver failure, and cardiorespiratory arrest. Diflunisal overdose resembles salicylate poisoning.

Treatment

There is no antidote. Maintain symptomatic treatment together with antacids for mild stomach problems; perform gastric lavage, followed by the administration of activated charcoal and a cathartic. Research suggests charcoal hemoperfusion may help in the treatment of phenylbutazone overdose, although it has not been proven.

Norwalk virus The most common cause of viral contamination in shellfish is the Norwalk virus, which can cause food poisoning when raw or improperly cooked food has been in contact with water contaminated by human excrement. The disease is mild and self-limiting and usually lasts for one or two days. Between July 1997 and June 2000, the Centers for Disease Control and Prevention (CDC) received 232 reports of norovirus outbreaks, 57 percent of which were foodborne, 16 percent were due to person-to-person contact, 3 percent were waterborne, and 23 percent were of unknown origin. The CDC estimates that 23 million cases of acute gastroenteritis are caused by norovirus infection.

Most foodborne outbreaks of the virus are likely to arise through direct contamination of food by a food handler immediately before it is consumed. Eating raw or poorly steamed clams and oysters also poses a high risk of infection. Outbreaks of gastroenteritis have been associated with oysters from contaminated waters as well. Other foods, including salads and raspberries, have been contaminated and their consumption has resulted in widespread illness.

Symptoms

Symptoms begin one to two days after eating contaminated food and include fever, weakness, appetite loss, headache, diarrhea, nausea and vomiting, and stomach pain. Dehydration is the most common complication and can be especially dangerous for young children and the elderly. Severe illness is very rare.

Treatment

Symptomatic; replace fluids and correct electrolyte disturbances using oral and intravenous fluids.

Prevention

Raw shellfish should be cooked for at least four minutes at 194°F. Patients with diarrhea or vomiting should not prepare food.

nutmeg *(Myristica fragrans)*　In small quantities this common spice is edible, but in large doses it can be fatal. Produced from the dried seeds of the nutmeg tree, it is found in the South Pacific and the East Indies. Mace, another popular spice and the extract used as a spray to discourage attackers, is also obtained from this tree.

Nutmeg has been used since the seventh century A.D. to treat asthma and fever. It takes up to three whole nutmegs or up to 15 g of the grated spice to become intoxicated.

Symptoms

Symptoms appear within two to six hours after ingestion and include sedation, euphoria, and hallucinations, which can last up to two days. The stimulation of the central nervous system may be accompanied by tachycardia, skin flushing, decreased salivation, and delirium, with nausea, vomiting, and abdominal cramps. Other symptoms, much like those of intoxication with PCP, can include belligerent behavior and hyperactivity. Occasionally, complications can lead to coma, shock, and death. In very high doses, nutmeg can cause liver damage and death.

Treatment

Gastric lavage; supportive treatment including a cathartic. Administer barbiturates or diazepam to control convulsions.

nux-vomica *(Strychnos nux-vomica)* **[Other names: strychnine.]**　Found in India and Hawaii, this "dog button plant" is actually a small tree, with oval leaves and yellow to white clusters of flowers. Its small, attractive fruit resembles a mandarin or Chinese orange and looks tempting to eat; the fruit contains seeds that look like gray velvet buttons.

Poisonous part

The entire tree contains strychnine, but the seeds contain the greatest concentration of the poison. The blossoms, which smell of curry powder, can be mistaken by a child as edible and are therefore a potential cause of poisoning.

Symptoms

Extreme irritability and restlessness followed by exhaustion, sweating, muscular rigidity, respiratory problems, and death. In severe cases, there are often generalized spasms that last from a few seconds to several minutes and are caused by external sensory stimuli. Metabolic acidosis may also appear.

Treatment

Establish an airway, provide oxygen if needed; convulsions may call for a general anesthetic and muscle relaxant; reduce fever and correct acidosis with intravenous sodium bicarbonate.

See also STRYCHNINE.

NONSTEROIDAL ANTI-INFLAMMATORY DRUGS		
Drug	Usual Daily Dose (adult)	Maximum Recommended Daily Dose (adult)
fenoprofen	900–2,400 mg	3,200 mg
ibuprofen	900–2,400 mg	2,400 mg
indomethacin	50–150 mg	200 mg
meclofenamate	200–400 mg	400 mg
mefenamic	1,000 mg	1,000 mg
naproxen	500–1,000 mg	1,250 mg
piroxicam	20 mg	20 mg
sulindac	300–400 mg	400 mg
tolmetin	1,200–1,800 mg	2,000 mg

octopus, blue-ringed *(Hapalochlaena maculosa)*
The only poisonous octopus, this small, harmless-looking marine animal seems playful and cute, but its bite can be fatal. The octopus is brown and speckled, with blue bands around its tentacles that glow just before the poison is released. Just 4 inches long, this unique octopod is usually found in shallow waters around the coast of Australia and can be deadly if provoked. It feeds on mollusks and crabs with its strong beak and can commonly be found under rocks at low tide.

Normally, both males and females are equally toxic, but when the female blue-ring begins brooding her eggs, her venom becomes even more potent. However, like most other female octopuses, she stops eating once she deposits her eggs and, soon after they hatch, she dies.

A relative, the Australian spotted octopus *(H. lunulata)*, lives near Queensland, New South Wales, Sydney, and Victoria, in the Indian Ocean, and Japan. Another relative, almost as deadly, is the North American west coast octopus *(Octopus apollyon)*, found from Alaska to Baja California.

Symptoms

The bite of the blue-ringed octopus is often not even noticed and usually occurs when the creature is picked up or played with, as it is generally shy and stays away from humans. Immediately after the bite, the poison begins to affect the central nervous system, causing severe pain and paralyzing muscles of the entire body until breathing stops. Its poison can kill in minutes.

Treatment

Immediately after the bite, it is important to maintain breathing through mouth-to-mouth resuscitation, since death usually occurs as a result of the neuromuscular poisons.

oleander *(Nerium oleander)*   Also known as Jericho rose, this extremely deadly poisonous plant is a native of Asia and is widely cultivated in the United States as an ornamental shrub and houseplant. It is widely planted in the South and Southwest because of its beautiful flowers and is widely found in the South planted along driveways and property lines as a colorful hedging. This plant's toxic reputation has been known since ancient times, although the general population today may not be aware of its deadly properties.

Oleander is a fragrant evergreen shrub with white, yellow, pink, or red blossoms and narrow leathery leaves that can reach 10 inches. Winged seeds are borne in long, narrow capsules.

Poisonous part

All parts of the oleander plant are poisonous; one leaf can kill an adult. Even the nectar from the flower, honey from the pollen, the smoke from the burning plant, and the water in which flowers are placed are poisonous. The clear, gummy sap contains cardiac glycosides, oldendrin and nerioside, which stop the heart. Serious poisoning cases have been reported from using oleander twigs to roast meat; children can be poisoned by chewing on a single leaf or flower.

Symptoms

Onset of symptoms may be immediate: pain in the mouth and throat, nausea, severe vomiting, stomach pain, bloody diarrhea, dizziness, altered state of consciousness, slow or irregular heartbeat, dilated pupils, drowsiness, slow respiration, coma, and death.

Treatment

Prompt gastric lavage is vital, together with cardiac depressants to control heart rhythm. The preferred antidote is dipotassium instead of calcium EDTA, since dipotassium chelates calcium in the body. Activated charcoal may be given later. Treatment is similar to that for digitalis poisoning.

See also CARDIAC GLYCOSIDES; FOXGLOVE.

oleander, yellow *(Thevetia peruviana)* While its action is the same as that of oleander and it is just as poisonous, its sap is milky. Growing to 20 feet tall, with leaves very similar to those of oleander, this plant has flowers that are yellow with a hint of peach. The small oval fruit contains up to four flat seeds. Yellow oleander is found in the southwestern United States, Florida, the West Indies, Hawaii, and Guam.

Poisonous part

All parts of the oleander plant are poisonous— especially its seeds, which contain a glycoside similar to digitalis.

Symptoms

Onset of symptoms may be immediate or appear later, depending on the amount of toxin ingested: nausea, severe vomiting, stomach pain, bloody diarrhea, dizziness, altered state of consciousness, slow or irregular heartbeat, dilated pupils, drowsiness, and slow respirations.

Treatment

Prompt gastric lavage is vital, followed by activated charcoal, together with cardiac depressants to control heart rhythm. Treatment is similar to that for digitalis poisoning.

See also CARDIAC GLYCOSIDES; FOXGLOVE.

olestra A fat-based substitute for conventional fats used in certain snack foods that, because of its unique chemical composition, adds no fat or calories to food. Potato chips, crackers, tortilla chips, or other snacks made with olestra (Olean) are lower in fat and calories than snacks made with traditional fats.

The U.S. Food and Drug Administration (FDA) found that olestra may cause abdominal cramping and loose stools in some people and that it inhibits the body's absorption of certain fat-soluble vitamins and nutrients. Products with olestra must carry a label stating that olestra is present and that the fat substitute "may cause abdominal cramping and loose stools. Olestra inhibits the absorption of some vitamins and other nutrients. Vitamins A, D, E and K have been added."

The two main producers of olestra-containing chips, Procter and Gamble and Frito-Lay, asked the FDA to drop its requirement for a warning notice on their products, stating that there was no proof olestra caused the symptoms reported. However, more than 20,000 consumers had filed complaints as of 2004, saying that olestra had caused problems ranging from gas to bloody stools to cramps so severe that they had to be treated in an emergency room, according to reports by the Center for Science in the Public Interest. In 2002, Procter and Gamble sold their factory in Cincinnati that produced olestra.

In 2003, researchers reported two cases of severe gastrointestinal conditions that developed in previously healthy children, which appear to have been caused by use of olestra. In one, an 11-year-old girl developed cramps, flatulence, and foul-smelling diarrhea over two weeks while eating olestra chips. Although these symptoms diminished when she stopped eating the chips, she then developed rectal bleeding and was found to have ulcerative colitis. In a 13-year-old boy, consumption of olestra chips appeared to be the cause of his constipation and abdominal distention, which then escalated into severe back pain, explosive diarrhea, gas, and abdominal cramps. After the boy lost 23 pounds within a few months, most of his colon was removed.

opium *(Papaver somniferum)* This sticky substance is found in the fruit and juices of the opium poppy, which grows throughout Europe, Asia, and the tropics and can be combined with other drugs to form laudanum, paragoric, and other medications.

It has been used in the Orient since 200 B.C., when it was mentioned in the writings of Theophrastus, a Greek philosopher who studied under Aristotle. At that time, opium was given through punctures in the skin or inhaled as a vapor into the nose and mouth, where it unpredictably produced either analgesia or death. In the second century A.D., the Greek physician Galen was treating his patients with opium, and in 700 years it had spread to Arabia.

In the 16th century, physicians figured out how to create laudanum from opium, but its use gradually evolved to include recreational abuse, and by the late 1600s opium smoking had spread everywhere. Opium was introduced as a medicine in Britain in 1680 by Thomas Syndenham, an English physician who proclaimed that opium was "universal and efficacious."

By 1729, however, its negative side was recognized in Asia, and opium smoking was outlawed in China and its import from India banned. Unfortunately, the British East India Company (which imported the drug) refused to stop and smuggled the drug into China—leading to the so-called opium wars between Great Britain and China in 1839 and again in 1856.

Opium's use reached a peak in popularity during Victorian times, when cities were honeycombed with opium dens and physicians prescribed laudanum for a variety of "female problems" (cramps, menstrual distress, etc.). Its use spread to the United States with the thousands of Chinese laborers imported to help build the western railroads in the middle of the 19th century.

Today, the extraction of morphine and the development of synthetic narcotics have rendered opium obsolete, and it is considered an old-fashioned remedy. It is used to treat infants who are born addicted because of their mothers' abuse of narcotics, usually in the form of paregoric, a mixture of opium, camphor, benzoic acid, and alcohol. Opium is classified as a Schedule II or III drug depending on its form.

Symptoms

Opium, which contains codeine, morphine, thebaine, papaverine, and narcotine, is a central nervous system depressant that restricts pupil size, slows breathing, and causes nausea, vomiting, constipation, weak pulse, low blood pressure, dehydration, and euphoria followed by cardiovascular depression, unresponsiveness, coma, respiratory failure, and death within two to three hours of ingestion of a large dose.

Treatment

Gastric lavage followed by activated charcoal and cathartics, with the administration of naloxone and other supportive and symptomatic treatment.

See also CODEINE; LAUDANUM; MORPHINE.

oral contraceptives   See BIRTH CONTROL PILLS.

organophosphate insecticides   These extremely potent insecticides interfere with nerve signal transmission and, if ingested, can cause serious systemic poisoning and death. The most common organophosphate insecticide is parathion. An outgrowth of nerve gas research done in Germany during the 1930s, these insecticides are often used by commercial growers to control insect pests and are the most common sources of insecticide poisoning in humans. The Environmental Protection Agency has reported that more than 80 percent of all pesticide poisoning hospitalizations were caused by the organophosphates, mostly involving children, laborers, and farmers.

Organophosphate insecticides like malathion and diazanon are also used by home gardeners to control spider mites, aphids, mealy bugs, and other pests. They continue to be popular because they are effective and don't remain in body tissues or the environment, due to their unstable chemical structure that disintegrates into harmless radicals within days of application. The organophosphates have largely replaced banned DDT as an agricultural insecticide.

Still, the use of organophosphate pesticides can result in a buildup of residue on leaves and stems and—if used inside the home—can result in the release of noxious vapor into the air. Individual organophosphates vary widely in their toxicity; probably the most dangerous is TEPP (tetraethylpyrophosphate), the oldest known organophosphate; malathion lies at the other end of the spectrum as the least toxic of the group.

The organophosphates interfere with the enzyme cholinesterase, which helps to regulate the amount of acetylcholine in the body; this causes a buildup of acetylcholine, which interferes with the central nervous system and the parasympathetic nervous system.

Toxic levels of organophosphates occur in children who ingest pesticides or animal flea and tick killers; they also occur in agricultural exposure by farm workers and suicide attempts (the largest number of cases).

For those occupations involving exposure to organophosphates, such as factory workers producing lubricants, fire retardants, and pesticides, it should be understood that these compounds are highly toxic and can penetrate the skin without producing sensations and can be fatal. These compounds are being investigated for delayed neurotoxicity.

Symptoms

Symptoms usually appear within 24 hours of exposure but vary according to the specific chemical, exposure and type of contamination. At first, symptoms include headache, cramps, vomiting, diarrhea, dizziness, weakness, sweating, and salivation. In cases of severe poisoning, symptoms include coma, pulmonary edema, psychosis, convulsions, bradycardia, cyanosis, twitching, and paralysis. Death usually occurs within 24 hours after complications occur in cases that have not been treated, or within 10 days in treated cases.

Treatment

Remove all contaminated clothes, wash thoroughly with soap followed by a second wash with alcohol. Administer syrup of ipecac (if victim is fully alert) and perform gastric lavage. Atropine is the antidote for organophosphate poisoning, with the possible administration of pralidoxime.

See also DDT; MALATHION; TEPP.

oven cleaner   See ALKALINE CORROSIVES.

oxalates   A class of compounds related to oxalic acid, named after the wood sorrel (Oxalidaceae) family, in which it was first identified. Oxalate salts and oxalic acid are found in philodendron, dieffenbachia, and other plants and can be very irritating to the skin and mucous membranes. In severe cases, exposure to calcium oxalate can cause the throat to swell shut, resulting in suffocation. In addition, oxalic acid and many of the oxalate salts can become concentrated in the kidneys and cause systemic poisoning.

See also DIEFFENBACHIA; PHILODENDRON.

oxycodone   A semisynthetic derivative of codeine marketed in the United States in liquid, tablet, extended-release tablet, capsule, and concentrated solution form. OxyContin is perhaps the most well-known form of this narcotic. Oxycodone is also an ingredient in many combination products, appearing with acetaminophen (Endocet, Percocet, and others), aspirin (Endodan, Percodan, Roxiprin, and others), and ibuprofen (Combunox). Oxycodone is a Schedule II drug (drug with high potential for abuse) capable of inducing a morphine-like dependence stronger than that associated with codeine. It has about the same painkilling ability as morphine when injected, and it retains half of its effectiveness when given by mouth.

Symptoms

Respiratory depression, stupor, cold and clammy skin, slow heartbeat, and low blood pressure. More severe overdoses can lead to apnea, circulatory collapse, coma, cardiac arrest, and death.

Treatment

The antidote is naloxone. Do not induce vomiting. Gastric lavage may be effective even after several hours following ingestion; administer activated charcoal and a saline cathartic. Give supportive and symptomatic treatment; seizures may be controlled with intravenous diazepam (Valium).

See also CODEINE; MORPHINE; NALOXONE; NARCOTICS; PERCODAN.

oxygen   This colorless, odorless gas is essential for all forms of life on earth, because it is necessary for the metabolic burning of foods to produce energy (aerobic metabolism). Oxygen is also used as a treatment following inhalation of toxic gases; 100 percent oxygen is indicated for carbon monoxide poisoning; hyperbaric oxygen (100 percent oxygen delivered to the victim in a pressurized chamber) is believed by some experts to more rapidly improve recovery from carbon monoxide poisoning.

See also CARBON MONOXIDE POISONING.

oxymorphone A semisynthetic derivative of oxycodone and a narcotic painkiller, oxymorphone has less of a depressing effect on the cough reflex; it is therefore used primarily as a painkiller for postsurgical patients. Reported to be more than 10 times stronger than morphine and almost twice as toxic, it is equally addictive.

Symptoms

Respiratory depression, stupor, cold and clammy skin, slow heartbeat, and low blood pressure. More severe overdoses can lead to apnea, circulatory collapse, coma, cardiac arrest, and death.

Treatment

The antidote is naloxone. Do not induce vomiting. Gastric lavage may be effective even after several hours following ingestion; administer activated charcoal and a saline cathartic. Give supportive and symptomatic treatment; seizures may be controlled with intravenous diazepam (Valium).

See also MORPHINE; NALOXONE; NARCOTICS; OXYCODONE.

paint removers   See HYDROCARBON.

paint thinner   See PETROLEUM DISTILLATES.

panther mushroom *(Amanita pantherina)*   Often confused with its close relative, fly agaric, the panther mushroom is a relatively small, squat plant with a cap surface colored from yellow to purple-brown and covered with white warts. Raised in the United States, it is found in spring and fall in conifer woods west of the Cascade Mountains in Oregon and Washington.

Poisonous part
Muscimol is a water-soluble toxin first isolated in the early 1960s from both the fly agaric and the panther mushroom. Both muscimol and its metabolic precursor, ibotenic acid, are believed to be the primary cause for the toxicity of these two mushrooms and a few related species.

Symptoms
Deaths from eating the panther mushroom have occasionally been reported in the United States. Within 20 to 90 minutes after ingestion, muscimol begins to affect the central nervous system, causing drowsiness, stupor, elation, hyperactivity, delirium, confusion, hallucinations, heartbeat problems, gastroenteritis, urinary retention, blurred vision, watery diarrhea, and convulsions.

Treatment
Induce vomiting and perform gastric lavage; administration of physostigmine and diazepam (Valium) may help control symptoms and convulsions. Stimulants are not advised.

See also AMANITA MUSHROOMS; FLY AGARIC; MUSCIMOL; MUSHROOM POISONING; MUSHROOM TOXINS.

paradichlorobenzene   One of two common ingredients in mothballs and toilet bowl cleaners (the other is naphthalene), this chemical has a pungent odor but is far less toxic than naphthalene. However, ingestion of large amounts can still cause stomach upset and central nervous system stimulation. Up to 20 grams have been well tolerated by adults.

Symptoms
Nausea and vomiting very soon after ingestion.

Treatment
There is no specific antidote. Administer activated charcoal and a cathartic. Treat coma or seizures if they occur.

See also NAPHTHALENE.

paralytic shellfish poisoning (PSP)   The most serious of all four forms of shellfish poisoning caused by toxic forms of plankton that produce a deadly neurotoxin (saxitoxin). Most cases of PSP have occurred when people ate raw tainted shellfish, although cooking will not destroy the toxin.

An incidence of PSP was recorded as early as 1689, and further outbreaks have been recorded many times since then. Traditionally, it has been considered a danger only to shellfish harvested in cold water, but the rate of incidence in tropical areas has been increasing. Oysters, clams, cockles and mussels are particularly prone to contamination because of their metabolic system, which pumps water across the gills to isolate plankton for their food. Crustacean shellfish (such as lobsters) only very rarely transmit PSP. In mussel, toxins are concentrated in the digestive glands and toxicity is usually lost within weeks, but the Alaskan butter clam can remain toxic for up to two years. However, the part of the mollusk that humans generally eat—the white meat, without the digestive glands—stores fairly small amounts of toxin.

Symptoms

Signs of shellfish poisoning develop within five to 30 minutes after eating contaminated crabs, clams, or mussels. Symptoms include gradual paralysis and trembling, with nausea, vomiting, and diarrhea. Later on, there may be shortness of breath, dry mouth, choking feeling, confused or slurred speech, and lack of coordination. Eating even a tiny amount of contaminated shellfish can be fatal, and survival usually depends on how much has been consumed.

Treatment

There is no known antidote for shellfish poisoning caused by saxitoxin, and no drug has proven effective, so treatment is supportive for infected patients. CPR may be needed as first aid. If the victim survives the first 12 hours, prognosis for complete recovery (within a few days to two weeks) is good; however, between 8 and 23 percent of PSP poisonings are fatal.

Prevention

You can't tell just by looking at the water whether toxic plankton are present. If you're not sure if the seafood you're eating is toxin-free, avoid eating it. To prevent outbreaks, samples of susceptible shellfish are tested for toxin by state health departments during certain times of the year. If contamination is found, affected growing areas are quarantined, and sale of shellfish prohibited. Warning signs are posted in shellfish growing areas, on beaches, and in the news. Fish and shellfish sold for human consumption must meet Food and Drug Administration standards of less than 80 micrograms of PSP toxin per 100 grams of shellfish tissue. You can't eliminate PSP from shellfish by cooking or freezing; even when pressure-cooked at 250°F for 15 minutes, it remains toxic.

Paraquat This powerful defoliant is not generally available on store shelves, as it can be toxic if inhaled, absorbed through the skin or ingested. Diquat, which is only half as toxic as Paraquat, is used much more widely as a defoliant; the two are contained together in a 2.5 percent granular formulation known as Weedol.

Solutions available for home use are generally extremely dilute (0.2 percent), but the commercial varieties may contain up to 21 percent Paraquat.

Symptoms

Appearing two to five days after ingestion, symptoms include burning mouth and throat, vomiting, abdominal pain, swelling, diarrhea, and fever. This is followed by liver and kidney damage and then respiratory problems, cyanosis, and fatal lung deterioration. Ingestion of as little as two to four grams (or 10 to 20 milliliters of concentrated 20 percent solution) has been fatal. Food in the stomach may bind Paraquat, preventing its absorption and reducing its toxicity.

Poisoning with Diquat may cause corrosive injury, with severe gastroenteritis, massive fluid loss, and kidney failure.

Treatment

There is no specific antidote. Induce vomiting with syrup of ipecac if gastric lavage is not possible or activated charcoal is not available (carefully, as paraquat can be corrosive). Immediately after vomiting, administer absorbent clay (or activated charcoal if clays are not available) plus a cathartic. Ingestion of any food or even plain dirt may give some protection if other absorbents are not immediately available. For skin contamination, remove clothes and wash thoroughly; in the event of eye contamination, wash eyes for 15 minutes and see an ophthalmologist. Avoid giving excessive oxygen and treat fluid and electrolyte imbalances.

See also HERBICIDES.

parasympathomimetic drugs These drugs, including physostigmine, pilocarpine, neostigmine, and methacholine, act on the parasympathetic nervous system and are administered by ingestion, injection, or application to mucous membranes. They are used to treat glaucoma, myasthenia gravis, bladder problems, and certain heart irregularities.

Symptoms

Overdose produces breathing problems, tremor, involuntary defecation and urination, pinpoint pupils, vomiting, low blood pressure, bronchial constriction, wheezing, twitching, fainting, slow pulse, convulsions, and death. Repeated small doses may mimic symptoms of acute poisoning.

Treatment

Prompt administration of atropine results in immediate recovery.

See also PHYSOSTIGMINE.

parathion (0,0-diethyl 0-p-nitrophenyl phosphorothioate) This brown-yellow liquid is used as an insecticide and also as a deadly nerve gas that is fatal upon contact. Most fatalities have occurred while spraying into the wind, cleaning equipment (and airplanes) used for spraying, or gathering produce that has been sprayed. Industrial poisonings have also occurred by workers who absorb the poison through the skin. It is also a common suicide choice in Europe.

Poisonous part

The toxic compound includes muscarine and other poisonous substances that have not yet been fully identified.

Symptoms

Parathion is highly toxic by skin contact, inhalation, or ingestion. It destroys enzymes needed for proper functioning of nerves and muscles, causing contraction of pupils, headache, sensitivity to light, spasms, abdominal pain, nosebleeds, nausea, muscle weakness, twitching, diarrhea, convulsions, heart block, paralysis, respiratory difficulty, and pulmonary edema, ending in fatal respiratory failure. Death is usually quite painful, with tremors, muscle spasms, and convulsions. Parathion used as a nerve gas is fatal upon skin contact, although it can also be absorbed by the lungs; it causes painful tremors, muscle spasms, convulsions, and death.

Treatment

The antidote is large doses of atropine for 48 hours plus treatment of symptoms.

See also MUSCARINE; ORGANOPHOSPHATE INSECTICIDES.

pavulon (pancuronium) See NEUROMUSCULAR BLOCKING AGENTS.

PCBs See POLYCHLORINATED BIPHENYLS.

PCP See PHENCYCLIDINE.

peach pit See *PRUNUS*.

penicillamine One of the derivatives of penicillin used not for fighting microbes, but for binding and removing heavy metals such as lead, mercury, arsenic, and copper from the body. It is often used following an initial treatment with calcium EDTA or dimercaprol. Penicillamine is easily absorbed in the body; the penicillamine and metal can then be excreted from the body.

See also ARSENIC; CALCIUM EDTA; DIMERCAPROL.

pennyroyal oil A volatile oil obtained from the pennyroyal plant *(Mentha pulegium),* one of a large number of plants belonging to the mint family. Pennyroyal has traditionally been used by American Indians to bring on menstrual periods and to cause abortions. A colorless liquid, pennyroyal oil readily evaporates at room temperature.

Symptoms

In large doses, pennyroyal oil induces a fatal reaction as a result of kidney failure.

Treatment

There is no known antidote for pennyroyal oil. Treatment is supportive and symptomatic.

See also VOLATILE OILS.

pep pills See AMPHETAMINES.

Percodan (oxycodone) This narcotic painkiller derived from morphine is used in the treatment of severe pain and is a combination of oxycodone and aspirin. Percodan depresses the central nervous system and its sedative qualities are strengthened when taken together with tranquilizers, antihistamines, antidepressants, sedatives, sleeping pills, alcohol, or narcotics. Combining this drug with phenytoin (Dilantin) can cause brain death.

Symptoms
When Percodan is taken in overdose, symptoms include drowsiness, clumsiness, lightheadedness, dizziness, sedation, nausea, and vomiting; severe overdose can produce weak muscles, stupor, coma, low blood pressure, respiratory depression, and cardiac arrest within 30 minutes.

Treatment
The antidote is naloxone.

See also MORPHINE; NALOXONE; NARCOTICS; OXY-MORPHONE; PHENYTOIN.

persistent organic pollutants POPs, or persistent organic pollutants, are a group of toxic chemicals that persist in the environment for long periods of time, and which biomagnify (increase in concentration, often to dangerous levels) as they move up the food chain. Persistent organic pollutants are often released into the environment through industrial, agricultural, and other human activities and carried around the world through the atmosphere, oceans, and other pathways, far away from their originating point. Because of their chemical makeup, POPs accumulate in fatty tissue in both humans and animals, including fish, fowl, meat, and dairy products. This global contamination process, along with the fact that POPs are associated with various harmful effects on human and animal health, including cancer, nervous system damage, reproductive disorders, and disruption of the immune system, prompted countries to begin limiting the production, use, and release of POPs into the environment. What started out as local

and then regional efforts soon became a global one, and the Stockholm Convention was created on May 22, 2001. This was a legally binding agreement, originally signed by 150 countries, entered into force in May 2004, and had 120 parties as part of the agreement as of March 2006.

The Convention on Persistent Organic Pollutants, which was signed by the United States in May 2001, is a commitment to reduce and/or eliminate the use, production, and/or release of the twelve POPs that are of the greatest concern to the world. The twelve POPs (known as the "dirty dozen") include aldrin, chlordane, DDT, dieldrin, endrin, heptachlor, hexachlorobenzene, mirex, polychlorinated biphenyls, polychlorinated dibenzo-p-dioxins, polychlorinated dibenzo-p-furans, and toxaphene.

There are three classifications of POPS based on how they enter the environment. Insecticides are purposefully introduced into the environment. Although most of the POPs have been banned, some developing countries still use them. Industrial chemicals, such as polychlorinated biphenyls (PCBs) leak into the environment, while the third category is by-products of manufacturing and combustion and enter the air, water, and soil through various means.

Symptoms
Certain POPs can result in a disease called porphyria, which may cause seizures. POPs may also increase the risk of infection and cancer, reproductive disorders, skin lesions, and disturbances in growth and development. Acute exposure to aldrin, dieldrin, and endrin can cause severe seizures, headache, nausea, anorexia, muscle twitching, and psychological illnesses, and possibly peripheral neuropathy and death. DDT can cause nausea and headache, irritation of mucous membranes, tremors, and other nervous system abnormalities. Heptachlor often causes hyperexcitation of the central nervous system, cerebrovascular disease, and death. Dioxins and furans reduce testosterone levels in males, and fetuses exposed to dioxins through the placenta and babies through breast milk exhibit dysfunctional muscle reflexes, while infants exposed to hexochlorobenzenes often develop arthritis and rashes.

Treatment

There is no way to eliminate POPs from the body. Treatment is supportive and symptomatic. If ingested, induce vomiting or perform gastric lavage followed by the administration of activated charcoal and a cathartic. If the skin has been contaminated, wash thoroughly.

See also ALDRIN; DIELDRIN; MIREX; POLYCHLORINATED BIPHENYLS; TOXAPHENE.

pesticides Also known as "crop protectants," pesticides are chemicals used in protecting crops from predators, competitors, and diseases that can cause major losses. Specific types of pesticides are used for different purposes: Insecticides control insects; fungicides control plant diseases; herbicides control weeds that compete with crops; and rodenticides control rodents that attack crops in storage.

American farmers use about 77 percent of all the pesticides in the United States, and these applications have a direct impact on the food supply. The remaining 23 percent is also important, however. In fact, 10 percent of the land area in the United States (including lawns, forests, and parks) is treated with pesticides. It's been estimated that the average homeowner in the United States uses two to six times more pesticides per acre than do farmers. Runoff from all pesticide use, including agricultural, industrial, and personal, has the potential to contaminate water and soil.

Various studies show a correlation between pesticide use and the development of cancer. In the Agricultural Health Study (*American Journal of Epidemiology,* 2003), for example, researchers found an association between use of agricultural pesticides and the risk of prostate cancer. A link between pesticide use and breast cancer has been reported by several research studies, including a 2007 study in the *American Journal of Epidemiology,* which was the first to suggest that self-reported use of residential pesticides may increase the risk of breast cancer.

Pesticide contamination on domestic and imported produce is monitored by the Food and Drug Administration (FDA) by testing selected samples. In 2003, the FDA tested 2,344 domestic and 4,890 imported produce items and found no residues in 62.7 percent of the domestic and

71.8 percent of the imported samples. Only 2.4 percent of domestic and 6.1 percent of imported samples had residue levels that violated the FDA's standards.

Acceptable levels of pesticides are set by the Environmental Protection Agency (EPA), based on current knowledge of the long-term effects of pesticide residues.

The alternative to buying conventionally grown produce (which has been treated with pesticides) is to buy organic food. For many years, the terms "organic" and "certified organic" had no federal legal definition, and organic farmers raised an outcry against the lack of national standards and the permissive rules that applied to organic foods. In 1998, for example, the United States Department of Agriculture (USDA) had proposed that food could be labeled "organic" even if it was irradiated to kill germs, genetically engineered, or subjected to sewage sludge or chemical sprays. These proposals were withdrawn by the USDA, and new rules were eventually put into effect.

Since 2002, organic certification in the United States has taken place under the authority of the USDA National Organic Program, which accredits organic certifying agencies and oversees the regulatory process. "Certified organic" refers to agricultural products that have been grown and processed according to uniform standards that are verified by independent state or private organizations, all of which must be accredited by the USDA. Anyone who sells products labeled or marketed as "organic" is required by law to be certified. For a farm to be certified, it must submit an organic system plan annually and submit to inspection of the fields and processing facilities. Inspectors verify that the farm is engaging in organic practices such as long-term soil management and buffering between organic farms and nearby conventional farms. Certified organic requires complete elimination of synthetic agrochemicals, irradiation, and genetically engineered foods or ingredients.

Rather than use pesticides, herbicides, fungicides, and other synthetic means to control diseases and pests, organic farmers build healthy soils by planting cover crops, using compost, and biologically based soil amendments. They use crop rotation, mechanical tillage, hand-weeding, cover crops, mulches, and other management methods to control weeds. Pests are controlled using beneficial insects, birds, soil organisms, traps, and barriers. As a last resort, certain botanical or other nonsynthetic pesticides can be used, as approved under the National Organic Program Rule.

Approximately 2 percent of the U.S. food supply is produced using organic methods. Since the mid 1990s, sales of organic products have increased annually by at least 20 percent. In 2005, retail sales of organic foods and beverages were about $12.8 billion, according to the Natural Marketing Institute (Health & Wellness Trends Database, March 2006). The Organic Farming Research Foundation reported that by 2007, there were approximately 13,000 certified organic producers in the United States. Organic foods are also becoming popular in foreign markets, with countries like Germany and Japan becoming important organic food markets.

See also ALAR; ALDICARB; ALDRIN; BACILLUS THURINGIENSIS (BT); BENZENE HEXACHLORIDE; BOTANIC INSECTICIDES; CARBAMATE; CARBARYL; CHLORDANE; CHLORINATED HYDROCARBON PESTICIDES; CHLOROBENZENE DERIVATIVES; CREOSOTE; DDT; DERRIS; DIELDRIN; ENDRIN; ETHYLENE DIBROMIDE; INDANE DERIVATIVES; INORGANIC CHEMICAL INSECTICIDES; INSECTICIDES; LINDANE; MALATHION; TEPP; TOXAPHENE.

pesticides, safety   Some of the most common poisoning problems are pesticides. According to the National Ag Safety Database (NASD), half the pesticide-related deaths in the United States are of children under the age of 10. Almost half of all households with children under age five have at least one pesticide stored in an unlocked cabinet less than four feet off the ground, according to a survey by the U.S. Environmental Protection Agency (EPA). The survey also found that 75 percent of households without children under age five also stored one pesticide within reach of children. This statistic matters because research shows that 13 percent of all pesticide poisonings occur away from the child's home.

Storing pesticides
Here are some quick and easy steps you can take to make sure you are storing your pesticides safely:

- Always store pesticides in a locked cabinet or garden shed away from a child's reach.
- Read the label before you use pesticides and follow all instructions, including precautions and restrictions.
- Before you apply indoor or outdoor pesticides, be sure there are no children or toys in the area: keep them away until the surfaces are dry (or until a recommended time has passed).
- Never leave pesticides out and open while you are using them (not even for a minute or two).
- Never put pesticides into another container; a child may think there is something to eat or drink in the container.
- Close the container tightly after you are finished using it.
- Make sure your child's other caregivers, grandparents, and so on follow these guidelines too.

Using pesticides safely
It is important not only to store your pesticides safely but to know how to use them properly as well. Follow these guidelines when using potentially toxic pesticide products:

- Always read the label before you use the product and follow the directions.
- Do not smoke while spraying or dusting; many of these chemicals are flammable.
- Wear protective clothing and masks. Keep your sleeves rolled down and your collar up.
- Wash immediately with soap and water if you spill pesticide material on your skin.
- Wash your hands immediately after spraying or dusting and before eating or smoking. Change your clothes as well.
- If you begin to feel sick while using a pesticide (or shortly thereafter), call your doctor immediately.
- Investigate organic alternatives: if you do use toxic pesticides, limit use and provide adequate ventilation. Keep children away from treated areas.

- If you use a bug bomb, keep children out of the treated area *at least overnight* and scrub areas where fumes may have settled.
- When treating your lawn with chemicals, close windows and keep your child indoors until treatment is over.
- Do not allow your child to play on chemically treated lawns at least until the chemicals have had a chance to seep into the soil; rain or a sprinkling from your hose will speed this process.

petroleum distillates A wide range of products are distilled from petroleum, including paint thinner, kerosene, gasoline, lighter fluid, petroleum-based insecticides, and mineral seal oils. All petroleum distillates are hydrocarbons, but not all hydrocarbons are petroleum distillates. Petroleum distillates are a specific type of hydrocarbons called aliphatics.

Ingestion of large amounts of hydrocarbons by young children is not common because these chemicals have a very foul taste. Aspiration also is usually unintentional. Among adolescents, however, aspiration of hydrocarbons ("huffing") is typically done to get high.

Between 1997 and 1999, an estimated 6,400 children younger than five years of age were seen in hospital emergency departments after they accidentally ingested hydrocarbons, with petroleum distillates being the most common ones taken. In 1998, unintentional ingestion of hydrocarbons caused the death of four children younger than 13 years of age and another 14 deaths by intentional ingestion.

Symptoms

Petroleum distillates in small doses cause nausea and vomiting, coughing, and spitting blood. Larger amounts can result in weakness, dizziness, slow, shallow breathing, and unconsciousness followed by convulsions and, sometimes, mild heart attack. Death from ingesting petroleum distillates is almost always a result of pulmonary problems.

Treatment

Gastric lavage only when preceded by insertion of endotracheal tube in comatose patients. *Do not induce vomiting* (unless an insecticide or other poison also has been ingested with the petroleum distillate). The victim's head should be kept lower than the hips to prevent vomitus from being aspirated into the lungs. Magnesium or sodium sulfate or citrate may be used as a cathartic. Oxygen and supportive therapy may also be needed.

See also INSECTICIDES; TURPENTINE.

pets, poisoning Pets are just as much at risk for common household poisoning as any curious two-year-old; curious pets can push and paw open cabinets, chew through child protective caps, and ingest toxic liquids in a very short time. Generally, any products that are considered poisonous to a young child should also be locked away from pets, including medications, household and garden chemicals, insect and rat killers, and automotive products.

According to experts at the National Animal Poison Control Center, it takes only a small amount of a potentially toxic substance to do serious harm to a pet. For example, one extra-strength acetaminophen tablet or one teaspoon of undiluted antifreeze can kill a seven-pound cat. An animal's medicine should never be given to another species (cat medicine for dogs, and vice versa). Flea and tick products can be toxic if used incorrectly, especially on cats, who are extremely sensitive to whole-house flea and tick treatments.

Among other common products that are poisonous is chocolate, which is toxic to dogs if eaten in sufficient quantities. Unsweetened baking chocolate is the most dangerous of all chocolate, as it contains 10 times the amount of theobromine and caffeine as white or milk chocolate. About one ounce of baking chocolate can be fatal to a 10-pound dog (or about one-fourth of an ounce for every two point two pounds). Although vomiting is the most common symptom, poisoning in animals may also cause diarrhea, anorexia, or sudden behavior change (such as depression). According to veterinarians at the National Animal Poison Control Center, if the pet has not ingested a caustic or oily substance, the best emergency treatment is to induce vomiting. But because vomiting on an empty stomach will make the animal retch without bringing up the toxic substance, owners should feed the pet a soft diet (such as canned pet food or milk) before giving an emetic. Possible emetics for pets can include syrup of ipecac, saline, or hydrogen peroxide.

A recent episode of massive pet poisoning occurred in 2007 and became evident early in the year when hundreds, and then thousands of dogs and cats in North America fell ill and died after eating contaminated pet food. The originating contamination point was the suppliers of wheat gluten and rice protein concentrate from China, which was then used in hundreds of different name brand pet foods. The first pet food recall began on March 16, 2007, and ultimately more than 130 different brand name pet foods for dogs and cats were pulled from the shelves as experts from the Food and Drug Administration (FDA), the American Association of Veterinary Laboratory Diagnosticians, experts from various veterinary schools, and others investigated the deaths. Experts believe that the contaminant was composed of two closely related chemicals—melamine and cyanuric acid, which then combined to form crystals in the kidneys of some animals. The crystals then blocked the microtubules through which urine flows, causing kidney damage, kidney failure, and sometimes death. The FDA reported that it appears the melamine was deliberately added to the ingredients in China to make them look like they were more protein-rich than they actually were.

It is difficult to know exactly how many animals were affected and died from the contaminated food. Many veterinarians reported that more cats than dogs were being brought to their clinics, which could be explained by the fact that cats' well-known susceptibility to kidney problems places them at higher risk for kidney damage than dogs. Because cats evolved in the African desert and got all their water from their prey rather than from drinking, they have the unique ability to highly concentrate their urine. Cats' kidneys are thus less adept at filtering out potentially dangerous waste, and they have too little water in their kidneys to dissolve the crystals. Dogs, however, drink more water and urinate more often, which helps them eliminate the crystals.

If you suspect poisoning

If your pet has ingested something that you suspect is toxic, call a veterinarian; do not wait for signs to develop. For poison treatment to be successful, immediate action is necessary, as many antidotes must be administered within 12 hours of toxin ingestion. If possible, bring a sample of the suspect substance with you to the veterinarian. Frequently veterinarians prescribe giving the animal one tablespoon of hydrogen peroxide to induce vomiting, so it is recommended to keep a bottle handy for emergencies. However, do not induce vomiting without first talking with a trained professional, as many chemicals (e.g., gasoline, kerosene) should not be eliminated through vomiting. If local expert help is unavailable, you may call the Animal Poison Control Center 24 hours a day for advice. Dial 888-426-4435 at a cost of $60 for a consultation fee.

Measures to Protect Your Pets against Poisoning

- Keep all prescription and over-the-counter medications out of your pets' reach. This also includes vitamins, herbs, and other natural supplements.

- Frequently check your vehicles for antifreeze and windshield wiper fluid leaks. These substances taste sweet and can be lethal in very small amounts to animals. Consider using animal-friendly antifreeze products that use propylene glycol instead of ethylene glycol.

- If you treat your garden or lawn with fertilizers or pesticides, do not let your pets have access to these areas until they have dried completely. If you are uncertain about the safety of any product, consult your veterinarian. Always store such items safely away from pets.

- Be aware of the plants you have in and around your home. Azalea, foxglove, laurel, oleander, easter lily, and many other plant species can be deadly if ingested.

- If you use any type of rodent or other pest control traps, place them in areas that are not accessible to your pets. Some traps contain ingredients that are very attractive to pets.

- Use pet products as instructed on the package or by your veterinarian. Failing to follow usage directions is one of the most common causes of pet toxicity.

- Do not give certain foods to your pets: alcohol, apple seeds, apricot pits, avocados (toxic to birds, mice, rabbits, horses, dairy goats), chocolate, coffee, grapes, macadamia nuts, moldy food, mushrooms, onions, potato leaves and stems, raisins, rhubarb leaves, salt, tea, tomato leaves and stems, walnuts, yeast dough.
- Secure your trashcans. Mixing food scraps with other waste items can be very toxic to rummaging animals.

phencyclidine (PCP) This former veterinary drug became popular as a cheap street drug during the late 1960s, when it was widely known as "angel dust." It may be snorted, smoked, ingested, or injected and is often substituted for other illicit drugs such as THC (tetrahydrocannabinol, the active ingredient in marijuana), mescaline, or LSD. It produces a dissociative state and inhibits pain perception in its street dosage of 1- to 6-milligram tablets; ingestion of 6 to 10 milligrams causes toxic psychosis. Overdose (150 to 200 milligrams) is fatal. Although classified as a stimulant, PCP can both excite and depress the central nervous system.

During 2003, a total of 785 exposures to phencyclidine were reported to the U.S. Poison Control Centers, which included eight deaths and 83 people who experienced severe morbidity. In that same year, the Drug Abuse Warning Network found that PCP was involved in nearly 0.75 percent of all drug-related emergency department visits (4,581 of a total of 627,923).

PCP was developed in 1957 as an analgesic and short-acting intravenous anesthetic, but the side effects were so toxic that the drug was withdrawn for human use; it was later reintroduced in 1967 only to veterinarians as an anesthetic under the trade name Sernyl or Sernylan. It became popular in the late sixties and was mixed with THC, LSD, psilocybin or mescaline. PCP is sprinkled onto parsley or marijuana for recreational smoking. There have been reports that users have been able to snap out of handcuffs and have attacked large groups of people and the police unarmed. The loss of fear may cause individuals to try to stop a train by standing in front of it or mutilating themselves.

Symptoms
Mild use produces lethargy, euphoria, hallucinations, and sometimes bizarre or violent behavior, with rapid swings between quietness and agitation. Severe overdose leads to high blood pressure, rigidity, high fever, rapid heartbeat, convulsions, and coma; the pupils are often small, and death may occur as a result of self-destructive behavior or as a result of high fever (kidney failure or brain damage).

Treatment
There is no specific antidote. Ammonium chloride is sometimes given to help remove the PCP from the central nervous system. Provide symptomatic treatment and sedation (benzodiazepines) to control agitated behavior; phenothiazines and other antipsychotics are ineffective and may induce low blood pressure or seizures. Do not induce vomiting because of the risk of rapid onset of seizures or coma. Perform gastric lavage only if ingestion has occurred during the past four hours, or when multiple agents have been ingested. Follow by activated charcoal and a cathartic. Mildly intoxicated persons should be managed with sensory isolation in a physically protected environment. Symptoms may last for several days as the drug empties into the stomach and is then reabsorbed through the intestines. Haloperidol or chlorpromazine are recommended for continued psychosis.

See also LSD; MEXICAN HALLUCINOGENIC MUSHROOM.

phenobarbital This barbiturate is used primarily to control convulsions as a side effect of poisoning, although it has generally been replaced by newer anticonvulsant drugs. Because there is a delay in onset of the beneficial effects of this drug, other anticonvulsants (diazepam or phenytoin) are generally tried first.

phenol Also known as carbolic acid, this is a white crystalline substance with a burning taste and a distinct acrid odor. It is used in the manufacture of fertilizers, paints, paint removers, textiles, drugs, and perfumes and is widely used in the dye, agricultural, and tanning industries. In addition, clove oil in clove cigarettes contains the phenol derivative eugenol and may cause severe breathing problems.

Phenol is equally deadly whether inhaled, absorbed through the skin or eyes or ingested. It was once used in households to kill germs but has been replaced today by less toxic compounds. Hexachlorophene is a chlorinated biphenol that was used throughout the United States as a topical antiseptic and scrub until its adverse effects on the brain were recognized. Other compounds of phenol include creosote, creosol, hydroquinone, eugenol, dinitrophenol, and pentachlorophenol.

Poisonous part

While the mechanism behind its toxicity on the central nervous system is not known, phenol can cause corrosive injury to the eyes, skin, and respiratory tract. There are no minimum toxic levels, although there have been reports of infants dying after repeated skin applications of small doses. Adult deaths have occurred after ingestion of 1 to 32 grams of phenol, although survival after ingesting 45 to 65 grams has also been reported. There have been reports of infant deaths with as small as 50 to 500 milligram doses.

Symptoms

Phenol is markedly corrosive on any tissue in which it comes in contact. Exposure to the eyes can cause blindness; contact with the skin (at even low vapor concentrations) can cause a delayed burning and gangrene, with paleness, weakness, sweating, high fever, shock, cyanosis, excitement, frothing, coma, kidney damage, and death. Ingesting large amounts of phenol can severely burn the mouth and throat and can cause abdominal pain, nausea, corrosion of the lips, mouth, esophagus, and stomach, cyanosis, muscle weakness, collapse, coma, and death. Death from phenol poisoning is most likely during hot weather when loss of body heat is inhibited.

Treatment

Do NOT induce vomiting, because phenol is corrosive and may induce seizures. Ingested poison can be treated with milk, olive oil, or vegetable oil followed by repeated gastric lavage. (Neither mineral oil nor alcohol should be used, since they speed up the absorption of phenol, although some medical texts still recommend them.) Castor oil dissolves phenols and interferes with absorption. Follow with activated charcoal and a cathartic.

For skin contact, wash the area for 15 minutes followed by the application on the skin of castor oil, olive oil, or petroleum jelly. For eye contact, immediately flush with tepid water or saline.

See also CREOSOTE.

phentolamine This vasodilator acts rapidly on both blood vessels and arteries (within two minutes) and is used to treat high blood pressure following overdose of phenylpropanolamine or stimulant drugs such as amphetamine, cocaine, or ephedrine.

See also AMPHETAMINES; COCAINE; DECONGESTANTS; EPHEDRINE.

phenurone See SLEEPING PILLS.

phenylpropanolamine See DECONGESTANTS.

phenytoin (Dilantin) This epileptic drug is used to prevent seizures and may easily cause an accidental overdose in persons in chronic therapy because of drug interactions or slight dosage adjustments. Poisoning may occur either by an acute overdose by mouth or by chronic overmedication. Poisoning may also occur following rapid intravenous administration. Persons with kidney problems may experience toxicity at lower levels.

Symptoms

Mild symptoms include nystagmus (involuntary movement of the eyeball), nause, vomiting, agitation, irritability, and hallucinations. At high levels of overdose, symptoms include stupor, coma, and respiratory arrest. The toxicity to the heart that occurs with rapid intravenous injection does not result from oral overdose.

Treatment

There is no specific antidote. Treat symptoms, induce vomiting or perform gastric lavage followed by the administration of activated charcoal and a cathartic orally or by gastric tube.

philodendron *(Philodendron)* This is the most popular houseplant in the United States, but eating the leaves can cause painful swelling and blisters in the mouth. This climbing vine has aerial roots and large, heart-shaped or notched leaves, sometimes with variegated patterns.

Poisonous part

The leaves contain raphides of calcium oxalate and other, unidentified proteins. The oxalates are insoluble and therefore do not cause systemic poisoning.

Symptoms

Pain and swelling of the lips, mouth, tongue, and throat; contact dermatitis is also possible.

Treatment

Pain and swelling fade by themselves, but keeping cold liquid in the mouth (such as milk) can help.
See also OXALATES.

philodendron, split leaf *(Monstera deliciosa)* **[Other names: breadfruit vine, cut leaf philodendron, fruit salad plant, hurricane plant, Mexican breadfruit, shingle plant, swiss cheese plant, window plant, windowleaf.]** This woody climber has thick leaves with irregular holes. Grown as an indoor plant in the United States and native to Mexico, it is also cultivated in the West Indies, Hawaii, and Guam.

Poisonous part

The leaves are toxic and contain raphides of calcium oxalates.

Symptoms

After eating, the lips, mouth, and tongue begin to burn and swell followed by an acute inflammatory reaction. Because eating the leaves of this plant is quickly painful, there is little danger that large amounts will be ingested.

Treatment

The pain and swelling will fade by themselves, but cool liquids (such as milk) held in the mouth, together with painkillers, may help ease the pain. The insoluble oxalates in these plants don't cause systemic poisoning.
See also OXALATES.

phosgene Once manufactured as a weapon for chemical warfare, phosgene is now used as an industrial gas to manufacture dyes, resins, and pesticides. In addition, it is often produced during fires or while welding metal that has been cleaned with chlorinated solvents.

An irritant, it does not immediately cause symptoms at low doses; for this reason, a person may unknowingly inhale the gas over a period of time, injuring the lungs.

Symptoms

Exposure to mild amounts causes cough and some irritation. After 30 minutes to eight hours (depending on how long the person was exposed) further symptoms develop: labored breathing and swelling in the lungs; and permanent lung damage may result because phosgene is changed in the alveoli into hydrochloric acid, causing damage and inflammation of the small airways and tissue.

Treatment

There is no specific antidote. Treat symptoms and give supplementary oxygen if needed.

phosphate esters A group of highly toxic compounds that are used as insecticides and are extremely poisonous to humans and animals; they are quickly absorbed from the skin, lungs, and gastrointestinal tract. The greatest hazard to humans from these insecticides is through breathing the compounds, which is three times more toxic than oral exposure and 10 times more toxic than skin absorption. These esters were discovered accidentally by the Germans during World War II in their search for poison gas.

Symptoms

Weakness, unsteadiness, blurred vision, vomiting, abdominal cramps, diarrhea, salivation, sweating, tremors, and problems in breathing.

Treatment

Administration of atropine, supportive therapy as required.

See also INSECTICIDES.

phosphine This colorless gas is heavier than air, and, while rarely causing poisoning in the general public, it does present a hazard to metal refiners, acetylene workers, fire fighters, and pest-control operators. Phosphine is a highly toxic gas of particular danger to the lungs, brain, kidneys, heart, and liver. Chronic exposure to less-than-lethal dosages can also produce toxic symptoms.

Symptoms

Inhalation causes severe lung irritation, cough, labored breathing, headache, dizziness, lethargy, and stupor followed by seizures, gastroenteritis, and kidney and liver problems. Symptoms usually appear fairly soon after inhalation, except in the case of chronic low-level exposure.

Treatment

There is no specific antidote. Treat symptoms, and provide supplemental oxygen if needed.

phosphorus A chemical used as an inorganic insecticide and also in the manufacture of fertilizers and fireworks. As a red, granular insoluble substance, phosphorus is nontoxic, but its yellow or white form is highly poisonous and ignites on contact with moist air and water, trailing white fumes and burning with an eerie green light. At one time, phosphorus was used on the tips of matches, but it has since been replaced because of its toxicity.

Phosphorus is highly corrosive and a general cellular poison; the fatal dose of white-yellow phosphorus is about one milligram per kilograms, although deaths have been reported from ingesting as little as 15 milligrams.

Symptoms

Immediately after ingestion, yellow phosphorus begins to affect the digestive tract, causing abdominal pain, nausea, vomiting luminescent material, and diarrhea. Cardiac collapse may occur because of fluid loss from vomiting and diarrhea and because of direct toxicity on the heart. It is possible that death may occur within 12 hours after ingestion. If not, there may follow one to three days with no symptoms, during which time phosphorus begins to damage the liver and muscle, heart, kidney, and nervous system; after about three days the symptoms will return, much more serious this time with liver enlargement, jaundice, delirium, convulsions, and coma.

Death may not occur until three weeks following ingestion. Phosphide (rat poison) ingestion causes jaundice, pulmonary edema, and cyanosis (blue skin color) and can be fatal within one week.

There is also a problem with skin contamination: If yellow phosphorus dries on the skin, it can cause a second- or third-degree burn.

If the phosphorus vapor is inhaled, symptoms appear within two days and include conjunctivitis, nausea, vomiting, fatigue, coughing, jaundice, tremors, numbness, low blood pressure, pulmonary edema, collapse, heart problems, convulsions, and coma. Inhalation may be fatal within four days to two weeks. The classic sign of chronic poisoning is called "phossy jaw," an aching and swelling of the jaw followed by deterioration of the jawbone, in addition to weakness, weight loss, anemia, and spontaneous fractures.

Treatment

There is no specific antidote. Eliminate exposure and give oxygen. With ingestion, perform gastric lavage followed by the administration of activated charcoal and a cathartic, although there is no evidence that charcoal absorbs phosphorus. Provide symptomatic and supportive treatment. Do not induce vomiting. For skin contamination, wash with plenty of water. For chronic poisoning causing jaw necrosis, surgical excision of affected jawbone may be required.

See also INSECTICIDES.

physostigmine A treatment used in poisoning cases with symptoms of agitated delirium, heart rhythm disturbances (sinus tachycardia), and high fever with no sweating. It is NOT used as an antidote for cyclic antidepressant overdose, nor at the same time as certain neuromuscular blockers (such as succinylcholine).

See also PARASYMPATHOMIMETIC DRUGS.

phytonadione See VITAMIN K.

phytotoxins Also called toxalbumins, these are extremely deadly protein molecules (similar to bacterial toxins) that are produced by a few plants, including the castor bean, rosary pea, and black locust. In a manner similar to that of bacterial toxins, the phytotoxins elicit an antibody response after ingestion. Eating just one seed from a plant containing these toxins can be fatal. Most phytotoxins are destroyed by heat.

Interestingly, however, different people will react differently to the presence of phytotoxins. Symptoms include gastrointestinal irritation, with lesions and swelling of organs.

See also BLACK LOCUST; CASTOR BEAN; ROSARY PEA.

pilocarpine See PARASYMPATHOMIMETIC DRUGS.

pit vipers Seventeen of the 19 venomous snakes in North America belong to this family of dangerous poison snakes, which includes about 290 species. There are three genera in the family: *Agkistrodon* (copperheads and cottonmouths), *Crotalus,* and *Sistrurus* (both rattlesnakes).

Pit vipers seem to be extremely highly evolved snakes very well designed for capturing, killing, and eating fairly large, warm-blooded prey. Most have stout bodies with wide heads, patterned with crossbands and blotches and with retractable hollow fangs in the front of the upper jaw. The fangs can be folded back and then positioned forward as the mouth opens to strike. The pit viper's name comes from the heat-sensitive pits located on each side of the head between the nostril and the eye, which is used to locate its prey.

Seriousness of the bite depends on a wide variety of variables, including the snake's size (usually the larger, the more venomous) and whether the snake is hungry or alert. The angle of the bite and its depth and length also affect the seriousness of the bite. In addition, the size of the victim can be important (children and infants are at greater risk), and the health of the victim at the time of the bite will also affect the outcome. Persons with diabetes, hypertension, or blood coagulation problems and the elderly are particularly sensitive to snake venom, and menstruating women may bleed excessively following the bite of a pit viper. Several cases of miscarriage have been reported when pregnant women have been bitten. Finally, the location of the bite itself is crucial to its seriousness; venomous snake bites on the head and trunk are twice as serious as those on the extremities, and bites on the arms are more serious than those on the legs.

Poisonous part
The venom of the pit vipers is a mixture of proteins that acts on a victim's blood. Even snakes that appear to have been killed by the side of the road have been reported to bite. The size of the snake can give an idea of its potential dangerousness and can be judged by the distance between the fang marks. Fang marks less than 8 millimeters apart would be a small snake; between 8 and 12 millimeters indicates a medium-size snake, and more than 12 millimeters suggests a large venomous snake. Even snakes that have been "defanged" can be dangerous, since all snakes grow new fangs from time to time.

Symptoms
Swelling, internal bleeding, changes in red blood cells, central nervous system symptoms including convulsions and sometimes psychotic behavior, muscle weakness, and paralysis. In addition, there are general systemic symptoms of fever, nausea, vomiting, diarrhea, pain, and restlessness. Tachycardia and bradycardia can develop, and kidney failure has been reported.

Treatment
Within the first 30 to 45 minutes after the bite of a pit viper, apply a venous tourniquet a few inches above the bite, loosening it every 15 to 30 min-

utes and reapplying it above the level of progressive swelling. Keep the victim quiet, lying down to decrease metabolic activity (which affects the spread of the venom). The wound area (especially if it is an arm or leg) should be kept lower than the heart. Within 30 minutes, trained individuals can incise the wound area and apply suction. Antivenin is available but should be administered within four hours; antivenin is rarely helpful if given more than 12 hours after the bite. Tetanus prophylaxis is advisable; other treatment might include blood transfusions, intravenous fluids, treatment for convulsions, and antihistamines to control itching. In addition, broad-spectrum antibiotics may be administered, since snakebites are notorious for becoming infected. If antivenin has not been administered (or was given hours after the bite), sloughing of the skin around the bite is common.

While certain anecdotal reports in the popular press have reported that some individuals become immunized after many bites of the pit viper, scientifically controlled attempts to develop immunity in human beings have failed.

See also COPPERHEAD SNAKE; RATTLESNAKE, CANEBRAKE; RATTLESNAKE, CASCABEL; RATTLESNAKE, EASTERN DIAMONDBACK; RATTLESNAKE, MEXICAN WEST COAST; RATTLESNAKE, RED DIAMONDBACK; RATTLESNAKE, SOUTH AMERICAN; RATTLESNAKE, TIMBER; RATTLESNAKE, WESTERN DIAMONDBACK; SNAKES, POISONOUS; WATER MOCCASIN.

plant safety Plants are a potential form of poisoning, especially for very young children who are likely to put plants—especially those with berries or other brightly colored parts—into their mouths. You are probably aware of some of the well-known poisonous plants, but did you know that a child can become seriously ill from biting into a daffodil bulb or drinking the water out of a vase holding lilies of the valley?

Teach your children from the very beginning that they should NEVER put a plant into their mouth without first checking with an adult. This must include ALL mushrooms found in the wild.

If, despite all of your precautions, your child has eaten a plant:

- Stay calm and check your child for adverse reactions.
- Determine how much of the plant and what parts (e.g., berries, flowers, leaves) have been eaten.
- Remove any uneaten plant material from the child's mouth; check for redness, blisters, swelling, irritation, and cuts
- Observe for allergic reactions: blotchy red skin, swelling, breathing problems, nausea, diarrhea
- Identify the plant: if someone else is in the house, send him or her to a nursery to identify the plant if you do not know its name
- Call the poison control center (see Appendix F for a list of regional centers). Report any adverse reactions and give the age and weight of the child.
- If told to go to a hospital, take the plant or a sample with you.
- If your child is too young to speak, retrace the child's steps and check for any damaged plants. If there is plant material in the mouth, try to match it with a plant in the area.

Child-safe plants

If you enjoy having plants and flowers in your home but have small children, you can still decorate with greens. Just choose safe plants that will not hurt your children even if they swallow the plant. Here is a list of safe plants:

African violet	dandelion
aluminum plant	Easter lily
aspidistra	gardenia
aster	impatiens
baby's tears	jade plant
begonia	kalanchoe
bird's nest fern	lipstick plant
Boston fern	magnolia
bougainvillea	marigold
California poppy	nasturtium
camellia	Norfolk Island pine
Christmas cactus	pepperomia
coleus	petunia
creeping Charlie	poinsettia
dahlia	prayer plant

purple passion	umbrella tree
rose	violet
sensitive plant	wandering Jew
spider plant	wax plant
Swedish ivy	wild strawberry
tiger lily	zebra plant

Plesiomonas shigelloides This bacterium is found in water, freshwater fish, and shellfish, and causes a type of gastroenteritis among people in tropical or subtropical areas. Because most infections are mild, people don't seek medical treatment. It is not commonly reported in the United States, but this may be becauses cases are included as a group of diarrhea diseases of unknown origin that respond to broad spectrum antibiotics. Many cases that may be reported in the United States involve people with preexisting health problems or very young patients. A cluster occurred in North Carolina in 1980, when 36 out of 150 people at an oyster roast experienced symptoms two days later. In June 1996, an outbreak occurred following a private party attended by 189 people, 30 of whom became ill. The offending food—macaroni salad, potato salad, and baked ziti—had been catered. The cause of the *P. shigelloides* outbreak was traced to contaminated well water used by the catering facility.

Most cases appear to be related to tainted water that is drunk or used to rinse vegetables eaten raw.

Symptoms

Symptoms usually appear within a day or two after eating or drinking tainted food or water and include fever, chills, abdominal pain, nausea, watery diarrhea, or vomiting. In severe cases, diarrhea may be foamy, greenish yellow, or tinged with blood. While the diarrhea is mild in most people, infants and young children may have high fever and chills; blood poisoning and death have occurred among those with faulty immune systems, or who are seriously ill with cancer or blood disorders.

Treatment

Most people recover on their own without treatment.

plum cherry pit See *PRUNUS.*

poinsettia *(Euphorbia pulcherrima)* This popular Christmas plant has a long-standing poisonous reputation, but there are only two cases of fatal poisoning by poinsettia in toxicological literature. All references to poinsettia as potentially lethal have been traced to one case in 1919 when a Hawaiian child was reported to have died after eating poinsettia. However, researchers in the 1970s found that poinsettia was not lethal; several rat studies showed that large amounts of poinsettia could be eaten without harm. While some authorities and many popular magazines still report poinsettia as poisonous, most experts now agree that it is virtually certain poinsettia is not.

In the 1988 annual report of the American Association of Poison Control Centers National Data Collection System, there were no serious poisonings reported out of 3,001 exposures during the rating period.

However, it may be possible that the plant's milky sap may cause mild abdominal pain with vomiting and diarrhea if ingested. Locally, this sap can cause skin and mucous membrane irritation.

poison control centers This network of more than 60 poison control centers across the country is available free of charge, 24 hours a day with poison treatment information. The idea had its roots in a report by the American Academy of Pediatrics in 1952, when an academy survey that year revealed that half of all household accidents involving children was due to some type of poisoning. The study noted that most of the poisonings were caused by common over-the-counter and prescription drugs, and cleaning products. Flavored children's aspirin, which had then been only recently introduced, was responsible for one-fourth of all poisoning cases in children under age five, resulting in about 400 deaths a year.

This report set off alarm bells at the academy and was responsible for the introduction of the first "child-proof" caps on aspirin bottles, responsible for the almost complete elimination of childhood aspirin poisoning cases.

A year after the academy's accident prevention study was completed, the first poison control center was established in Chicago under the leadership of the Illinois chapter of the American Academy of Pediatrics. A few months later, the Duke University Poison Control Center was begun in North Carolina.

With the appearance of these two centers, the idea of poison control centers spread across the country. In 1957, the Food and Drug Administration established the National Clearinghouse for Poison Control Centers in order to coordinate activities at poison control centers across the United States. The clearinghouse collected and standardized product toxicology data, reproduced this information on large file cards and distributed them nationwide to poison control centers.

At about the same time, the American Academy of Pediatrics and the American Pediatric Health Association established the American Association of Poison Control Centers. See Appendix F for a list of regional poison control centers.

poisoning, emergency You may never need to handle a poisoning emergency, but you should be prepared for the possibility. Here are the guidelines:

- Post the number of your nearest poison control center on your phone. The number should be listed on the inside front cover of your local telephone directory. Regional numbers are listed in Appendix F of this volume.

- If you suspect or know that poisoning has occurred, call your nearest poison control center immediately. If you have not placed the number by the phone or cannot find it, call 911, the operator, or your local emergency number.

- When you reach someone at the poison control center or a doctor, be prepared to offer the following information:
  - Your name
  - Victim's name, age, and weight
  - Name or kind of poison (name on bottle, ingredients, type of plant, etc.)
  - How much of the poison was consumed

- When the poison was consumed
- Symptoms
- Other medical problems the victim may have, such as diabetes, heart problems, asthma, epilepsy, or high blood pressure
- Any drugs (including over-the-counter) that the victim may take regularly
- Whether the victim has vomited
- Whether you have given the victim anything to eat or drink

The personnel at the poison control center will tell you whether or not to induce vomiting. Some poisons, such as acids or alkalies, should not be brought up. If you do not know the identity of the substance that was swallowed, DO NOT induce vomiting.

Poison control may recommend that you use activated charcoal, Epsom salts, or specific products to neutralize the poison. Always follow the instructions given by a poison control center. DO NOT trust antidote information given on product labels, and do not use mustard or salt to induce vomiting. These old-fashioned methods do not work well. First aid procedures differ according to the kind of poison involved and how it entered the body, the victim's weight, how long the poison has been working, and other factors. Only expert medical personnel can determine the correct procedures. If you try to treat the victim yourself without expert advice, you may do further harm.

Other tips to remember when there is a poisoning emergency:

- Do not give a saltwater solution, especially to children. Use of saltwater was a recommendation from the past, but it can be potentially dangerous and if given repeatedly it can cause salt intoxication, seizures, and death.

- Do not administer fruit juice or vinegar to neutralize an alkali. Studies show that if you give an acid to neutralize a base it produces heat, which increases the possibility of a burn injury.

- Do not use sodium bicarbonate, chalk, or soap to treat an acid poisoning. Studies suggest that giving a base to neutralize an acid can release carbon dioxide gas, stretch the stomach, and even cause it to rupture.

- Do not give milk to coat the digestive tract. Milk may bind syrup of ipecac and interfere with vomiting. If the victim consumed a petroleum substance, milk may cause vomiting, which could introduce the substance into the lungs.

- Dilution with water or milk should be done only when a corrosive poison has been swallowed. For other types of poison, milk or water will actually increase the rate of absorption by causing the substances to dissolve more rapidly. A stomach filled with water or milk will force its contents through the sphincter between the stomach and the small intestines, where they will be absorbed faster. However, water can be given when using ipecac syrup.

poisonings, in home   You may think of your home as an oasis of safety in an unsafe world, and for the most part that may be true. But your home can be a very dangerous place for youngsters when it comes to accidental poisoning, where even one tablet of certain medications can kill a young child.

More than 2.4 million cases of poisoning are reported to poison centers across the United States each year. Among those, most accidental poisonings occur among children under the age of six because this age group is especially curious about everything in their environment, and their bodies are small enough so that a relatively small amount of a toxin can be fatal.

Common poisons

The substances most often consumed by children under age five, according to the Poison Control Centers, are:

Plants
Soaps, detergents, cleaners
Perfume, cologne, toilet water
Antihistamines, cold medications
Vitamins, minerals
Aspirin
Household disinfectants, deodorizers
Insecticides
Miscellaneous painkillers
Fingernail preparations
Liniments
Household bleach
Miscellaneous external medicines
Cosmetic lotions, creams

Other common, potentially dangerous products found in nearly every home and garage include polishes and waxes, alcohol, hair dyes, garden products (roach powders, rat pellets, weed killers, lime, sprays), and garage products (antifreeze, kerosene, gasoline, pain thinners, and strippers).

Prevention

Parents should make a rule that all hazardous items be kept in high cupboards, on tall shelves in closets or in locked drawers or cabinets. All toxic products should be returned to their secure cabinets after every use.

- In the kitchen, keep all household chemical products out of sight and locked up when they are not being used. Do not keep chemicals stored under the sink and on the counters because they are within easy reach of most youngsters.

- Make sure all harmful products have child-resistant caps.

- Keep all harmful products in their original containers. Original labels often give first aid information in the event of poisoning, and products stored in other containers may look like food to a child.

- Keep harmful products stored in a place separate from food.

- In the garage and utility rooms, keep the following items in a locked cabinet with childproof latches: antifreeze, windshield washing fluid, gasoline, kerosene, and other automobile fluids; also pesticides and other garden products (see "Pesticide Safety").

poison ivy (*Toxicodendron radicans*)   Poison ivy is one of the most common plants in the United States that are poisonous to touch; it causes a contact dermatitis in most people—as many as 87 million Americans.

The leaves of the poison ivy plant are glossy green, may be notched or smooth and almost always grow in groups of three—two leaves opposite each other and one at the end of the stalk. However, according to some experts there are exceptions, and leaves may sometimes appear in fives, sevens, or even nines. In early fall, the leaves may turn bright red. Although it usually grows as a long, hairy vine—often wrapping itself around trees—it can also be found as a low shrub growing along fences or stone walls. Poison ivy has waxy yellow-green flowers and greenish berries that look rather like a peeled orange. These berries can help in identification of the plants in late fall, winter, and early spring before the leaves appear.

Poison ivy is found throughout the United States, but it is most common in the eastern and central states.

Poisonous part

Poison ivy, poison oak, and poison sumac are closely related species, all three containing a colorless or slightly yellow resin called urushiol, which comes from a Japanese word meaning "lacquer." Skin contact with urushiol causes an allergic reaction known as contact dermatitis in many individuals. While each of these three plants contains a slightly different type of urushiol, they are so similar that individuals sensitive to one will react to all three. The entire plant contains urushiol and is therefore poisonous: leaves, berries, stalk, and roots.

Urushiol is easily transferred from an object to a person, so anything that touches poison ivy—clothing, gardening tools, a pet's fur, athletic equipment, sleeping bags—can be contaminated with urushiol and cause poison ivy in anyone who then touches the object. Urushiol remains active for up to one year, so any equipment that touches poison ivy must be washed. Even the smoke from burning poison ivy is toxic and can irritate the skin of the face, eyes and lungs, since urushiol can be carried in smoke. It can irritate the throat if eaten. Individuals should never burn poison ivy plants as a way to get rid of them, since the smoke given off by these burning plants is particularly dangerous and can enter the nasal passages, throat, and lungs of anyone who breathes it.

As the leaves die in the fall, the plant draws certain nutrients and substances (including the oil) into the stem. But the oil remains active, so that even in winter it may cause rash if the broken stems are used as firewood kindling or vines on a Christmas wreath.

Symptoms

While not every person is allergic to poison ivy, about seven out of 10 Americans are sensitive to urushiol and will develop contact dermatitis if exposed to a large enough dose.

Symptoms vary from one person to the next; some people exhibit only mild itching, while others experience severe reactions, including severe burning and itching with watery blisters. The skin irritation, swelling, blisters, and itching may appear within hours or days, usually developing within 24 to 48 hours in a sensitized person. The skin becomes reddened followed by watery blisters, peaking about five days after contamination and gradually improving over a week or two, even without treatment. Eventually, the blisters break, and the oozing sores crust over and then disappear.

About 15 percent of the people who are allergic to poison ivy, poison oak, and poison sumac are so highly sensitive that they react within four to 12 hours instead of 24 to 48. These individuals often experience swollen eyes, rapidly developing blisters that ooze pus, and fever.

Despite common misconception, poison ivy is *not* spread by scratching open blisters or skin-to-skin contact but by the oil (urushiol) found in the plant. Anything that brushes against this oil is contaminated and can pass on poison ivy if it brushes the skin. Poison ivy is not spread from person to person, by touching blisters, since only the oil spreads the rash. For this reason, doctors recommend not scratching blisters because any remaining urushiol that hasn't been washed off can be transmitted to another part of the body. In addition, scratching blisters may cause infection from germs on the fingernails. Animals can also transmit poison ivy from their fur to their owners' skin. Any animal suspected of coming in contact with poison ivy should be given a bath; wear protective gloves when bathing affected animals.

In addition, allergy to poison ivy, oak, and sumac may also mean a person is allergic to related plants, including cashews, pistachios, mangos, and Chinese or Japanese lacquer trees.

Treatment

The best treatment is to wash the affected area immediately after contact (within 10 minutes, if possible) with yellow laundry soap and *cold* water, or water from a shower. Do not bathe in a tub, as this could spread the oil. Do not scrub with a brush. If contaminated while in isolated areas, wash in a cold running stream. Any clothing that might have come in contact with urushiol must be washed several times. If the urushiol is washed off, there is little further treatment needed of mild cases of the rash. Remove rings, watches, bracelets, etc., before washing hands. Wash contaminated jewelry.

Early application of topical steroids minimizes the severity of dermatitis; systemic steroids given during the first six hours after exposure are the most effective.

Itching can be treated with compresses soaked in cold water. A calamine lotion spread over the rash will help relieve the itching and burning and dry the area. Products containing local anesthetics (such as benzocaine) or irritants (camphor or phenol) should be avoided. Systemic antihistamines do not work against the rash, although their sedative action may help the person sleep. In the case of a severe reaction, a physician may prescribe corticosteroid drugs by mouth or injection.

Prevention

New barrier creams (bentoquatam) may offer some protection; these have been recently approved by the U.S. Food and Drug Administration. Cream should be applied 15 minutes before exposure and every four hours afterward. It should not be used if a rash is already present, nor by children under age six. Dermatologists are also working on a skin treatment to prevent the oil from penetrating the skin.

Most people could be immunized against poison ivy through prescription pills, which contain gradually increasing amounts of active extract from the plants. However, this procedure can take four months to achieve a reasonable degree of "hyposensitization," and the medication must be continued over a long period of time. In addition, it often causes uncomfortable side effects such as skin problems, stomach problems, fever, and inflammation. Convulsions have occurred in children following oral doses of the plant's extract.

This procedure is recommended only if the doses are given before contact with the plant, and only for people (such as firefighters) who must live or work in areas where they come into constant contact with poison ivy. Consult your dermatologist for his or her advice on whether you should consider this type of immunization. Allergy shots also are available to help prevent recurring episodes of poison ivy, poison oak, and poison sumac. Because these shots are often ineffective, however, they should be used only by people who are extremely sensitive to urushiol.

See also POISON OAK; POISON SUMAC; URUSHIOL.

poison oak *(Toxicodendron diversilobum)*   A plant poisonous by touch, this is one of three closely related species containing similar forms of the resin urushiol. Urushiol causes a contact dermatitis in seven out of 10 Americans who come in contact with it. The leaves of poison oak occur in groups of three and are very similar to oak leaves, from which the plant gets its name. The underside of the leaves are much lighter green than the tops because of the thousands of tiny fine hairs that cover them. Berries may be greenish or creamy white, although not all plants bear fruit. Poison oak usually grows as a low shrub on the west coast from Mexico to British Columbia.

Symptoms

Symptoms vary from one person to the next, ranging from mild itching to severe burning and itching with watery blisters, and usually develop within 24 to 48 hours in a sensitive person. Symptoms usually peak about five days after contamination and gradually improve over a week or two even without treatment. Eventually, the blisters break, and the oozing sores crust over and then disappear. Poison oak is *not* spread by scratching open blisters but by the urushiol found in the plant. Anything that brushes against this oil is contaminated and can pass on poison oak if it brushes the skin. For this reason, doctors recommend not scratching blisters, since any remaining urushiol that hasn't been washed off can be transmitted to another part of the body. Animals can also transmit poison oak from their fur to their owners' skin. Any animal suspected of coming in contact with poison oak should be given a bath (gloves should be worn).

Treatment

The best treatment is to wash the affected area immediately after contact with yellow laundry soap and *cold* water, lathering several times and rinsing the area in running water after each sudsing. Do not scrub with a brush. If contaminated while in isolated areas, wash in a cold running stream. Any clothing that might have come in contact with urushiol must be washed several times. If the urushiol is washed off the skin, there is little further treatment needed in mild cases. Itching can be treated with compresses soaked in cold water, and calamine lotion spread over the rash will help relieve the itching and burning. In the case of a severe reaction, a physician may prescribe corticosteroid drugs by mouth or injection.

See also POISON IVY; URUSHIOL.

poisons, by symptom   Sometimes it is not so easy to figure out exactly what poisonous substance someone has ingested—especially if the person is a young child. If all you have to go on is a symptom, it can help to have a way to link symptoms to poisonous substances.

Remember that most poisons cause more than one symptom, and that the severity of the symptoms differs depending on how much of the poison was ingested.

Aggression

atropine, belladonna, ketamine, PCP, Preludin

Anxiety

amphetamines, barium, bronchial tube relaxers, camphor, carbon monoxide, ecstasy, mercury, Minipress, PCP, potassium, sodium fluoroacetate, Thyrolar, water hemlock, yellow jessamine

Blood problems

Many poisons can cause a variety of blood-related symptoms, including anemia, hemorrhages (excessive bleeding), high or low blood sugar, or a low red blood count.

Anemia   Dilantin, pathalene, rattlesnake, trinitrotoluene

Bleeding   aspirin, atophan, Depakene, warfarin

Blood Sugar—High   Lasix, Vacor

Blood Sugar—Low   akee, *Amanita* mushroom, Dilantin, Inderal, insulin, phosphorus

Hemorrhage   adder, aspirin, atophan, castor bean, chlordane, cinchona bark, cottonmouth, Depakene, fer-de-lance, isopropanol, paternoster pea, potassium permanganate, rhubarb, savin, Vacor, warfarin

Low Red Blood Count   carbon monoxide, ethinamate, warfarin

Bruises

See SKIN PROBLEMS.

Collapse

A variety of poisonous substances are serious enough that, when ingested, they can trigger a total collapse. The following poisons may cause collapse:

adder, ammonia, bromates, cantharidin, castor bean, cationic detergents, chloramine-T, cinchona bark, cottonmouth, ethylene chlorohydrin, formaldehyde, Haldol, Indian tobacco, ipecac, lead, narcissus, nicotine, nitroglycerin, privet, procaine, silver nitrate, stingray, Vacor

Coma

akee, aldrin, amphetamines, aniline, antimony, arsenic, aspirin, atropine, barbiturates, belladonna, boric acid, bromates, bryony, cantharidin, cassava, castor bean, Catapres, celandine, chloral hydrate, cinchona bark, cinchophen, cocaine, codeine, columbine, corn cockle, *Cortinarius* mushroom, croton oil, daphne, death camas, dieldrin, Elavil, epinephrine, ergot, ethyl alcohol, GHB, *Gyromitra* mushroom, Haldol, heroin, hydrogen sulfide, Inderal, Indian tobacco, insulin, isopropanol, jimsonweed, lead, lithium, Lomotil, LSD, mandrake, marijuana, morphine, nicotine, nitroglycerin, opium, panther mushroom, paral, paternoster pea, PCP, Percodan, Permitil, petroleum distillates, phenol, potato, procaine, rhododendron, savin, selective serotonin reuptake inhibitors, silver nitrate, Sinequan, sodium fluoroacetate, Stelazine, tetrachloroethane, Thorazine, toxaphene, Vacor, Valium, valproic acid, yew

Confusion

amphetamines, aniline, atropine, barbiturates, carbon monoxide, carbon tetrachloride, chloral hydrate, DDT, Dilantin, endrin, flunitrazepam, Inderal, lithium, nicotine, opium, Preludin, selective serotonin reuptake inhibitors, sodium thiocyanate, Tagamet, Tylenol

Convulsions or Seizures

akee, aldrin, amphetamines, aniline, arsenic, aspirin, atropine, barium, belladonna, benzene, benzene hexachloride, benzylpiperazine, betel nut seed, boric acid, boron, bromates, bronchial tube relaxers, bryony, caffeine, calcium, camphor, cassava, castor bean, cationic detergents, cinchophen, cobra, cocaine, columbine, *Cortinarius* mushroom, cyanide, daffodil, daphne, DDT, dieldrin, dyphylline, Elavil, elderberry, endrin, epinephrine, ethyl alcohol, fool's parsley, gelsemium, grounsel, *Gyromitra* mushroom, hydrangea, Inderal, Indian tobacco, ipecac, jimsonweed, ketamine, oleander, Lomotil, LSD, meadow saffron, monkshood, monoamine oxidase (MAO) inhibitors, moonseed, mountain laurel, narcissus, nicotine, panther mushroom, parathion, paternoster pea, PCP, Permitil, persistent organic pollutants, Phenergan, physostigmine, pokeweed, potato, procainamide, procaine, pyrethrum, quaalude, Ritalin, rhododendron, rotenone, scorpion fish, scorpions, selective serotonin reuptake inhibitors, silver nitrate, sodium fluoroacetate, sodium thiocyanate, spindle tree, Stelazine, stingray, stonefish, strychnine, tansy, TEPP, Thorazine, toxaphene, turpentine, water hemlock, yellow jessamine, yew

Delirium

atropine, benzene, brown recluse spider, cinchophen, corn cockle, ethylene chlorohydrin, foxglove, henbane, horse chestnut, Inderal, iodine, jimsonweed, ketamine, lead, meadow saffron, panther mushroom, Tagamet, tetrachlorethane, Vacor, white snakeroot

Depression

amphetamines, ecstasy, ketamine, mountain laurel

Dizziness or Vertigo

A wide range of poisonous substances can lead to either dizziness or vertigo (a sensation in which the person feels he or his surroundings are constantly spinning or moving).

Aldomet, aldrin, amphetamines, aniline, arsenic, aspirin, baneberry, Barbados nut, barbiturates, benzene, bloodroot, bronchial tube relaxers, camphor, carbon tetrachloride, chloral hydrate, codeine, *Cortinarius* mushroom, daffodil, dieldrin, Dilantin, elderberry, ethylene chlorohydrin, fly agaric, gelsemium, geography cone, Gila monster, hydrogen sulfide, jimsonweed, Lasix, methanol, monkshood, morphine, nicotine, nitroglycerin, Norflex, panther mushroom, Percodan, Persantine, petroleum distillates, Phenergan, phenol, Preludin, procaine, propane, quinidine, Sinequan, sodium fluoroacetate, stingray, Tagamet, Thorazine, toxaphene, trichloroethane, turpentine, Vacor, Valium

Euphoria/Excitement

amphetamines, benzene, Halcion, heroin, LSD, marijuana, nitrous oxide, opium, Preludin

Hair Loss

A few substances, including arsenic or boric acid, may lead to hair loss (alopecia). Medications that cause this symptom include Depakene (valproic acid), a central nervous system antidepressant, or the high blood pressure medicine Minipress (prazosin hydrochloride). Polonium-210 can also cause hair loss.

Hallucinations

amphetamines, atropine, belladonna, betel nut seed, bronchial tube relaxers, cocaine, Elavil, ethyl alcohol, GHB, Haldol, Inderal, lily of the valley, LSD, marijuana, mercury, PCP, Preludin, selective serotonin reuptake inhibitors, toxaphene, Valium

Headache

Aldomet, aldrin, aniline, arsenic, barbiturates, *Bacillus anthracis*, benzene, boron, bronchial tube relaxers, cadmium, camphor, carbon monoxide, corn cockle, DDT, dieldrin, dyphylline, elderberry, ergot, ethylene chlorohydrin, foxglove, galerina mushrooms, GHB, hydrogen sulfide, Inderal, jimsonweed, Lasix, lily of the valley, malathion, methyl alcohol, Minipress, naphthalene, nicotine, nitroglycerin, nitrous oxide, panther mushroom, parathion, persantine, persistent organic pollutants, potato, Preludin, quinidine, stibine, Tagamet, TEPP, tetrachloroethane, Thyrolar, trichloroethane, tularemia, yellow jessamine

Hearing Problems

Deafness/Hearing Loss aspirin, bromates, quinine

Tinnitus aspirin, cinchona bark, Elavil, endrin, Gila monster, nicotine

Heart Problems

Many poisons act directly on the heart and are capable of causing a range of adverse effects.

Cardiac Arrest bloodroot, calcium, Catapres, cocaine, Elavil, ergot, insulin, oleander, Percodan, potassium, sodium, Stelazine, Valium

Chest Pain beryllium, cadmium, carbon monoxide, ergot, foxglove, jellyfish, monkshood, Portuguese man-of-war, sea anemone, TEPP, turpentine, Vacor

High Blood Pressure amphetamines, bronchial tube dilators, cadmium, Demerol, ecstasy, ketamine, monoamine oxidase (MAO) inhibitors, PCP, Preludin, scorpion, Sinequan, Thyrolar, yellow jessamine

Irregular Heartbeat *Bacillus anthracis* (anthrax), barbiturates, benzylpiperazine, black hellebore, bloodroot, caffeine, Dilantin, Elavil, epinephrine, ether, formaldehyde, foxglove, *Inocybe* mushroom, ipecac, nitrous oxide, phosphorus, Portuguese man-of-war, sodium fluoroacetate, stingray, Tylenol, valproic acid

Low Blood Pressure acid, alkalies, aniline, arsenic, barbiturates, boric acid, bromates, cantharidin, carbon tetrachloride, Catapres, chloral hydrate, cobra, curare, cyanide, dyphylline, Elavil, ethylene chlorohydrin, false hellebore, flunitrazepam, fly agaric, Haldol, heroin, Inderal, insulin, ipecac, Lasix, monkshood, monoamine oxidase (MAO) inhibitors, nitroglycerin, opium, panther mushroom, Percodan, Permitil, Phenergan, phy-

sostigmine, procainamide, procaine, quinidine, rhododendron, scorpions, sodium azide, sodium thiocyanate, Stelazine, stingray, Tagamet, TEPP, Thorazine, trichloroethane, Tylenol, Vacor

Rapid Heartbeat acid, amphetamines, atropine, baneberry, belladonna, bromates, caffeine, camphor, cocaine, *Cortinarius* mushroom, croton oil, cyanide, digitoxin, dyphylline, ecstasy, elderberry, epinephrine, fool's parsley, foxglove, Halcion, Haldol, hemlock, insulin, ipecac, marijuana, Minipress, monoamine oxidase (MAO) inhibitors, morphine, nicotine, paral, paraquat, paternoster pea, Phenergan, selective serotonin reuptake inhibitors, Sinequan, tansy, Thorazine, turpentine

Slow Heartbeat/Pulse black locust, bloodroot, carbon tetrachloride, Catapres, codeine, curare, dog mercury, false hellebore, fly agaric, foxglove, Inderal, larkspur, lily of the valley, monkshood, morphine, panther mushroom, physostigmine, rhododendron, yellow jessamine

Weak, Irregular Pulse black locust, hemlock, *Inocybe* mushroom, monkshood, valproic acid

Hyperactivity

cocaine, cottonmouth, PCP, Preludin, Thyrolar

Insomnia

amphetamines, bronchial tube relaxers, caffeine, dyphylline, Elavil, endrin, Inderal, Phenergan, Preludin, Reglan

Irritability

barbiturates, carbon monoxide, cottonmouth, dieldrin, lily of the valley, propane

Itching

See SKIN PROBLEMS.

Kidney/Liver Damage

It's the job of your liver and kidneys to help filter poisons from the body; some substances may cause kidney damage or complete organ failure.

Liver Damage arsenic, botulism, Catapres, chlordane, Depakene, Dilantin, formaldehyde, methanol, monoamine oxidase (MAO) inhibitors, potassium permanganate

Kidney Damage botulism, daphne, Dilantin, galerina mushrooms, methanol, naphthalene, phenol, potassium permanganate, privet, rhubarb, tansy, Tylenol

Kidney Failure cadmium, colocynth, ecstasy, excessive fluid intake, mercury, mountain laurel, PCP, sodium, turpentine

Lung Problems

In overdose or inappropriate dosage, many medicines and poisons can affect the lungs, causing swelling, coughing and breathing problems, and even leading to respiratory failure.

Breathing Problems aldrin, anaphylaxis, aniline, antimony, atropine, *Bacillus anthracis* (anthrax), Barbados nut, barbiturates, barium, belladonna, benzene, beryllium, betel nut seed, bloodroot, bronchial tube relaxers, cadmium, calcium, camphor, carbon monoxide, carbon tetrachloride, cassava, Catapres, chloral hydrate, cobra, cocaine, codeine, curare, death camas, dimethyl sulfate, Elavil, elderberry, ergot, fer-de-lance, gelsemium, geography cone, Gila monster, hemlock, heroin, horse chestnut, Inderal, insulin, ipecac, isopropanol, jellyfish, larkspur, Lasix, Lomotil, malathion, meadow saffron, mercury, Minipress, morphine, mountain laurel, nicotine, opium, paral, parathion, PCP, percodan, petroleum distillates, Phenergan, phosgene, pokeweed, potassium, pufferfish, physostigmine, rattlesnake, rhubarb, scorpion, shellfish poisoning, sodium, sodium fluoroacetate, stibine, TEPP, trichloroethane, turpentine, Valium, valproic acid, water hemlock, yellow jessamine

Bronchitis dimethyl sulfate, lead dust, malathion, mold

Cough acid, ammonia, *Bacillus anthracis* (anthrax), cadmium, hydrogen sulfide, mercury, mold, paral, petroleum distillates, potassium permanganate, trinitrotoluene, tularemia, turpentine

Coughing Blood aspirin, castor bean, warfarin

Pulmonary Edema ammonia, aspirin, antimony, bronchial tube relaxers, cadmium, epinephrine, formaldehyde, hydrogen sulfide, isopropanol, malathion, methanol, parathion, petroleum distillates, phosgene, quaalude, scorpion, sodium fluoroacetate, turpentine

Respiratory Failure anectine, blue-ringed octopus, bryony, cantharidin, cinchona bark, corn cockle, ether, fool's parsley, geography cone, Gila monster, heroin, meadow saffron, monkshood, nicotine, nitroglycerin, oleander, opium, Pavulon, procaine, star of Bethlehem, strychnine, Thorazine, toxaphene, tubarine, Vacor, water hemlock

Mouth Problems

Some plants and other substances can cause symptoms by direct contact with the mouth.

Drooling cadmium, columbine, death camas, fly agaric, Haldol, *Inocybe* mushroom, lily of the valley, malathion, mercury, mountain laurel, panther mushroom, PCP, Phenergan, rhododendron, silver nitrate

Foaming acid, ammonia, chloramine-T, phenol, tansy, water hemlock

Gum Problems adder, cobra, Dilantin, fer-de-lance, lead, mercury, polonium-210

Swelling black hellebore, dimethyl sulfate, *Inocybe* mushroom, potassium permanganate

Muscle Problems

Weak or stiff muscles, spasms, or cramps may all be caused by some poisons.

Cramps (leg) Barbados nut, potassium

Flaccidity calcium, chloral hydrate, marijuana, potassium, Percodan, Valium

Rigidity ammonia, black widow spider, camphor, gelsemium, Haldol, ketamine, PCP

Spasms aldrin, amphetamines, benzene, boric acid, caffeine, camphor, cocaine, DDT, dieldrin, Dilantin, Elavil, epinephrine, Lasix, lithium, LSD, mercury, nicotine, parathion, physostigmine, pokeweed, Preludin, procaine, pyrethrum, Reglan, rotenone, scorpion, sodium fluoroacetate, sodium thiocyanate, strychnine, tansy, TEPP, Thorazine, Thyrolar, Vacor, white snakeroot, yellow jessamine

Stiffness atropine, black widow spider, marijuana, Permitil, strychnine

Weakness acid, Aldomet, aldrin, barium, beaked sea snake, benzene, beryllium, bloodroot, cadmium, corn cockle, *Cortinarius* mushroom, daphne, death camas, dieldrin, endrin, false hellebore, gelsemium, Gila monster, hemlock, Indian tobacco, Lasix, lead, meadow saffron, Minipress, morphine, Norflex, parathion, Persantine, petroleum distillates, potassium, phenol, pokeweed, rhubarb, sodium thiocyanate, stibine, stingray,

Thyrolar, tularemia, Vacor, Valium, white snake-root, yellow jessamine, yew

Paralysis

Some poisonous substances act on the central nervous system, causing paralysis. These include: atropine, benzene, blue-ringed octopus, botulism, bryony, calcium, cobra, croton oil, curare, gelsemium, geography cone, hemlock, jimsonweed, monkshood, mountain laurel, narcissus, parathion, Pavulon, potassium, pufferfish, pyrethrum, rattlesnake, rhododendron, scorpion fish, sea anemone, sodium, stonefish, TEPP

Psychosis

atropine, camphor, cocaine, Depakene, Dilantin, epinephrine, ergot, ethyl alcohol, Halcion, Haldol, LSD, marijuana, mercury, Preludin

Restlessness

amphetamines, aspirin, black widow spider, heroin, horse chestnut, LSD, Preludin, selective serotonin reuptake inhibitors, water hemlock

Shock

ammonia, baneberry, cadmium, fer-de-lance, insulin, iodine, Lasix, malathion, moonseed, phenol, Portuguese man-of-war, potassium permanganate, rattlesnake, sea anemone, silver nitrate, stingray, yew

Skin Problems

Bleeding   adder, black widow spider, brown recluse spider, cobra, rattlesnake

Bruises   aspirin, Depakene, Lasix, polonium-210, warfarin

Discoloration—Black   silver nitrate

Discoloration—Blue (cyanosis)   acid, *Amanita* mushroom, amphetamines, aniline, aspirin, boric acid, brown recluse spider, castor bean, chloral hydrate, chloramine-T, curare, cyanide, dimethyl sulfate, epinephrine, ether, ethinamate, Gila monster, heroin, hydrangea, *Inocybe* mushroom, jellyfish, larkspur, nitroglycerin, paral, paraquat, phenol, phosgene, procaine, TEPP, tetrachloroethane, trinitrotoluene

Discoloration—Brown   acid, potassium permanganate

Discoloration—Red   ammonia, atropine, belladonna, bronchial tube relaxers, brown recluse spider, cyanide, *Inocybe* mushroom, insulin, lily of the valley, nitroglycerin, persantine, procaine, pufferfish, turpentine

Discoloration—Yellow   Indian tobacco, nicotine, trinitrotoluene

Irritation   acid, Aldomet, antimony, arsenic, atropine, belladonna, benzene hexachloride, boric acid, brown recluse spider, cadmium, cantharidin, Catapres, croton oil, DDT, dog mercury, ethylene chlorohydrin, formaldehyde, hydrogen sulfide, larkspur, Librax, malathion, Minipress, narcissus, paraquat, parathion, phosphorus, pyrethrum, sodium azide, Tagamet, tansy, tetrachloroethane, trinitrotoluene

Itching   larkspur, opium

Necrotic Tissue   acid, alkalies, aniline, benzene, brown recluse spider, cantharidin, cobra, cottonmouth, ergot, ether-chloroform, iodine, jellyfish, mercury, phenol, phosphorus, potassium permanganate, rattlesnake, sea anemone, Tylenol

Paleness   malathion, phenol, trinitrotoluene, yew

Swelling   adder, anaphylaxis, blue-ringed octopus, brown recluse spider, cobra, jellyfish, rattlesnake, scorpion fish

Speech Problems

blue-ringed octopus, chloral hydrate, codeine, curare, ethyl alcohol, gelsemium, GHB, Haldol, ketamine, lithium, marijuana, pufferfish, Thorazine, yellow jessamine

Stomach or Intestinal Problems

Abdominal Pain   alkalies, *Amanita* mushroom, ammonia, arsenic, aspirin, baneberry, barium, bloodroot, bromates, cantharidin, carbon tetrachloride, cassava, cinchophen, cocaine, colocynth, corn cockle, daffodil, daphne, fool's parsley, formaldehyde, hydrangea, iodine, isopropanol, jellyfish, lead, lily of the valley, meadow saffron, mercury, methanol, Minipress, mountain laurel, paraquat, parathion, Portuguese man-of-war, potato, privet, rhubarb, rotenone, scorpions, spindle tree, stibine, stingray, tetrachloroethane, Thyrolar, turpentine, Vacor, water hemlock, yew

Appetite Loss   *Bacillus anthracis* (anthrax), Preludin

Bloating   Barbados nut

Constipation   opium, Percodan, Vacor, white snakeroot

Cramps   arsenic, castor bean, colocynth, elderberry, heroin, panther mushroom, pokeweed, scorpions, stingray, TEPP

Diarrhea (bloody)   acid, *Amanita* mushroom, antimony, *Bacillus anthracis* (anthrax), baneberry, colocynth, croton oil, daphne, fool's parsley, meadow saffron, mercury, moonseed, oleander, tetrachloroethane, warfarin

Diarrhea   alkalies, amphetamines, arsenic, Barbados nut, barium, benzene hexachloride, betel nut seed, black hellebore, boric acid, boron, bromates, bryony, cadmium, cantharidin, cinchophen, daffodil, digitoxin, false hellebore, fly agaric, formaldehyde, foxglove, *Gyromitra* mushroom, hemlock, horse chestnut, Inderal, iodine, lead, malathion, mandrake, Minipress, mold, naphthalene, nicotine, panther mushroom, paraquat, parathion, paternoster pea, phosphorus, poinsettia, pokeweed, polonium-210, potato, privet, pyrethrum, quinidine, rhododendron, silver nitrate, spindle tree, Tagamet, TEPP, Thyrolar, tularemia, turpentine, water hemlock, yew

Nausea   akee, aldrin, *Amanita* mushroom, amphetamines, antimony, arsenic, *Bacillus anthracis* (anthrax), baneberry, barium, benzene, black locust, black widow spider, boron, botulism, brown recluse spider, bryony, cadmium, camphor, cantharidin, carbon monoxide, carbon tetrachloride, cassava, castor bean, Catapres, cationic detergents, celandine, cinchona bark, cobra, columbine, corn cockle, *Cortinarius* mushroom, daffodil, daphne, Depakene, dieldrin, digitoxin, dyphylline, ecstasy, elderberry, endrin, epinephrine, ergot, ethyl alcohol, ethylene chlorohydrin, false hellebore, fly agaric, foxglove, Gila monster, grounsel, Halcion, hydrangea, hydrogen sulfide, Inderal, Indian tobacco, ipecac, isopropanol, larkspur, Lasix, lily of the valley, malathion, mercury, methanol, Minipress, monkshood, monoamine oxidase (MAO) inhibitors, morphine, mountain laurel, naphthalene, narcissus, nicotine, Norflex, opium, panther mushroom, parathion, paternoster pea, Percodan, Permitil, Persantine, persistent organic pollutants, phosphorus, pokeweed, polonium-210, privet, pyrethrum, quaalude, quinidine, rattlesnake, Reglan, rhododendron, rhubarb, Ritalin, rotenone, selective serotonin reuptake inhibitors, shellfish poisoning, stibine, stingray, Talwin, tanghin, tetrachloroethane

Stool (dark)   lead

Vomiting   acid, akee, aldrin, alkalies, *Amanita* mushroom, ammonia, amphetamines, antimony, arsenic, atophan, baneberry, Barbados nut, barium, benzene, benzene hexachloride, betel nut seed, black locust, black widow spider, bloodroot, blue ringed octopus, boric acid, boron, bromates, bronchial tube relaxers, brown recluse spider, bryony, cadmium, caffeine, camphor, cantharidin, carbon tetrachloride, cassava, castor bean, celandine, cinchona bark, cocaine, columbine, *Cortinarius* mushroom, croton oil, daphne, DDT, dieldrin, digitoxin, dog mercury, dyphylline, epinephrine, ergot, ethyl alcohol, ethylene chlorohydrin, false hellebore, formaldehyde, foxglove, grounsel, *Gyromitras* mushroom, Halcion, hemlock, horse chestnut, Inderal, Indian tobacco, insulin, iodine, ipecac, ketamine, larkspur, Lasix, lead, lily of the valley, malathion, mandrake, meadow saffron, mercury, Minipress, monkshood, monoamine oxidase (MAO) inhibitors, mountain laurel, naphthalene, narcissus, nicotine, nitroglycerine, Norflex, oleander, opium, paraquat, Percodan, petroleum distillates, phosphorus, physostigmine, poinsettia, pokeweed, polonium-210, potato, privet, pyrethrum, quaalude, rattlesnake, rhododendron, rhubarb, Ritalin, rotenone, savin, selective serotonin reuptake inhibitors, shellfish poisoning, silver nitrate, sodium fluoroacetate, spindle tree, stingray, Tanghin, TEPP, toxaphene, turpentine, Tylenol, Vacor, water hemlock, white snakeroot, yew

Stupor

aniline, black locust, castor bean, Indian tobacco, *Inocybe* mushroom, iodine, monoamine oxidase (MAO) inhibitors, PCP, Percodan, potato, rotenone

Unconsciousness

benzene, camphor, carbon fumes, carbon monoxide, carbon tetrachloride, chloral hydrate, cocaine, codeine, cyanide, Dalmane, endrin, ether, ethyl alcohol, ethylene chlorohydrin, formaldehyde, heroin, hydrangea, hydrogen sulfide, *Inocibe* mushroom, marijuana, Minipress, morphine, oleander, opium, petroleum distillates, stonefish, trichloroethane, turpentine, Valium

Urinary Tract Problems

Lack of Urine atropine, belladonna, black widow spider, bromates, colocynth, cort mushrooms, Elavil, ergot, iodine, meadow saffron, rhubarb, savin, silver nitrate, tansy, trinitrotoluene

Dark Color flagyl, phenol

Painful Urination Barbados nut, naphthalene, turpentine

Frequent Urine Lasix, Vacor

Urinary Retention aspirin, atropine, belladonna, benzylpiperazine, black widow spider, bromates, colocynth, flunitrazepam, isopropanol, lead, naphthalene, paraquat, savin, trinitrotoluene

Uremia aldrin, aspirin, brown recluse spider, cantharidin, carbon tetrachloride, castor bean, cort mushrooms, dieldrin, iodine, mercury, naphthalene, savin, turpentine, warfarin

Yellow Urine atophan

Visual Problems

Blindness ammonia, atropine, hemlock, jimsonweed, methanol, phenol, propane

Blurry/Double Vision alkalies, atropine, beaked sea snake, belladonna, benzene, betel nut seed, botulism, cinchona bark, digitoxin, dimethyl sulfate, ecstasy, Elavil, epinephrine, ethyl alcohol, false hellebore, fool's parsley, foxglove, Haldol, hemlock, henbane, heroin, hydrogen sulfide, jimsonweed, Lasix, Librax, malathion, methanol, Minipress, monkshood, nicotine, Norflex, panther mushroom, Permitil, Tanghin, TEPP, Vacor

Dilated Pupils atropine, belladonna, benzylpiperazine, bloodroot, cocaine, Elavil, epinephrine, ethyl alcohol, heroin, horse chestnut, Indian tobacco, lily of the valley, parathion, tansy, water hemlock, yellow jessamine, yew

Pinpoint Pupils morphine, opium, physostigmine, TEPP

Reddened Eyes dimethyl sulfate, hydrogen sulfide

Sensitivity to Light atropine, Lasix, parathion

Teary Eyes dimethyl sulfate, fly agaric mushroom, formaldehyde, malathion, mountain laurel, panther mushroom, rhododendron, TEPP

poison sumac (*Toxicodendron. vernix* [L.] Kuntzel [= *Rhus vernix* L.]) This poisonous tree, a relative of poison ivy and poison oak, has seven to 13 long, narrow leaves growing in pairs with a single leaf at the end of the stem. In the spring, the leaves are bright orange and look something like velvet; as the season progresses, they become dark green and glossy on the upper surface of the leaf and light green on the underside. In the fall, the leaves turn red or orange. Poison sumac can be differentiated from nonpoisonous sumacs by its drooping clusters of green berries—nonpoisonous sumacs have red, upright clusters of berries. Poison sumac can grow to be 25 feet tall, although it more often reaches heights of five to six feet. It is found in swampy areas throughout eastern United States.

Symptoms

Symptoms vary from one person to the next, ranging from mild itching to severe burning and itching with watery blisters, and usually develop within 24 to 48 hours in a sensitive person. Symptoms usually peak about five days after contamination and gradually improve over a week or two even without treatment. Eventually, the blisters break, and the oozing sores crust over and then disappear. The poison sumac rash is *not* spread by scratching open blisters but by the urushiol found in the plant. Anything that brushes against this oil is contaminated and can pass on the rash if it brushes the skin. For this reason, doctors recommend not scratching blisters, since any remaining urushiol that hasn't been washed off can be transmitted to another part of the body. Animals can also transmit poison sumac from their fur to their owners's skin. Any animal suspected of coming in contact with poison sumac should be given a bath; gloves should be worn while bathing.

Treatment

The best treatment is to wash the affected area immediately after contact with yellow laundry soap and *cold* water, lathering several times and rinsing the area in running water after each sudsing. Do not scrub with a brush. If contaminated while in isolated areas, wash in a cold running stream. Any clothing that might have come in contact with urushiol must be washed several times.

If the urushiol is washed off the skin, there is little further treatment needed in mild cases. Itching can be treated with compresses soaked in cold water, and calamine lotion spread over the rash will help relieve the itching and burning. In the case of a severe reaction, a physician may prescribe cortico-steroid drugs by mouth or injection.

See also POISON IVY; URUSHIOL.

poisonwood (Metopium toxiferum) One of a group of plants that are poisonous on contact, poisonwood is found in southern Florida to the Bahamas, Honduras, and the West Indies. It is related to poison oak and poison sumac, which places it in the Anacardiaceae family. Anyone who lives or works in southern Florida should learn to recognize poisonwood because any contact with it causes a negative reaction. Poisonwood is found in pinelands, sandy dunes near salt water, and in hammocks. The plant has a yellow-orange fruit that is enjoyed by many birds and animals.

Poisonous part

The sap contains alkaloids that cause a toxic effect on contact with the skin. Since any part of this tree can carry the sap, contact with any part of the poisonwood tree can be poisonous.

Symptoms

Upon contact, the individual's skin turns black and a rash and blisters develop. Smoke from a burning tree can cause temporary blindness.

Treatment

Symptomatic. According to folk medicine, the sap of another tree indigenous to the same area, the gum elemi or gumbo-limbo tree *(Bursera simaruba)*, is an antidote to the sap of the poisonwood.

pokeweed (Phytolacca americana) [Other names: American nightshade, cancer jalap, crow berry, Indian polk, inkberry, pigeon-berry, pocan bush, poke, pokeberry, red ink plant, red weed, scoke.] This unpleasant-smelling plant is found in damp, woodsy areas from Maine to Minnesota, south to the Gulf of Mexico, Florida, and Texas and also in California and Hawaii; it can also be found in parts of Canada, Europe, and southern Africa. It is commonly found along fields and fences, growing 12 feet tall with white to purple drooping flowers, black berries, and a large perennial rootstock. Young leaves and stems are sometimes eaten as cooked greens, and these can be eaten safely if cooked twice in two different pans of water.

Poisonous part

All parts of the pokeweed plant contain the poison laccine, saponins, and glycoproteins, especially the roots and leaves—and the seeds are almost as toxic as the roots. Only two or three unripe berries can be fatal if eaten by a child, although mature berries are relatively nontoxic. Poisonings usually occur from eating uncooked leaves in salads or by mistaking the roots for parsnips or horseradish.

Symptoms

Symptoms begin about two hours after ingestion and include burning and bitterness in the mouth, nausea, vomiting and diarrhea; occasionally, spasms, convulsions, and death occur.

Treatment

Gastric lavage; replacement of fluids and electrolytes.

See also SAPONIN.

polonium-210 At the end of the 19th century, Marie Curie discovered polonium-210, a radioactive material that occurs in nature at very low levels as part of the decay of uranium and from lead-containing wastes from uranium, radium, and vanadium refining. Polonium-210 also can be produced artificially in nuclear reactors, which requires highly skilled individuals and sophisticated equipment to do so. Nearly all of the world's legal polonium-210 is produced in Russia.

Polonium-210 emits alpha particles that are 5,000 times more radioactive than radium. These particles carry high amounts of energy that can damage or destroy genetic material in the body. Industrially, polonium-210 is used to eliminate static electricity in processes such as manufacturing sheet plastics, spinning synthetic fibers, and rolling paper. It is also used to make nuclear weapons, power supplies in satellites, and in the oil industry.

Polonium-210 poses a radiation hazard only if it enters the body, either through eating, a break in the skin, or through breathing. Once inside the body it irradiates the internal organs, which can result in life-threatening symptoms or death. Polonium-210 is not harmful if it touches unbroken skin or membranes, although it is recommended to wash any areas that have been exposed.

Polonium-210 hit headlines around the world in 2006 when Alexander Litvinenko, a former officer of the Russian Federal Security Service who had received political asylum in Great Britain, was poisoned with the material while dining at a British eating establishment. He died within three weeks of ingesting the polonium and was the first known victim of lethal polonium-210 caused acute radiation syndrome.

Symptoms

Within 48 hours of exposure, symptoms include nausea, vomiting, and diarrhea. If a large dose enters the gut, it can cause bone marrow failure which manifests as nosebleeds, bleeding gums, bruising, and sudden hair loss two to four weeks after exposure. At high doses, polonium-210 can damage tissues and organs such as kidneys, spleen, liver, and bone marrow. As it travels throughout the body in the blood it damages all cells it encounters, eventually leading to death.

Treatment

There is no antidote or cure for polonium-210 poisoning. Treatment is symptomatic. At lower doses, intense antibiotic therapy, bone marrow transplant, and chelation may be beneficial if the poisoning is diagnosed quickly.

polychlorinated biphenyls (PCBs) This group of up to 209 individual chlorinated compounds (called congeners) are no longer produced in the United States, as the Environmental Protection Agency (EPA) banned their manufacture in 1977 because of evidence that they may cause cancer and other serious health problems in humans. They are known to produce cancer in animals.

PCBs are either oily liquids or solids that are colorless to light or dark amber. Some PCBs exist as vapor in air. Although PCBs were banned decades ago, they continue to cause problems in the environment because they have a long half-life, are very stable, and are readily taken up by living organisms. Before 1977, PCBs were used as coolants and lubricants in transformers, capacitors, and other electrical equipment because they are good insulators. Many of these items that once contained PCBs have leaked the substance into the environment, making PCB contamination almost universal. PCBs also entered the environment from accidental spills, from fires in products that contained the toxins, and from leaks that occurred during their transport. Today these toxins are still being released from hazardous waste sites, from improper or illegal disposal of consumer and industrial products, and from the burning of some waste in incinerators.

Once PCBs reach the environment, they can exist for many years and they can travel great distances in the air and by water. PCBs in water usually stick to organic particles and sediment and also bind strongly to soil. Fish and other marine mammals take up PCBs and accumulate the toxins in their bodies, passing them along to other animals or humans who eat them. For these and other reasons, PCBs are still found in human milk, in human fat tissue, and in the brain and liver of young children.

In 2008, the French-owned waste management company, Veolia Environmental Services, in Port Arthur, Texas, petitioned the EPA for permission to burn 40 million pounds of PCBs from Mexico in its plant. The plant has been disposing of PCB waste from the United States since 1992. The EPA gave tentative approval to the proposal in March 2008, and a final decision was expected by the second half of 2009.

Currently, the EPA has set a limit of 0.0005 milligrams of PCBs per liter of drinking water. Any spill, discharge, or accidental release of one pound or more of PCBs into the environment must be reported to the EPA. The acceptable amount of PCBs in food is determined by the Food and Drug Administration, which states that no more than 0.2–0.3 parts of PCBs per million parts (0.2–0.3

ppm) can be contained in infant foods, eggs, milk and other dairy foods, fish, shellfish, poultry, and red meat. Many individual states have fish and wildlife consumption advisories for PCBs.

Symptoms

PCBs are readily taken up by the body, when inhaled, ingested, or absorbed through the skin. They are also well absorbed from the gastrointestinal tract and are stored in fat. Both skin contact and ingestion cause the skin disease chloracne, liver damage, skin hyperpigmentation, blindness, swelling, nausea, vomiting, and abdominal pain. PCBs are far more likely to cause poisoning as a result of long-term exposure rather than with a single acute overdose. Chronic exposure may cause symptoms as much as six weeks or longer after the onset of exposure.

Treatment

There is no way to remove PCBs once they have entered the body. Treatment is supportive and symptomatic, aimed at preventing liver damage. If inhaled, give supplemental oxygen. Wash contaminated skin or eyes; if ingested, induce vomiting or perform gastric lavage followed by the administration of activated charcoal and a cathartic.

See also SAPONIN.

Portuguese man-of-war *(Physalia physalis)* A well-known member of the jellyfish family, the Portuguese man-of-war (also known as a bluebottle) gets its name from the floating portion of its body that appears above the surface of the ocean and resembles the rigging of a caravel. Technically, the Portuguese man-of-war is not a jellyfish but a hydroid—a colony that consists of four types of polyps: a pneumatophore, or float; dactylozooids, or tentacles; gastrozooids, or feeding zooids; and gonozooids, which produce reproductive cells.

Poisonous part

The tentacles of the Portuguese man-of-war trail several feet below its body, floating on the surface of the water; some tentacles will be markedly longer than the others and are called "fishing tentacles." These poisonous tentacles may extend from the central float bag for 50 feet or more. All the tentacles are covered with many thousands of stinging cells that emit a coiled hollow thread that can penetrate skin. Venom in these coils is injected through the thread. The man-of-war is found throughout the world in warm waters, and its sting is far more severe than those from the more common jellyfish.

Symptoms

Toxicity depends on the sensitivity of the victim and the number of stings. Symptoms include immediate and intense stinging or throbbing, a radiating sensation similar to being stung by hornets, causing wheals and blisters, severe chest and abdominal pain, shock, and collapse. The pain has been compared to an electric shock, with the sensation extending up the extremity. More generalized symptoms include headache, shock, cramps, nausea, and vomiting, and recent reports have noted the possibility of acute kidney failure.

Treatment

There is no known specific antidote. At one time, the recommended way to deactivate the tentacles was to pour alcohol, ammonia, vinegar, or salt water over the stings, after which they could be scraped off with a towel. Now, however, it's been discovered that vinegar causes the nematocysts (coiled threadlike structures) to discharge a toxin. In smaller species of jellyfish, vinegar inhibited some nematocysts but discharged others. Alcohol also has been shown to cause a massive discharge of toxin in a similar species of jellyfish and so is no longer recommended. Studies that have looked at the effectiveness of baking soda, papain, meat tenderizer, and commercial sprays that contain aluminum sulfate and detergents have been inconclusive, and it is possible that these substances can cause further damage.

The suggested course of treatment includes: (1) gently pick off any visible tentacles using a stick, gloved hand, or anything that does not promote further injury; (2) rinse the sting thoroughly with fresh or salt water; (3) apply ice to control pain; (4) for rash or persistent itching, use 1 percent hydrocortisone ointment four times daily and one or two 25-mg diphenhydramine tablets every six hours.

Because the tentacles will continue to discharge their nematocysts as long as they remain on the skin, it is critical to remove them. Stung individuals should be watched carefully for signs of shock or breathing difficulties.

See also JELLYFISH.

potassium hydroxide   See ALKALINE CORROSIVES.

potassium or sodium thiocyanate   This drug, traditionally given for high blood pressure, has been replaced by safer drugs, although sodium thiocyanate is still prescribed by a few physicians.

Symptoms
Almost immediately upon ingestion of large amounts, the drug begins to depress cellular activity of the heart and brain, causing disorientation, weakness, low blood pressure, confusion, psychotic behavior, convulsions, and death. Even when the victim begins to recover from thiocyanate poisoning, death can still occur after a sudden relapse as much as two weeks after poisoning.

Treatment
Perform peritoneal dialysis.

potassium permanganate   A disinfectant and mild antiseptic with astringent properties that can be used to treat skin inflammation and wounds, potassium permanganate may be applied to a dressing or directly to the skin. It is sometimes used to treat strychnine, nicotine, and quinine poisoning, although it is always hazardous to use. Care needs to be taken when mixing the crystals in water, because if the mixture is too concentrated (greater than one to 5,000 parts strength), the solution will cause corrosive burns and destroy the mucous membranes. Potassium permanganate tablets (400 mg, 1:1,000) are commonly used in clinical practice, and they are diluted in four liters of water to reach a safe dilution of 1:10,000.

Some women have used potassium permanganate to induce abortion by inserting it into the vagina, and the result has been massive hemorrhaging and serious injury to the vaginal walls.

Symptoms
While symptoms vary depending on the dose, low concentrations cause a burning feeling in the throat, nausea, vomiting, difficulty in swallowing, and some gastroenteritis. In stronger concentrations (2 or 3 percent solutions), symptoms will also include swollen throat and dry mouth, making swallowing difficult. At even greater concentrations (4 to 5 percent), kidney damage will occur and there may be possible disorientation, low blood pressure, and rapid, shallow pulse; death may follow from circulatory failure or pulmonary complications.

Treatment
In cases of skin contamination, wash affected area repeatedly with warm tap water, and treat perforations surgically. For ingestion, do NOT induce vomiting; perform gastric lavage cautiously. Activated charcoal and cathartics are not useful. Give large amounts of fluid and supportive therapy. Cold milk is also suggested as a way to oxidize organic material.

See also NICOTINE; QUININE; STRYCHNINE.

potato   This cousin of deadly nightshade is a popular vegetable throughout the world, but it can be poisonous if eaten raw and unripe. Although the skin of a potato has more fiber, iron, potassium, and B vitamins than the flesh, skins that have a greenish tinge should be avoided, as this signals the presence of chlorophyll, a sign that the potato was exposed to too much light after harvest. Chlorophyll alone is harmless, but in potatoes, the green indicates the presence of glycoalkaloids, and in this case, a toxin called solanine. Ultraviolet and visible light in the blue-violet region promotes the formation of glycoalkaloids. High levels of solanine cause affected potatoes to taste bitter after they are cooked. Solanine formation in potatoes is limited to the skin and usually no deeper than an eighth of an inch into the flesh.

Poisonous part
The leaves, stems, skin, and sprouts of potatoes with greenish skin contain solanine, a naturally occurring glycoalkaloid, and other toxins. Although undamaged potatoes contain some solanine, the

concentration is very low and a person would have to eat about 12 pounds of them to be poisoned. If a potato has greenish skin, pare away the green areas and gouge out all sprouts. Solanine has a stronger effect on children.

Symptoms

A fast-acting toxin, solanine causes symptoms including burning and rawness in the throat, headache, vomiting, abdominal pain, diarrhea, swelling of the brain, stupor, coma, convulsions, and death (usually in children).

Treatment

Gastric lavage, cathartics, and fluid and electrolyte monitoring.
   See also NIGHTSHADE, DEADLY.

pothos (Epipremnum aureum) [Other names: devil's ivy, golden Ceylon creeper, golden hunter's robe, golden pothos, ivy arum, Solomon Island ivy, taro vine, variegated philodendron.]   This popular indoor plant often found in hanging baskets grows outdoors throughout subtropical climates of southern Florida, Hawaii, Guam, and the West Indies, where it twines on trees up to 40 feet high.

Poisonous part

The entire plant is toxic and contains calcium oxalate raphides and other, unidentified irritants.

Symptoms

Skin contact causes dermatitis, and ingestion by children results in diarrhea.

Treatment

There is no specific treatment, but guard against dehydration in children with diarrhea.
   See also OXALATES.

pralidoxime   This drug is used as an antidote to organophosphate insecticide poisoning and is most effective if treatment is begun within 24 hours after exposure. Its use in the treatment of carbamate poisoning is still controversial; it may not be harmful, but it is not often used because of its short duration.

See also CARBAMATE; ORGANOPHOSPHATE INSECTICIDES.

Preludin (phenmetrazine hydrochloride)   One of the appetite-suppressant drugs of high toxicity, Preludin is a white water-soluble powder and is available in tablets or injectables. Similar to amphetamines, Preludin activates the central nervous system and raises blood pressure; rapid heartbeat and addiction are quite common. Within a few weeks or using this drug, tolerance begins to develop.

Symptoms

Appetite suppression, impaired judgment, incoordination, palpitations, high blood pressure, restlessness, dizziness, dry mouth, euphoria, insomnia, tremors, confusion, headache, hallucinations, panic, fatigue, and depression. Psychotic episodes are possible even at recommended doses, together with an unpleasant taste in the mouth, diarrhea or constipation, and other stomach problems. Overdose may cause circulatory collapse, coma, high or low blood pressure followed by death. Abruptly stopping the drug causes depression, fatigue, irritability, hyperactivity, and psychosis (sometimes confused with schizophrenia).

Treatment

Sedation with barbiturates.
   See also AMPHETAMINES.

privet (Ligustrum vulgare)   This common hedge plant is a deciduous shrub with small, white clustering flowers and blue or black waxy berries that appear throughout the winter. Native to the Mediterranean, privet hedges are grown throughout the United States and Canada.

Poisonous part

The entire plant, including the berries, contains the irritant glycoside syringin (ligustrin), nuzhenids, and secoiridoid glucosides.

Symptoms

A large number of berries can cause diarrhea, colic, and gastroenteritis; poisoning can be fatal in young children.

Treatment

Fluid replacement to prevent dehydration.

procaine A local anesthetic and related to cocaine, this drug is a synthetic version of the coca bush alkaloids. It is used to control possible irregular heartbeat following poisoning by a variety of cardioactive drugs and toxins (such as digoxin, cyclic antidepressants, stimulants, and theophylline). It is also used to relieve pain and irritation caused by sunburn or hemorrhoids, to numb tissues before minor surgery and as a nerve block. It is used topically to relieve pain when inserting needles, and it is given intravenously as an antiarrhythmic agent following a heart attack to reduce the danger of ventricular arrhythmias (irregular heartbeat).

Although procaine is used to treat poisoning by other drugs, it is also toxic itself if used excessively.

Symptoms

Immediately upon ingestion, procaine causes giddiness followed by dizziness, blue color, low blood pressure, tremors, irregular and weak breathing, collapse, coma, convulsions, and respiratory arrest. Procaine is considered to be the most dangerous of all the cocaine derivatives; even a small amount can cause fatal shock.

Treatment

Efforts to remove the drug after 30 minutes are useless. The ingested drug must be removed immediately and absorption from the injection site limited by tourniquet and wet cloths. Give oxygen and artificial respiration until the nervous system depression lifts. If the victim survives for one hour, recovery outlook is good.

See also ANESTHETICS, LOCAL; COCAINE; DIGOXIN; LIDOCAINE.

propane The principal ingredient in bottled gas in northern states, which (in low concentrations) is physiologically inert. However, high concentrations of the gas may cause narcosis (a state of sleep or drowsiness). A concentration of 10 percent propane causes slight dizziness in a few minutes; displacement of air by this gas can cause shortness of breath, unconsciousness, and death. The principal toxic effects from gases are from carbon monoxide.

See also CARBON MONOXIDE.

propranolol This beta adrenergic blocker is used to control heart irregularities caused by overdose of theophylline, caffeine, amphetamines, ephedrine, or cocaine.

See also AMPHETAMINES; CAFFEINE; COCAINE; EPHEDRINE; THEOPHYLLINE.

Prunus A genus of trees and shrubs that includes apricot, cherry, choke cherry, peach, plum, and sloe, whose chewed pits are poisonous and possess cyanogenic glycosides. The *Prunus* species have white or pink flowers and a fleshy fruit over a stone or pit. They are widely cultivated throughout the northern temperate zone, and a large number of these fruit trees are available commercially.

Poisonous part

The kernel of the pit is poisonous, as it contains the cyanogenic glycosides (amygdalin) that liberate hydrocyanic acid on hydrolysis. Of all the poisonings associated with the entire genus, the most fatal cases involve ingestion of apricot pits.

Symptoms

Hours may pass between ingestion of the pit and toxic symptoms, because the glycosides must be hydrolyzed in the gastrointestinal tract before cyanide is released. Once this occurs, symptoms include abdominal pain, vomiting, lethargy, and sweating. Cyanosis (blueness of the skin) may or may not occur. In severe cases, the victim may lapse into a coma and experience convulsions, flaccid muscles, and incontinence.

Treatment

If the patient is conscious, perform gastric lavage. Although activated charcoal absorbs cyanide, it releases it slowly during its passage through the intestine; instead, give a 25 percent solution of sodium thiosulfate after lavage. If unconscious, correct acidosis, treat for shock and administer oxygen; administer cyanide antidote.

See also CYANOGENIC GLYCOSIDES.

Psilocybe mexicana   See MEXICAN HALLUCINOGENIC MUSHROOM.

psilocybin   One of the active substances found in a range of hallucinogenic mushrooms such as *Psilocybe cubensis, Panaeolus subbalteatus,* and *Gymnopilus spectabilis.* Psilocybin primarily affects the levels of a brain transmitter known as serotonin; this effect is similar to the activities of mescaline or LSD. It commonly has an impact on the senses, particularly intensifications of color perception and "kaleidescope effects" with eyes closed. Mood alteration is also common, ranging from elation to anxiety, as are feelings of paranormal occurrences, such as the sensation of leaving the body or traveling through time. The sensations usually last between four and 10 hours, and there are no lingering effects.

See also HALLUCINOGENIC MUSHROOMS; MEXICAN HALLUCINOGENIC MUSHROOM.

ptomaine poisoning   Ptomaines are substances produced by decaying animal or vegetable proteins; ptomaine poisoning is not the same as food poisoning. Foods that contain ptomaines are far from appetizing; they look, smell, and taste completely unpleasant and therefore are not usually a danger to humans. Most ptomaines aren't harmful; most ptomaine poisoning is actually staphylococcal poisoning. Ptomaine poisoning is also an obsolete term for food poisoning caused by bacterial poisons.

pufferfish   This exotic food fish, considered a delicacy in Japan where it is known as "fugu," can cause poisoning if improperly prepared and cooked. It can also inflict a painful sting. There are more than 120 species of puffer, all belonging to the family Tetraodontidae; they are considered to be one of the most poisonous fish in the world,

with a 60 percent fatality rate even with treatment. In Japan, there are about 50 deaths a year; at least three have been reported in Florida. Pufferfish is still the primary cause of death from food poisoning in Japan. From 1955 to 1975, 3,000 Japanese were poisoned by eating fugu and 1,500 died.

Three cases of tetrodotoxin poisoning occurred among chefs in California in April 1996, when they shared contaminated pufferfish brought from Japan by a coworker as a prepackaged, ready-to-eat product. The amount that each chef ate was very small, ranging from about a quarter to half an ounce. Symptoms began between three and 20 minutes after eating the fish, and all three people were transported by ambulance to a local emergency department.

In Japan, cooks and restaurants that serve fugu must have a special license and training to prepare this sometimes deadly dish. Still, about 10 Japanese diners die each year from eating the wrong parts of the fish. Fugu lovers say that the fish tastes like chicken and that it produces a mild intoxication, feelings of warmth, and euphoria. In the United States, one species of puffer (called the blowfish) is served in restaurants under the name of "sea squab."

Pufferfish get their name from their ability to inflate themselves when threatened, puffing themselves up to several times their normal girth until they are almost spherical. Puffers are most toxic just before and during their reproductive season, because of the interaction between gonad activity and toxicity, although the same species found in different locations at the same time could vary widely in its toxicity. They are commonly found in warm or temperate regions around the world, including the west coast of Central America, throughout the Indo-Pacific, Japan, and from Australia to South America.

Puffers are very territorial and seek rocky crevices to hide in. A close relative is the deadly porcupine fish, which not only inflates when threatened but also erects sharp quills all over its body.

Although it is against the law for an individual to bring pufferfish into the country, the U.S. Food and Drug Administration has allowed pufferfish to be imported and served in Japanese restaurants by certified fugu chefs on special occasions. A cooperative agreement with the Japanese Ministry of Health and Welfare ensures fugu is properly processed and certified safe for consumption before export by the government of Japan. If cleaned and dressed properly, the puffer flesh or musculature is edible.

Although arriving travelers are required to declare all food products brought into the United States, control measures rely primarily on the traveler. People who travel to countries where puffer is served should be aware of the potential risk of eating this fish.

Poisonous part

The liver, gonads, intestines, and skin of these fish contain tetrodotoxin, a powerful neurotoxin that can cause death in approximately 60 percent of persons who ingest it. Other animals, such as the California newt and the eastern salamander also have tetrodotoxin in lethal quantities. Tetrodotoxin is a basic compound that does not deactivate when heated. This nerve poison is 150,000 times more deadly than curare. There is evidence that the toxin is included as part of the Haitian voodoo potion used in the zombie ritual.

Symptoms

While death from a puffer *sting* is rare, it causes an immediate severe throbbing pain that may stay at the site of the wound or spread throughout the body and last for several hours or days. There may be redness and swelling at the site of the sting, and the area may become numb.

Improperly preparing or cooking this fish causes a far more serious type of poisoning. Within minutes to hours, symptoms include numbness and tingling beginning in the extremities and spreading over the body together with a floating feeling. Other symptoms include fatigue, headache, tightness in throat and upper chest, speech problems, flushing, shaking, nausea, and vomiting. Paralysis in an ascending pattern appears, and the victim finds it difficult to breath, which progresses to coma, convulsions, respiratory arrest, and death. The first 24 hours after ingestion are critical; there is a high fatality rate. Severe poisoning causes symptoms of low blood pressure, slow heart rate, and fixed dilated pupils.

Diagnosis

Tetrodotoxin poisoning is diagnosed based on symptoms and a history of recent consumption of pufferfish.

Treatment

For a puffer sting, contact medical help immediately; flush the wound with fresh or salt water and then soak the affected area in hot water or put hot compresses on it. The water should be very hot (122°F), so that the heat will deactivate the poison. Continue applying hot water for 30 minutes to an hour.

There is no antidote to tetrodotoxin ingestion, and there is great controversy over the relative benefits of the administration of atropine, edrophonium, or pyridostigmine. Otherwise, treatment is supportive. Induce vomiting or perform gastric lavage if ingestion occurred within the preceding hour, followed by the administration of activated charcoal. Intravenous fluids may be helpful.

See also TETRODOTOXIN.

pyrethrin The active chemical derived from pyrethrum (extracted from chrysanthemums grown in the Democratic Republic of Congo and Kenya), pyrethrin is one of the oldest known botanic insecticides. It was used hundreds of years ago in China, and the plants were cultivated in Europe more than a century ago. Pyrethrin and pyrethrum come from two strains of chrysanthemum (roseum and carneum). To make the insecticide, pyrethrum flowers are ground and then used either undiluted or mixed with inert ingredients or other insecticides to kill a variety of garden and household insect pests.

While pyrethrin has largely been replaced by more toxic insecticides, it is still often found in pesticide preparations for fighting fleas in dogs. Both pyrethrum and pyrethrin are the most widely used natural insecticides because they are deadly to a wide range of insects—possibly as effective in controlling pests as Sevin (carbaryl), a popular synthetic pesticide.

Pyrethrin is stronger than its dried flower source, since it has been strengthened to prevent insects from recovering from the effects of the poison. These substances are somewhat controversial today because in large quantities they can affect the human nervous system. They can kill or incapacitate beetles, caterpillars, flies, wasps, bees, moths, fruit flies, butterflies, borers, whiteflies, chafers, leaf rollers, and many other insects.

Symptoms

Breathing pyrethrin causes the most toxic reaction because of its highly allergic properties; skin contact can cause dermatitis in about half of those sensitive to ragweed. Severe poisoning with pyrethrin is unusual, although it can cause nausea, vomiting, gastroenteritis, excitability, incoordination, muscular paralysis, and death from respiratory failure. Symptoms may last between two days and two weeks. Less serious poisoning results in reddened skin, burning, and itching, swollen cheeks, headache, stomach problems, and numb lips and tongue.

Treatment

Atropine therapy may control gastroenteritis. Wash pyrethrin from eyes and skin, as it can cause a severe local dermatitis. Treat symptoms.

See also BOTANIC INSECTICIDES; PYRETHRUM.

pyrethrum   A wide-spectrum botanic insecticide used for hundreds of years in China, pyrethrum is a powder made from one of two forms of chrysanthemums (roseum and carneum). Pyrethrin is the active chemical derived from pyrethrum and is also used as an insecticide.

Pyrethrum is a widely used natural insecticide because it can kill a wide variety of insects while posing little harm to humans and animals. Pyrethrum is more benign than its chemical ester pyrethrin and breaks down much faster (usually within 24 hours). It does not kill some insect pests but only stuns them for a period of time.

See also BOTANIC INSECTICIDES; PYRETHRIN.

pyridoxine (Vitamin B$_6$)   See VITAMINS.

Quaalude (methaqualone) An antianxiety drug introduced in 1965 as a safe barbiturate substitute, helpful in relieving anxiety and tension and as a sleeping pill. Experience showed, however, that Quaalude was very addictive and the severity of withdrawal symptoms was similar to that of barbiturates. By 1972, "luding out" (taking methaqualone with wine) was a popular college pastime.

In the United States, the marketing of methaqualone pharmaceutical products stopped in 1984, and methaqualone was transferred to Schedule I of the Controlled Substance Act, the highest designation of abuse potential. They are still available on the street as a drug of abuse.

Symptoms

Within five to 30 minutes, depending on whether the drug was injected or taken as a pill, symptoms of overdose appear; they include nausea and vomiting, stomach irritation, pulmonary edema, convulsions, and death.

Treatment

Overdose is more difficult to treat than barbiturate overdose, and deaths have frequently occurred. Gastric lavage and treatment of symptoms are the only treatment.

See also NARCOTICS.

quicklime (calcium oxide) Also called unslaked lime, this very powerful caustic is a component of portland cement and liberates heat in contact with water. It can cause serious damage if ingested, inhaled, or allowed to contact the eyes. Note: Slaked lime (calcium hydroxide) is a simple alkali, and because of its low solubility in water, it is not greatly corrosive.

Symptoms

Contact with the skin may product first-, second-, or third-degree chemical burns; eye contact may produce severe conjunctivitis as well as damaged corneas. Ingestion produces burning pain from mouth to stomach, with marked difficulty in swallowing. Mucous membranes are soapy and white and then turn brown and become ulcerated. Vomit is bloody and may contain shreds of mucous membrane. Pulse is feeble and rapid, breathing is rapid, and collapse may follow. Death may result from shock, asphyxiation from swelling and intercurrent infections; pneumonia may occur in 48 to 72 hours. Esophageal stricture may develop within weeks, months, or even years after ingestion.

Treatment

Cold milk, water, or tea should be given immediately. Irrigate the mouth with water; the damage to the esophagus from caustic alkalies occurs within the first minute, and therefore first aid measures after that are of doubtful value. DO NOT give carbonated beverages, and DO NOT induce vomiting or attempt gastric lavage (the small amount of alkali that usually reaches the stomach is quickly neutralized by the acid gastric juice). Olive oil may temporarily ease pain but should not be given in large amounts.

See also ALKALINE CORROSIVES.

quinidine This is one of a group of antiarrhythmic drugs commonly used to control heartbeat irregularities and malaria and other infections. Acute ingestion of one gram of quinidine should be considered potentially lethal.

Symptoms

This drug primarily affects the cardiovascular and central nervous systems. Symptoms include heart problems, dry mouth, dilated pupils, delirium, seizures, coma, and respiratory arrest. In addition, there may be nausea, vomiting, and diarrhea after acute ingestion, and with chronic doses there may be tinnitus (ringing in the ears), vertigo, deafness, and visual disturbances.

Treatment

Most therapies have proven ineffectual, and there is no known antidote. The primary goal is to keep the heart functioning until the drug is eliminated, which usually occurs within a few hours. Heart problems are treated with hypertonic sodium bicarbonate. Do not induce vomiting; perform gastric lavage followed by the administration of activated charcoal and a cathartic. Quinidine is not effectively removed by dialysis. Treat low blood pressure, heart rhythm irregularities, coma, and seizures as they occur; treat recurrent rapid heartbeat with lidocaine or phenytoin.

See also ANTIARRHYTHMIC DRUGS.

quinine A former drug treatment for malaria, quinine has largely been replaced by chloroquine but is still used for cases resistant to the newer drug. It is still prescribed for the treatment of nocturnal muscle cramps and has also been used to induce abortions. The chief alkaloid of cinchona bark, quinine also contains related drugs (including quinidine).

The quinine content of "tonic" water is usually no larger than 30 milligrams per 100 milliliters, although this small amount can produce symptoms in very sensitive people. Dubonnet contains seven milligrams per 100 milliliters.

The mechanism behind quinine's toxicity is believed to be similar to that of quinidine, although quinine is much less toxic to the heart. It is available in capsules and tablets of 130 to 325 milligrams; the minimum toxic dose for an adult is 3 to 4 grams (one gram has been fatal to a child), although some people have taken much larger doses and survived.

Symptoms

Quinine depresses the cell function throughout the body, affecting the heart, kidney, liver, and central nervous system. Quinine toxicity causes a syndrome called cinchonism, which causes tinnitus (ringing in the ears), blurred vision, weakness, nausea, vomiting, low blood pressure, and heart problems. Evidence of the drug's effect on the brain can be seen in the resulting apprehension, confusion, and excitement. Convulsions and respiratory arrest have also been reported, and death occurs from respiratory or circulatory collapse in a few hours to a few days.

If the victim recovers, there may be residual damage to the eyes and ears—even causing deafness.

Treatment

There is no antidote to quinine. Perform gastric lavage, followed by the administration of magnesium sulfate or activated charcoal. Do not induce vomiting. Give hypertonic sodium bicarbonate for heart problems.

See also QUINIDINE.

radiation poisoning   Although excessive exposure to radiation is rare, it is a potentially catastrophic possibility in the nuclear age. Radiation poisoning may occur from internal or external contamination and from particle-emitting solids, liquids, or gases (including beta and alpha particles, neutrons, protons, and positrons) and electromagnetic sources (such as X-rays or gamma rays).

Radiation interferes with the function of the body and damages RNA and DNA. Cells that turn over quickly, such as those found in the skin or gastrointestinal tract, are affected first. While contact with electromagnetic sources of radiation does not make the victim radioactive or dangerous to others, exposure to particle-emitting sources can be very contaminating to anyone who comes in contact with the victim.

Radiation dose is expressed in various terms, but rad (radiation absorbed dose) is the most common.

Symptoms

Symptoms are dose related: Exposure to 100 to 200 rads causes nausea, vomiting, abdominal cramps, and diarrhea; 200 rads is potentially fatal, and 600 rads is nearly always fatal within a few days, causing severe gastroenteritis and marked dehydration. Brief exposure to excessive amounts (5,000 rads or more) causes confusion and lethargy followed within minutes to hours by convulsions, coma, cardiovascular collapse, and death.

In addition, exposure from anywhere between 200 and 1,000 rads often depresses the bone marrow function, opening the way to infections. Other symptoms include skin burns and hair loss.

Treatment

For expert assistance in evaluation and treatment, contact the federal Oak Ridge Radiation Emer-
gency Assistance Center and Training Site (available 24 hours a day) at (865) 576-3131. Chelating agents may be useful for ingestion or inhalation of certain particles. Treat symptoms, maintain airway and replace fluid losses.

For particulate exposure, move the victim from the area, remove all clothing, and wash the skin with soap and water; all water and clothing must be properly destroyed. Rescuers and hospital personnel should wear protective gear. Induce vomiting or perform gastric lavage in cases of ingestion.

radon   This invisible, odorless radioactive gas is created by the natural decay of radium and uranium found in rocks and soil. It is relatively harmless out of doors; it is most dangerous once it has seeped inside a house, where it breaks down into harmful elements that attach to dust particles that can enter the lungs. Once in the lungs, the elements decay in minutes, releasing alpha radiation. This radiation can cause cell damage possibly leading to lung cancer, and is among the most dangerous of toxic substances because of the number of cases of cancer it is estimated to cause each year.

According to EPA estimates, radon is the number one cause of lung cancer among nonsmokers and the second leading cause of lung cancer. Experts believe radon is responsible for about 21,000 deaths by lung cancer every year, and that about 2,900 of these deaths occur among nonsmokers.

According to the Environmental Protection Agency (EPA), it is estimated that one in 15 American homes has levels of radon high enough to pose a health risk. And another study of 552 homes suggested that there are about one million homes in the United States where the chances of developing lung cancer from radon are at least as great as one in 40 over a lifetime.

But in a 1991 survey by the American Lung Association, only 11 percent of Americans had tested their homes for radon. Further, animal studies suggest that in an average home in the United States, an individual has about a one in 300 chance of developing lung cancer in his or her lifetime from indoor radon—or that about 10 percent of all cases of lung cancer in this country are caused by this gas. (It must be remembered, however, that smokers are more susceptible to cancer from radon than nonsmokers.)

Radon is able to enter a building because of the small difference between inside and outside air pressure, which draws in the radon in much the same way as a fire draws heated air up a chimney: A heated house draws cool air from the basement or ground floor, where the pressure is low, and sends it to the upper floors, where the pressure is higher.

There are two main types of radon test kits available (see Appendix A), and both types are simple, inexpensive, and available at local hardware stores. Short-term tests remain in your home for two to 90 days. These tests come in the form of charcoal canisters, alpha tracks, electret ion chambers, continuous monitors, and charcoal liquid scintillation detectors. Because radon levels vary from day to day and season to season, short-term tests are less likely to give you an accurate picture of your yearly exposure. Short-term tests are usually used when you need results quickly, such as when you are selling your home.

Long-term tests remain in your home for more than 90 days. The most commonly used tests for this purpose are alpha track and electret detectors. The results of long-term tests provide a more accurate annual average radon level than a short-term test. Because there is no known safe level of radon exposure, the EPA recommends that homes with radon levels of 2.0 to 4.0 picocuries per liter or greater should be remedied. The average radon concentration in the indoor air of homes in the United States is 1.3 picocuries per liter, while the average concentration of radon in outdoor air is 0.4 picocuries per liter.

If radon is found in the home, there are several options to deal with it. The basement or crawl spaces of most houses have a slightly lower air pressure than the soil beneath, and this speeds the rate at which the gas can enter the house through the foundation. One way to cut down on the problem is to install pipes to the outdoors that ventilate the soil beneath the house. Or, consumers could pressurize the basement or crawl space with an air blower, flushing out the radon. Sealing cracks in the foundation and basement floor has not been shown to be an effective way to reduce the inflow of radon.

ragwort *(Senecio)* **[Other names: butterweed, squaw weed, stinking willie, tansy ragwort. In the United States, groundsel, ragwort, and butterweed are commonly applied to many different varieties of** *Senecio***.]** There are about 3,000 species of *Senecio,* including threadleaf groundsel *(S. longilobus)* and common groundsel *(S. vulgaris);* many of the varieties contain poisonous alkaloids.

Ragwort is a four-foot-tall biennial or perennial herb with yellow flower clusters that has become naturalized in parts of Canada south to Massachusetts and in Washington and Oregon west of the Cascades.

Threadleaf groundsel is a shrubby perennial with white flowers found in Colorado and Utah south to western Texas and northern Mexico.

Common groundsel is a smaller annual with soft, fleshy leaves and yellow flowers that has become naturalized in Alaska and throughout Canada south to North Carolina and west to Wisconsin; it is also found in California, New Mexico, and Texas.

Poisonous part

The entire plant is poisonous; honey made from the nectar and milk from animals who have grazed on these plants also contain the poisonous pyrrolizidine alkaloids. In general, poisonings have occurred from excessive drinking of herbal teas made from this plant. Ragwort's toxins can also be absorbed through the skin or inhaled as pollen. Once inside the body, the poisons damage liver cells in a slow and irreversible process that results in cirrhosis months or even years later. For grazing animals, new research indicates that the seedlings may be more toxic than the mature plants. While horses and other grazing animals typically avoid the mature plant, the seedlings often go undetected and are eaten along with grasses.

Symptoms

Abdominal pain; anorexia with nausea, vomiting, and diarrhea. Chronic use of tea made from these plants can result in fatal cases of cirrhosis.

Treatment

There is no treatment for this type of liver disease caused by the pyrrolizidine alkaloids.

See also ALKALOIDS.

rat poison Most rat poisons (or rodenticides) that are the most toxic to humans and pets are restricted for use only by commercial exterminators and government agencies. Inorganic rat poison compounds include arsenic, thallium, phosphorus, barium carbonate, zinc phosphide, and Vacor. Organic compounds include sodium fluoroacetate, alphanaphthylthiourea, warfarin, red squill, strychnine sulfate, and dicarboximide.

There are two types of rodenticides: single dose (or acute) compounds and chronic varieties, such as the anticoagulant rat poisons. Acute poisons kill rats after a single feeding and usually include red squill, zinc phosphide, strychnine, arsenic, phosphorus, and thallium sulfate. Chronic rat poisons, on the other hand, are preferred, since they do not produce symptoms in the rat that make it stop eating before acquiring a fatal dose, and anticoagulants are less toxic to humans and animals.

Poisoning with anticoagulant rodenticides is extremely rare, since huge doses would be needed in order to be toxic. When it occurs, the treatment is the administration of vitamin K_1 or blood transfusions.

See also ARSENIC; PHOSPHORUS; RED SQUILL; THALLIUM; VACOR; WARFARIN.

rattlesnake, canebrake (Crotalus horridus atricaudatus) This snake is one of a number of species of rattlesnakes known as pit vipers because of their heat-sensing pits behind the eyes and nose, with tail rattles that hiss before striking. The canebrake is the southern United States' version of the timber rattler.

Symptoms

Symptoms appear within 15 minutes and include excessive thirst, nausea, vomiting, shock, paralysis, respiratory problems, anemia, necrosis, kidney problems, and sometimes death. The bite of a rattlesnake is painful. Indications of a serious bite include swelling above the elbows or knees within two hours, hemorrhages, numbness at the puncture site, tingling around the mouth, yellow vision, vomiting, and violent spasms.

Treatment

Antivenin is available. Local care of the bite site is essential. Antibiotics and tetanus vaccine should be given.

See also MASSASAUGA; PIT VIPERS; RATTLESNAKE, CASCABEL; RATTLESNAKE, EASTERN DIAMONDBACK; RATTLESNAKE, MEXICAN WEST COAST, RATTLESNAKE, RED DIAMONDBACK; RATTLESNAKE, TIMBER; RATTLESNAKE, WESTERN DIAMONDBACK; RATTLESNAKES; SIDEWINDER; SNAKES, POISONOUS; VIPER, GABOON; VIPER, JUMPING; VIPER, MALAYAN PIT; VIPER, RUSSEL'S; VIPER, SAWSCALED; VIPER, WAGLER'S PIT; VIPERS; WATER MOCCASIN; WUTU.

rattlesnake, cascabel (Crotalus durissus) Also known as the tropical or South American rattler, the cascabel is one of the two most deadly rattlesnakes in the world and is found in tropical South America.

Poisonous part

Crotamine, a toxin that causes convulsions, is found in the venom of this snake, which also relaxes the victim's neck muscles, causing the head to flop and adding to this snake's reputation as a neck breaker.

Symptoms

Symptoms appear within 15 minutes and include excessive thirst, nausea, vomiting, shock, paralysis, respiratory problems, anemia, necrosis, kidney problems, and sometimes death. The bite of a rattlesnake is painful. Indications of a serious bite include swelling above the elbows or knees within two hours, hemorrhages, numbness at the puncture site, tingling around the mouth, yellow vision, vomiting, and violent spasms.

Treatment

Antivenin is available.

See also MASSASAUGA; PIT VIPERS; RATTLESNAKE, CANEBRAKE; RATTLESNAKE, EASTERN DIAMONDBACK; RATTLESNAKE, MEXICAN WEST COAST; RATTLESNAKE, RED DIAMONDBACK; RATTLESNAKE, TIMBER; RATTLESNAKE, WESTERN DIAMONDBACK; RATTLESNAKES; SIDEWINDER; SNAKES, POISONOUS; VIPER, GABOON; VIPER, JUMPING; VIPER, MALAYAN PIT; VIPER, RUSSELL'S; VIPER, SAWSCALED; VIPER, WAGLER'S PIT; VIPER, WATER MOCCASIN; WUTU.

rattlesnake, eastern diamondback *(Crotalus adamanteus)* Also called the Florida diamondback, this snake is considered to be the most dangerous in North America, with a venom highly destructive to blood tissue. The largest of all the rattlesnakes and heavier than its western relative, the eastern diamondback has large dark brown or black diamonds with light centers on a body color of olive, brown, or black and grows to be eight feet long. There are also prominent light diagonal lines on the side of its head. It has a heavy body with a large, sharply distinct head.

It is found in sparse woodland, dry pine flatwoods, abandoned farms and lowland coastal regions of the southeastern Gulf states of the United States and throughout Florida. However, the population has been reduced by hunters and land development.

Symptoms

Symptoms appear within 15 minutes and include excessive thirst, nausea, vomiting, shock, paralysis, respiratory problems, anemia, necrosis, kidney problems, and sometimes death. The bite of a rattlesnake is painful. Indications of a serious bite include swelling above the elbows or knees within two hours, hemorrhages, numbness at the puncture site, tingling around the mouth, yellow vision, vomiting, and violent spasms.

Treatment

Antivenin is available.

See also MASSASAUGA; PIT VIPERS; RATTLESNAKE, CANEBRAKE; RATTLESNAKE, CASCABEL; RATTLESNAKE, MEXICAN WEST COAST; RATTLESNAKE, RED DIAMONDBACK; RATTLESNAKE, TIMBER; RATTLESNAKE, WESTERN DIAMONDBACK; RATTLESNAKES; SIDEWINDER; SNAKES, POISONOUS, VIPER, GABOON; VIPER, JUMPING; VIPER, MALAYAN PIT; VIPER, RUSSELL'S; VIPER, SAWSCALED; VIPER, WAGLER'S PIT; VIPERS; WATER MOCCASIN; WUTU.

rattlesnake, horned See SIDEWINDER.

rattlesnake, Mexican west coast *(Crotalus basiliscus)* The world's second most deadly rattlesnake, the Mexican west coast rattlesnake is found in western Mexico.

Symptoms

Symptoms appear within 15 minutes and include excessive thirst, nausea, vomiting, shock, paralysis, respiratory problems, anemia, necrosis, kidney problems, and sometimes death. The bite of a rattlesnake is painful. Indications of a serious bite include swelling above the elbows or knees within two hours, hemorrhages, numbness at the puncture site, tingling around the mouth, yellow vision, vomiting, and violent spasms.

Treatment

Antivenin is available.

See also MASSASAUGA; PIT VIPERS; RATTLESNAKE, CANEBRAKE; RATTLESNAKE, CASCABEL; RATTLESNAKE, EASTERN DIAMONDBACK; RATTLESNAKE, RED DIAMONDBACK; RATTLESNAKE, TIMBER; RATTLESNAKE, WESTERN DIAMONDBACK; RATTLESNAKES; SIDEWINDER; SNAKES, POISONOUS; VIPER, GABOON; VIPER, JUMPING; VIPER, MALAYAN PIT; VIPER, RUSSELL'S; VIPER, SAWSCALED; VIPER, WAGLER'S PIT; VIPERS; WATER MOCCASIN; WUTU.

rattlesnake, red diamondback *(Crotalus ruber)* This rattler looks very much like the western diamondback rattlesnake, but its body color is more reddish or pinkish and its markings less distinct.

It has diamond shapes down its midline, usually edged in lighter colors. Black and white rings circle the tail.

This snake prefers arid and semidesert, cold coastal regions in the foothills and mountains in southern California, Baja California, and northern Mexico. It is most often seen during the spring sheltering in the sun or crossing the road at night.

Symptoms

Symptoms appear within 15 minutes and include excessive thirst, nausea, vomiting, shock, paralysis, respiratory problems, anemia, necrosis, kidney problems, and sometimes death. The bite of a rattlesnake is painful. Indications of a serious bite include swelling above the elbows or knees within two hours, hemorrhages, numbness at the puncture site, tingling around the mouth, yellow vision, vomiting, and violent spasms.

Treatment

Antivenin is available.

See also MASSASAUGA; PIT VIPERS; RATTLESNAKE, CANEBRAKE; RATTLESNAKE, CASCABEL; RATTLESNAKE, EASTERN DIAMONDBACK; RATTLESNAKE, MEXICAN WEST COAST; RATTLESNAKE, TIMBER; RATTLESNAKE, WESTERN DIAMONDBACK; RATTLESNAKES; SIDEWINDER; SNAKES, POISONOUS; VIPER, GABOON; VIPER, JUMPING; VIPER, MALAYAN PIT; VIPER, RUSSELL'S; VIPER, SAWSCALED; VIPER, WAGLER'S PIT; VIPERS; WATER MOCCASIN; WUTU.

rattlesnake, South American See RATTLESNAKE, CASCABEL.

rattlesnake, timber *(Crotalus horridus)* The only rattler found in the populated northeastern United States, the timber rattlesnake has a range extending into much of the central and southern states except for Florida. As a result of urban pressure, this species has been exterminated in many parts of its range.

There are two distinct races of the timber rattler: *C. h. horridus,* found in the northern part of the species' range in pine forests and wooded slopes; and the canebrake rattlesnake, *C. h. atricaudatus,* found in southern lowlands in cane thickets and swamps. The timber rattler is large, with a robust body and a large, flat unmarked head. Its color is yellow brown or dark brown, with darker crossbands; completely black snakes are not uncommon. The canebrake rattler is more brightly marked, with a pink buff or brown color with bold black crossbands and an orange or red dorsal stripe. Both types have a black tail.

The timber rattler is often seen coiled up and motionless waiting for prey in the daytime during spring and fall, and on summer nights. In the north, large groups of timber rattlers can be seen in rocky dens, sometimes with copperheads.

Symptoms

Symptoms appear within 15 minutes and include excessive thirst, nausea, vomiting, shock, paralysis, respiratory problems, anemia, necrosis, kidney problems, and sometimes death. The bite of a rattlesnake is painful. Indications of a serious bite include swelling above the elbows or knees within two hours, hemorrhages, numbness at the puncture site, tingling around the mouth, yellow vision, vomiting, and violent spasms.

Treatment

Antivenin is available.

See also MASSASAUGA; RATTLESNAKE, CANEBRAKE; RATTLESNAKE, CASCABEL; RATTLESNAKE, EASTERN DIAMONDBACK; RATTLESNAKE, MEXICAN WEST COAST; RATTLESNAKE, RED DIAMONDBACK; RATTLESNAKES.

rattlesnake, tropical See RATTLESNAKE, CASCABEL.

rattlesnake, western diamondback *(Crotalus atrox)* Also called a coon tail rattler, this is the largest rattlesnake of the North American West. The western diamondback has a heavy body, with a large, spade-shaped head that is distinct from the neck. The body color is gray-brown or pink, with light-bordered, dark diamond blotches on the back. The diamonds are often covered with small dark spots, which are often faded and dusty looking. The tail is distinctive, ringed boldly with black and white. There are two light diagonal lines on the side of its face, and the stripe behind the eye meets the upper lip in front of the jaw angle.

The western diamondback is found in the semidesert and dry arid areas, rocky canyons, river bluffs, and some cultivated areas in much of the southwestern parts of the United States from southeastern California east to central Arkansas, and as far south as central Mexico. Toxicologists consider this snake to be the most dangerous snake in the United States.

When threatened, the western diamondback stands its ground, lifts up its head and sounds a "rattling" warning. It is most active late in the day during the hot summer months.

Symptoms

Symptoms appear within 15 minutes and include excessive thirst, nausea, vomiting, shock, paralysis, respiratory problems, anemia, necrosis, kidney problems, and sometimes death. The bite of a rattlesnake is painful. Indications of a serious bite include swelling above the elbows or knees within two hours, hemorrhages, numbness at the puncture site, tingling around the mouth, yellow vision, vomiting, and violent spasms.

Treatment

Antivenin is available.

See also MASSASAUGA; PIT VIPERS; RATTLESNAKE, CANEBRAKE; RATTLESNAKE, CASCABEL; RATTLESNAKE, EASTERN DIAMONDBACK; RATTLESNAKE, MEXICAN WEST COAST; RATTLESNAKE, RED DIAMONDBACK; RATTLESNAKE, TIMBER; RATTLESNAKES; SIDEWINDER; VIPER, GABOON; VIPER, JUMPING; VIPER, MALAYAN PIT; VIPER, RUSSELL'S; VIPER, WAGLER'S PIT; VIPERS; WATER MOCCASIN; WUTU.

rattlesnakes Rattlesnakes resemble any other viper except that they almost all have a rattle at the end of the tail formed by a series of dry, horny segments that vibrate with a rattling sound when shaken by the snake as a warning of its presence. Each time the snake loses its skin, a new segment is added to the rattle. More than 98 percent of the snakebites in the United States are from rattlesnakes, which are found in two separate snake families: the Crotalidae (the eastern and western diamondbacks, the timber rattler, the canebrake rattler, the pacific rattler, and the mojave rattler), and the Viperidae (the sidewinder, or horned, rattler, and two types of pygmy rattlers—the massasauga and the pygmy). They are all considered pit vipers because of the heat-sensing pits between each nostril and eye.

Outside the United States, the cascabel rattler (also known as the tropical or South American rattler) is found in tropical South America and is one of the two most dangerous rattlers. The Mexican west coast rattler is the second most dangerous rattler and is found in western Mexico. The Brazilian rattler is found in southeastern Brazil, Argentina, and Paraguay.

Although rattlesnake are poisonous, fatalities in the United States are rare because antivenin is usually available immediately.

Poisonous part

Rattlesnake venom includes the toxin acetylcholinesterase, and in some tropical varieties the convulsion-inducing toxin crotamine also appears.

Symptoms

Within 15 minutes to an hour after being bitten, the victim will begin to experience thirst, nausea, vomiting, paralysis, shock, respiratory distress, and drooping eyelids. Death follows malfunction of the kidneys. Tingling around the mouth, yellow vision, and a numbed wound site all are indicative of a serious bite with a large amount of venom. In cases of severe poisoning, there will be swelling caused by hemorrhages above the elbows or knees within two hours.

Treatment

Antivenin is available.

See also MASSASAUGA; PIT VIPERS; RATTLESNAKE, CANEBRAKE; RATTLESNAKE, CASCABEL; RATTLESNAKE, EASTERN DIAMONDBACK; RATTLESNAKE, MEXICAN WEST COAST; RATTLESNAKE, RED DIAMONDBACK; RATTLESNAKE, TIMBER; RATTLESNAKE, WESTERN DIAMONDBACK; SIDEWINDER; SNAKES, POISONOUS; VIPER, GABOON; VIPER, JUMPING; VIPER, MALAYAN PIT; VIPER, RUSSELL'S; VIPER, SAWSCALED; VIPER, WAGLER'S PIT; VIPERS; WATER MOCCASIN; WUTU.

red squill This botanic rat poison is one of the least toxic of all the organic rodenticides available. When ingested in large doses, it can interfere with the function of the heart; it is also an irritant and central-acting emetic.

Symptoms

Acute poisoning causes nausea, vomiting, diarrhea, abdominal pain, cardiac irregularities, convulsion, and death from ventricular fibrillation.

Treatment

Induce vomiting with syrup of ipecac followed by gastric lavage. Administer lidocaine or phenytoin; monitor electrolytes.

See also RAT POISON.

rescue, procedures for smoke and fumes Poisoning by smoke, gas, or chemical fumes requires special rescue methods. It is CRITICALLY IMPORTANT that you do not light a match, turn on a light switch, or produce a flame or spark in the presence of gas or fumes.

If you are alone, call for help before attempting to rescue the victim. To avoid poisoning yourself, hold your breath. Before you enter the affected area, take several breaths of fresh air, then inhale deeply as you go in. If smoke and fumes are visible in the upper part of the room, stay below them by crawling. If auto exhaust or other heavy fumes are visible near the floor, keep your head above them. Remove the victim immediately. Do not perform first aid until you reach fresh air.

resins Also called resinoids, these compounds are made up of a wide variety of substances that are both resinous and semisolid at room temperature, and include potent toxins such as those found in rhododendron and laurel. Symptoms of resin poisoning include stomach irritation, vomiting, diarrhea, headache, weakness, irregular heartbeat, convulsions, coma, and, sometimes, death.

See also LAUREL, MOUNTAIN; RHODODENDRON.

rhododendron *(Rhododendron)* Once considered as belonging to two separate genera, rhododendron and azalea are now both considered to be in the *Rhododendron* genus. There are about 800 *Rhododendron* species, which are subdivided into eight subgenera.

This extremely common evergreen, semievergreen, and deciduous shrub is found everywhere throughout Canada, Britain, and the United States (except for the north central states and subtropical Florida). Rhododendrons are odorless, with bell-shaped flowers that come in a variety of colors; azaleas are sweet smelling with funnel-shaped flowers. Both are deadly narcotics said to have poisoned Xenophon's army from honey made from the flowers' nectar.

Poisonous part

All parts of the plant are poisonous and contain carbohydrate andromedotoxin—the same poison found in mountain laurel. Honey made from the plant's nectar has also caused poisoning. Children who have chewed on the leaves have become seriously poisoned.

Symptoms

Burning in the mouth, followed within six hours of ingestion by increased salivation, vomiting, tearing eyes, nasal discharge, prickling skin, difficulty in breathing, slow heartbeat, muscle weakness progressing to paralysis, convulsions, coma, and death.

Treatment

Fluids and electrolyte replacement; atropine for slow heart rate; ephedrine for low blood pressure.

See also LAUREL, MOUNTAIN.

rhubarb (*Rheum rhabarbarum;* sometimes incorrectly referred to as *R. rhaponticum*) [Other names: pie plant, wine plant.] This common perennial, grown for its tasty stalk, has poisonous leaves that can be fatal if mistakenly cooked along with the rhubarb stalks or eaten raw.

Several feet tall at maturity, the plant has large, wavy oval leaves and is cultivated across the United States for its edible stalk.

Poisonous part

The leaves are the only poisonous part of the rhubarb plant and contain oxalic acid, potassium and calcium oxalates, and anthraquinone glycosides. They must be removed before eating or cooking.

Symptoms

Several hours after ingestion, the digestive irritant in the leaves can cause stomach pain, nausea, vomiting, hemorrhage, respiratory problems, burning mouth, and possibly cardiac or respiratory arrest following a drop in the calcium content of the blood. Without treatment, death or permanent kidney damage may occur. It is believed that symptoms are almost completely caused by the anthraquinone cathartics in the leaves.

Treatment

Gastric lavage, together with calcium salts, calcium gluconate, and other forms, helps remove the oxalate. Fluids must be replaced to prevent kidney malfunction.

See also OXALATES.

ringhals *(Hemachatus hemachatus)* One of the spitting cobras, this brick-red snake is found in South Africa and prefers to spray venom toward the eyes rather than bite. The openings of the venom ducts are on the front of its fangs, so that when faced with an enemy the ringhals can apply muscular pressure on the gland to force the liquid in a stream straight at the enemy's eyes. The aim of the ringhals is absolutely deadly, and they are a real threat because they have a range of up to 10 feet. Spitting cobras can also bite, but they seem reluctant to do so.

Symptoms

When contact is made with the eyes, there is excruciating pain and sometimes permanent blindness; there is also weakness, respiratory distress, collapse, and death.

Treatment

Antivenin is available, but only the specific antiserum for the type of cobra involved should be used, and victims are often tested for sensitivity before being treated. If the eyes are contaminated, they should be immediately flushed out and treated or blindness may result.

See also COBRA; COBRA, SPITTING; SNAKES, POISONOUS.

Ritalin Known chemically as methylphenidate, this drug is a stimulant but is ironically given to hyperactive children to calm them down. In adults, it acts as a central nervous system stimulant and, if taken with monoamine oxidase (MAO) inhibitors, can drastically increase blood pressure. It is well absorbed when taken by mouth and is metabolized extensively by the liver. It has a low therapeutic index (that is, toxicity occurs at levels only slightly above the usual doses). A high degree of tolerance can occur after continued use.

Symptoms

Overdose can cause agitation, nausea, vomiting, hyperthermia, tremors, seizures, hypertension, coma, and convulsions; if taken with anticonvulsants, it may change seizure pattern. An overdose can be fatal.

Treatment

Treat symptoms if they occur. There is no specific antidote for Ritalin; hypertension may be treated with a vasodilator such as phentolamine. Do not induce vomiting; perform gastric lavage and administer activated charcoal.

rosary pea *(Abrus precatorius)* [Other names: bead vine, black-eyed Susan, coral bead plant, crab's eyes, Indian licorice, jequirity bean, licorice vine, love bean, lucky bean, mienie-mienie Indian bean, paternoster pea, prayer bead, precatory bean, red bead vine, rosary bean, Seminole bead, weather plant, wild licorice.] This climbing, woody vine is found in tropical regions in Africa and Asia, and in Florida, Hawaii, Guam, Central America, southern Europe, and India. Its leaves have short leaflets that droop at night and in cloudy weather, and its pea-shaped fruit pod holds five scarlet, pea-sized seeds with hard seed coats and a small black spot. Its seeds are used in rosaries, bracelets, leis, good luck charms, and children's toys, but the seeds are harmless unless chewed.

Poisonous part

Seeds, or beans, if chewed. If swallowed whole, the hard seed coat prevents absorption and poisoning. The toxalbumin called abrin, one of nature's most poisonous substances, is the poison in rosary pea; the tetanic glycoside abric acid is found in the seeds. Abrin interferes with the protein synthesis in cells of the intestinal wall.

Symptoms

The severity of symptoms, which appear from several hours to several days after eating, depends on the number of beans eaten and how much they were chewed. Symptoms include mouth irritations, nausea, vomiting, severe diarrhea, acute gastroenteritis, chills, weakness, clammy skin with perspiration, weak, rapid pulse, and convulsions ending in death from heart failure. One seed chewed by a child can be fatal despite intensive care.

Treatment

The long time between ingestion and symptoms allows for the removal of the poisonous substance; convulsions are treated as they occur, together with a high carbohydrate diet to head off liver damage.

See also GLYCOSIDE; PHYTOTOXINS.

roseum A variety of chrysanthemum used in the production of the botanic insecticide pyrethrum.

See also PYRETHRUM.

rotenone Also known as derrin or derris, rotenone is a broad-spectrum botanic insecticide derived from the derris root and used in lotions and ointments to treat chiggers, scabies, and head lice; in dusts, washes, and dips against animal parasites; and in insecticide sprays for home and agricultural use. Once believed to be harmless, it is now known to be more toxic than pyrethrin. While it has been used for many years, it has regained popularity in the last decade because it kills a wide variety of insects and is easy to make. This white, odorless crystal is sold in a 1 percent and 5 percent powder or spray.

Symptoms

Rotenone affects the nervous system and is most toxic when inhaled; skin contamination can cause a local irritation, and ingestion will cause stomach irritations but it is rarely fatal. If inhaled, it can cause vomiting, abdominal pain, tremors, and incoordination and can lead to convulsions and death from respiratory failure. Skin contact causes local irritation and dermatitis; ingestion produces nausea and vomiting. Chronic poisoning can cause kidney and liver damage.

Treatment

Symptomatic.

See also BOTANIC INSECTICIDES; DERRIS; PYRETHRIN.

rubbing alcohol See ISOPROPYL ALCOHOL.

rust remover See ALKALINE CORROSIVES.

S

saccharin Saccharin is an artificial sweetener discovered by accident in 1878 that is 400 times as sweet as sugar; American consumers ate or drank more than 5 million pounds of it a year before it was banned. Although the Food and Drug Administration banned saccharin in March 1977 because it is mutagenic and causes cancer in laboratory animals, it is still an ingredient in many low-calorie and sugar-free foods, including soft drinks, baked goods, jams, canned fruit, candy, dessert toppings, and salad dressings, and in almost all toothpastes in the United States. It is also the major ingredient in Sweet'n Low, the sweetener in the pink packets, which (like all foods that contain saccharin) carries a mandatory warning label that might be removed should saccharin ever lose its classification as a suspected carcinogen.

A Canadian scientist first identified it as a possible carcinogen in 1977 and the FDA proposed a ban. But the public was outraged at the FDA's plan, since another artificial sweetener (cyclamate) had already been taken off the market after studies had cited it as a cause of cancer. Diabetics, who rely on artificial sweeteners, argued that they needed saccharin.

In a compromise, Congress passed a law preventing the ban but requiring the warning labels. In 1981, saccharin went on the government's list, which now has 169 suspected carcinogens and 29 known carcinogens. Its name is derived from the Latin word *saccharun,* meaning "sugar"; pure saccharin is an odorless white powder that easily dissolves in warm water but is destroyed by high heat. It has been criticized almost from the beginning of its use, first because it offered no food value and later because of its animal carcinogenicity.

Symptoms

Ingestion of large amounts can produce toxic symptoms such as vomiting, diarrhea, abdominal pain, frothing, muscle spasms, convulsions, and stupor. In hypersensitive persons, even small doses may cause gastrointestinal symptoms such as vomiting and diarrhea, and allergic skin reactions.

Treatment

Gastric lavage or induced vomiting for large overdoses, followed by a saline cathartic; symptomatic treatment.

See also SWEETENERS, ARTIFICIAL.

salicylates Widely valued for their painkilling and anti-inflammatory properties, the salicylates are found in a wide variety of over-the-counter preparations and cold products. The substance is an ingredient in aspirin and in most other analgesic preparations, and before the introduction of child-resistant caps, salicylate poisoning was one of the leading causes of accidental death in children. Oil of wintergreen, found in many skin ointments, is also high in salicylate content and can be fatal if ingested.

Aspirin should never be taken with acetaminophen (Tylenol), since it increases the liver toxicity of the Tylenol. Aspirin also increases the activity of blood thinners. Vitamin C in large doses taken with aspirin can cause poisoning, but this is not usually fatal. Aspirin also interferes with the utilization of vitamin K in the liver.

Symptoms

Salicylate poisoning causes a wide range of symptoms depending on the person's age and the amount swallowed. Two distinct syndromes may occur depending on whether the exposure is chronic or acute: acute ingestion of 150 to 200 milligrams per kilogram will produce a mild reaction; ingestion of 300 to 500 milligrams per kilogram will produce a more serious response. Chronic intoxication may occur with ingestion of 100 milligrams per kilogram for two or more days.

Onset of symptoms may be delayed for 12 to 24 hours. In cases of acute poisoning, vomiting is followed by ringing in the ears and lethargy; severe poisoning causes coma, seizures, low blood sugar, high fever, and pulmonary edema followed by death due to central nervous system failure and cardiovascular collapse.

Chronic poisoning may result with older persons who have become confused over their dosage, or with young children. Symptoms include confusion, dehydration, and acidosis, which may often be misdiagnosed. With chronic poisoning, death rates are much higher and cerebral and pulmonary edema are more common.

Treatment

There is no specific antidote for salicylate poisoning, but sodium bicarbonate is often given to help the kidneys eliminate the drug. Treat symptoms, replace fluid, and maintain electrolyte balance; induce vomiting or perform gastric lavage followed by the administration of activated charcoal and a cathartic. With very large ingestions of salicylate, very large doses of activated charcoal are also needed to absorb the salicylate. Hemodialysis can be effective in removing salicylate. The victim should be treated for shock until medical care is available.

See also ASPIRIN.

Salmonella Bacteria (including *S. enteritidis, S. cubana, S. aertrycke, S. choleraesius*) that multiply rapidly at room temperature and cause salmonellosis, an illness characterized by nausea, vomiting, and diarrhea. Salmonella is found in raw meats, poultry, eggs, fish, raw milk, and foods made from them, as well as in pet turtles and marijuana.

See also SALMONELLOSIS.

salmonellosis One of the most common types of food poisoning, typically associated with a very wide range of foods. It is caused by one of the more than 2,300 strains of *Salmonella* that multiply rapidly at room temperatures; *Salmonella enteritidis* and *S. typhimurium* are the most common. According to the FDA *Bad Bug Book,* 2 million to 4 million cases of salmonellosis occur in the United States each year, yet only about 40,000 cases are reported, as many mild cases are not diagnosed or reported. An estimated 1,000 people die of the condition each year.

Salmonellosis occurs in raw or undercooked poultry and eggs, raw meats, fish, nonpasteurized milk, and any foods made from them. Most recently, a large outbreak (more than 1,300 people affected as of August 2008) that covered 43 states involved jalapeno and Serrano peppers imported from Mexico. Originally this outbreak, which was caused by a rare strain of Salmonella called *S. saintpaul,* was attributed to tomatoes, and tomato sales slumped dramatically. However, further investigation by the Food and Drug Administration and others uncovered the pepper connection and dismissed the case against the tomatoes. An outbreak of salmonellosis in Oregon in March 2008 involved cantaloupe, while another in 2002 affected 650 people from all 50 states and was linked to a Dallas hotel food worker who contaminated the salsa the hotel served.

Symptoms

From six to 48 hours after eating contaminated food, symptoms appear, including severe headache, nausea, fever, stomach cramps, diarrhea, vomiting, and sometimes a rash. Symptoms usually last two to seven days, and the infection may be mild to severe. It can be fatal, especially in very young or very old patients, or those with underlying impaired immune systems.

Treatment

Treatment is symptomatic, including a bland diet (liquids and soft solids) and fluids to offset dehydration. Antibiotic treatment (chloramphenicol, ampicillin, or a tetracycline) should be administered only in cases of severe infection, or for people at high risk for complications.

Complications

Meningitis, blood poisoning, bone/joint infections.

Cooks should be sure to prepare and cook chicken, eggs, and other poultry and meats completely, and to promptly refrigerate leftovers. Consumers also should refrigerate eggs and not use them raw (such as in eggnog). Raw chicken should never touch any other food or utensils during preparation, and cooks should wash their hands after touching it.

saponin   One of the toxic glycoside compounds that vary in strength in any particular plant depending on the plant part and time of the year. While saponins are not easily absorbed by a healthy digestive tract, in the presence of other substances irritating to the digestive tract they can be absorbed, causing pain, vomiting, and diarrhea similar to gastroenteritis. There is still much to be learned about the saponins, and many of the plants whose toxicity is a result of this compound have not been extensively studied. The saponin content of any one plant changes according to the part of the plant, its stage of growth, and the season.

Plants that contain saponins include the corn cockle, tung tree, beech, English ivy, and pokeweed.

See also CORN COCKLE; GLYCOSIDE; IVY; POKEWEED.

savin *(Juniperus sabina)*   This extremely common shrub is found throughout the world and is an ancient abortifacient (abortion-inducer); oil made from the shrub is used to counteract overdose of cardiac medications like digitalis.

Poisonous part

The entire savin plant is toxic.

Symptoms

In small doses, ingestion causes water loss and starts menstruation; in large doses, it causes gastroenteritis with hemorrhages, vomiting, polyuria (excessive urine), oliguria (reduced urine) and anuria (absence of urine), and convulsions. Topically, savin oil cause blisters. Death from respiratory arrest occurs from 10 hours to several days later.

Treatment

Castor oil followed by gastric lavage or emesis; follow immediately with a saline cathartic. Treat symptoms; give milk and plenty of fluids.

saxitoxin   A deadly neurotoxin that is produced by plankton and causes paralytic shellfish poisoning (PSP). This poison gets its name from the Alaskan butter clam *(Saxidomus giganteus),* from which it is extracted; it blocks nerve impulses, causes paralysis of the respiratory muscles and can be fatal if even one contaminated shellfish is eaten. It has minimal effects on the cardiovascular system. Although there is no antidote to saxitoxin, it is readily absorbed by activated charcoal.

See also DINOFLAGELLATE; PARALYTIC SHELLFISH POISONING; SHELLFISH POISONING.

scombroid poisoning   A type of poisoning caused by eating any of a group of scombroid fish (including mackerel, swordfish, moray eel, mahimahi, tuna, bluefish) that have begun to spoil when histamine in the flesh interacts with certain types of bacteria. When these fish are allowed to stand at room temperature for several hours, the bacteria produce a histaminelike substance called saurine.

Scombroid fish are more susceptible to the development of saurine than are most other kinds of fish; all of the species that are potentially toxic live in temperate or tropical waters (especially around California and Hawaii). Even commercially canned tuna can become toxic, although the most common fish responsible is mahimahi.

In annual reports, scombroid poisonings still rank among the top four most often reported seafood food poisonings. No doubt consumer mishandling in recreational and home settings can contribute to the incidence, and food service establishments must be better advised in product selection and handling.

Studies have shown that toxic histamine levels can be generated within less than six to 12 hours exposure without ice or refrigeration. This problem is of particular concern immediately after catch aboard a commercial or recreational boat. Likewise, the recreational catch lying on a warm dock or beach is prone to histamine production in certain species.

Symptoms

Symptoms of saurine poisoning resemble those of a severe allergy: Soon after eating, the victim begins to experience headache, throbbing blood vessels in the neck, nausea and vomiting, burning throat, and massive welts and itching. Recovery begins between eight and 12 hours later.

Treatment

Antihistamines are usually prescribed.

Prevention

The potential toxins are not destroyed by freezing, cooking, smoking, curing, or canning. Chemical testing is the only reliable way to evaluate a potentially contaminated product.

scorpion Looking like a little crab with eight legs (in fact, scorpions are cousins to the sea-dwelling crustaceans), the scorpion has a segmented tail that curls over the body and ends in a poison reservoir and stinger. This tail is so flexible that it is almost impossible to pick up a scorpion with the bare hands and avoid a sting. The scorpion of the Southwest inflicts severe pain with its neurotoxic venom and is especially dangerous to children.

Because of its eight legs, it belong to the Arachnida family (as do tarantulas and spiders). Most of the more than 700 species are about 3 inches long, are either black or yellow and are found in most warm regions of the world.

Some of the most poisonous species are found in Mexico, North Africa, South America, parts of the Caribbean, and India. About 40 species live in the United States, and though the stings of most scorpions are more or less harmless, the venom of one found in the southern states—the sculpturatus scorpion *(Centruroides exilicauda)*—contains a neurotoxin and can be lethal. Other poisonous scorpions in the United States include the brown scorpion *(C. gertschii)* and the common striped scorpion *(C. vittatus).*

Poisonous scorpions in Mexico and Brazil are the *Tityus bahiensis* and *T. serrulatus;* the most deadly scorpions in North Africa, India, and Pakistan are *Androctonus asutralis* and *Buthus occitanus.*

While scorpions don't attack humans, they like dark, moist places and hide in clothing or shoes, where they will sting if stepped on. Because of their fondness for the dark and the wet, they often crawl into shoes at night, where they present a dangerous hazard. In areas with heavy infestations of scorpions, residents spread out a wet burlap sack at night; scorpions crawl in and can then be easily located and destroyed in the morning.

Poisonous part

In equal amounts, scorpion venom is proportionately more poisonous than snake venom; however, scorpions inject a smaller amount of venom when they sting. The pale yellow desert scorpion is about 2 inches long and is more lethal than the big black scorpion, and the red scorpions are not deadly. The poison of the scorpion carries a neurotoxin that destroys nerve tissue and disturbs the heart.

Symptoms

The first symptom is a severe, sharp, and burning pain, similar to a bee sting. If the sting was of a nonlethal scorpion, the area of the sting will become swollen and discolored and may form a blister; symptoms will last for eight to 12 hours. If the sting was of the lethal species, the sharp pain produced by the sting is quickly followed by a pins-and-needles sensation at the sting site. The area of the sting will not become swollen or discolored; within one to three hours the following symptoms will appear: itchy eyes, nose, and throat; tightness of jaw muscles and difficulty in speaking; extreme restlessness and muscle twitching; muscle spasms with pain; nausea, vomiting, and incontinence (caused by stimulation of the autonomic nervous system); drowsiness, difficulty in breathing, and irregular heartbeat.

Because scorpion toxicity is dose related, fatalities are uncommon in adults; the smaller the victim, the greater the danger of death. Therefore, children and the elderly are at higher risk. Symptoms appearing within two to four hours after a lethal scorpion sting indicate a serious medical problem. Fatalities have occurred as much as four days after a scorpion sting. However, it is not true that any scorpion sting brings death, since very few species are toxic enough to be fatal. Only one out of a thousand stings is fatal. Interference with the absorption of venom will head off serious symptoms.

Treatment

Contact medical help immediately whether or not it is a lethal scorpion sting. Have the person lie still, with the bitten part immobile and lower than the heart. Apply ice packs to the wound, and apply a constricting band two to four inches above the bite, snug but loose enough to allow a pulse farther out on the limb. If swelling reaches the band, tie another band two to four inches higher up, and then remove tthe first one. After 30 minutes, remove the band. If pain is the only symptom, a cold compress and painkillers may be enough. More severe cases call for local anesthetics and powerful painkillers, plus an antivenin to deactivate the venom. Antivenins against the venoms of local, deadly species of scorpion are available in most parts of the world where the creatures are found. *Not recommended:* hot packs, alcohol, morphine, or incisions.

See also SCORPION, BROWN; SCORPION, COMMON STRIPED; SCORPION, SCULPTURATUS.

scorpion, brown *(Centruroides gertschii)*   One of three species of poisonous scorpions in the United States, the brown scorpion lives primarily in the Southwest—especially in Arizona.

Poisonous part

The sting of the brown scorpion carries a deadly neurotoxin far more lethal than snake venom, which can destroy nerve tissue and cause heart problems.

Symptoms

Intense pain, numbness, and hemorrhage of the intestines and stomach; lung and seizure activities. There is generally only a mild tingling at the wound site, followed by throat spasms, restlessness, muscular spasms, stomach cramps, convulsions, blood pressure abnormalities, pulmonary edema, and respiratory failure. Symptoms usually

begin in one to two days, but death can come as much as four days after a sting. Still, only one of a thousand stings is fatal.

Treatment

Antivenin is available.
See also SCORPION.

scorpion, common striped *(Centruroides vittatus)* One of three poisonous scorpions living in the United States, the common striped scorpion lives primarily in Arizona and other areas of the American Southwest. Scorpions live near homes and like the dark warmth of shoes and closets; they are not aggressive toward humans unless suddenly disturbed. When attacking, the scorpion's front pincers grab on and its tail flings forward to sting (once or repeatedly).

Poisonous part

The sting of the common striped scorpion carries a deadly neurotoxin far more lethal than snake venom, which can destroy nerve tissue and cause heart problems.

Symptoms

Intense pain, numbness, and hemorrhage of the intestines and stomach; lung and seizure activities. There is generally only a mild tingling at the wound site, followed by throat spasms, restlessness, muscular spasms, stomach cramps, convulsions, blood pressure abnormalities, pulmonary edema, and respiratory failure. Symptoms usually begin in one to two days, but death can come as much as four days after a sting. Still, only one of a thousand stings is fatal.

Treatment

Antivenin is available.
See also SCORPION.

scorpion, sculpturatus *(Centruroides exilicauda)* One of three poisonous scorpions found in Arizona, New Mexico, and parts of California. The bite from the sculpturatus scorpion contains a powerful neurotoxin that can be lethal. Scorpions live near homes and like the dark warmth of shoes and closets; they are not aggressive toward humans unless suddenly disturbed. When attacking, the scorpion's front pincers grab on and its tail flings forward to sting (once or repeatedly).

Poisonous part

The sting of the sculpturatus scorpion carries a deadly neurotoxin far more lethal than snake venom, which can destroy nerve tissue and cause heart problems.

Symptoms

Intense pain, numbness, and hemorrhage of the intestines and stomach; lung and seizure activities. There is generally only a mild tingling at the wound site, followed by throat spasms, restlessness, muscular spasms, stomach cramps, convulsions, blood pressure abnormalities, pulmonary edema, and respiratory failure. Symptoms usually begin in one to two days, but death can come as much as four days after a sting. Still, only one of a thousand stings is fatal.

Treatment

Antivenin is available.
See also SCORPION.

scorpion fish   The family of scorpion fish includes about 350 species, some of them as venomous as a cobra, that are found in oceans throughout the world. The scorpion fish proper is closely related to other poisonous members of the Scorpaenidae family, including the zebra fish, waspfish, butterfly fish, rockfish, stonefish, and lionfish.

The scorpion fish is found in the reefs and coral caves of the Pacific Ocean and is about four to eight inches long with a large head and big mouth, colored in red-brown and white bands. Scorpion fish look so much like stones that they can be almost unnoticeable and can be easily stepped on when a person walks in shallow water. Most scorpion fish stings, however, are reported after handling of the fish when taking them off the hook or out of a net; there are about 300 cases of scorpion fish poisoning reported yearly in the United States. Depending on the species, scorpion fish have 17 or 18 venomous spines that are covered by a layer of skin called the integumentary sheath. As each spine enters a person's skin, its sheath is pushed down, releasing the venom from a gland that lies hidden beneath it. This venom is the deadliest poison of any fish, lethal enough to kill a swimmer or beachcomber in two hours.

There are about 60 species of rockfish in the scorpion fish family, mostly found in the cool waters of the Pacific Ocean. Rockfish have a hard protective covering around their heads, as well as the needle-sharp spines common to all scorpion fish.

The most exotic of all the scorpion fish are the zebra fish, which usually swim in pairs in the open, marked with a striking pattern of stripes and feathery fins. Among those fins are 18 long, slender, pointed spines that deliver a venom that can cause a painful and swollen wound leading to gangrene, delirium, convulsions, cardiac failure, and even death. The zebra fish is found in the Red Sea and the Indian Ocean, and in the waters surrounding China, Japan, and Australia. Swimmers in these areas should avoid approaching a zebra fish, especially from the side, which irritates this fish. When frightened, it moves around so its spine is aimed directly at the intruder, stinging with a darting, lightning-fast jab.

Symptoms

The sting of the scorpion fish causes an immediate severe stinging or throbbing pain, which may stay at the site of the wound or spread throughout the body and last for several hours or days. There may be redness and swelling at the site of the sting, and the area may become numb. The more dangerous varieties can cause loss of consciousness, paralysis, delirium, and convulsions, leading to fatal cardiac arrest. The profound pain, convulsions, paralysis, and unconsciousness—which can be immediate—can cause drowning. In addition, there is often a secondary infection and a fluctuating fever.

Treatment

There is no known antidote, although stonefish antivenin may be administered. Contact medical help immediately; flush the wound with fresh- or salt water and then soak the affected area in hot water or put hot compresses on it. The water should be very hot (120°F) so that the heat will deactivate the poison. Continue applying hot water for an hour. Recovery from a scorpion fish sting may take months and leave a permanent scar.

See also LIONFISH; STONEFISH.

sea cucumber (Holothurioidea class)   Although sea cucumbers under most circumstances are safe to eat, there are toxic species that are difficult to identify. In addition, some species of sea cucumbers produce a poison that is quite toxic and can cause burning and inflammation on human skin and blindness if it comes in contact with the eyes.

The toxin is located in tubules within the creature's body, from which it can be excreted, forming long, sticky threads that can capture and trap an attacker.

Poisonous part
The toxin is called holothurin.

Symptoms
While little is known of the symptoms produced by poisonous sea cucumbers, eating the toxic species can be fatal. However, such intoxications are rare. Contact with liquid ejected from some sea cucumbers may cause rash or blindness.

Treatment
There is no known antidote. Treatment is symptomatic.

sea snake (Hydrophidae)   Considered by the *Guinness Book of World Records* to be the most venomous snake in the world, the sea snake has highly toxic venom—in some cases, more than 50 times as deadly as that of the king cobra. Of the 50 cataloged species of sea snakes, all are venomous, and as many as 25 percent of their victims will die.

Sea snakes inhabit the Pacific and Indian Oceans and are widely found around the Ashmore Reef in the Timor Sea off the coast of northwestern Australia. None have ever been found in the Atlantic Ocean or the Mediterranean or Red Seas. Huge clumps of many thousands of sea snakes may sometimes be found at sea; some experts believe

this is because small fish often swim in shoals beneath floating debris.

True snakes, the Hydrophidae have lidless eyes and a forked tongue, growing an average of four feet long. They are very well adapted to life in the sea, with a streamlined body, nostrils on top of their heads and special glands that excrete salt. Reports conflict as to whether these snakes are considered to be docile or aggressive. They have long been killed for their leather.

Fortunately, however, the mechanism for injecting poison is not well developed in the sea snakes, and their fangs are very small. While it is often believed that these snakes have small mouths and can only bite a human's tender skin at the base of the thumb, this is not true. Many pearl divers in the Persian Gulf who weren't wearing goggles have died after accidentally grabbing sea snakes.

Poisonous sea snakes include the banded, or annulated, sea snake (*Hydrophis cyanocinctus*); beaked sea snake (*Enhydrina schistosa*); yellow-lipped sea krait (*Laticauda colubrina*); olive-brown sea snake (*Aipysurus laevis*); yellow sea snake (*Hydrophis spiralis*); Hardwicke's sea snake (*Lapemis hardwickii*); and the pelagic sea snake (*Pelamis platurus*). The largest species is *Laticauda semifasciata;* the sea snakes of this species gather together in groups numbering in the thousands to breed in the large coastal caves of Gato north of Cebu. Some species, such as the *Laticauda colubrina,* live partly on land, entering the water occasionally, although they are well equipped for life in the sea.

Of all the sea snakes, the beaked sea snake is the most venomous and is responsible for more fatalities than all other sea snakes combined. The yellow sea snake and the Hardwicke's sea snake are not nearly as venomous, although both have caused several fatalities. The pelagic sea snake is the most common and least toxic, found on the west coast of the American tropics.

In general, however, sea snakes are fairly inoffensive and pose no great threat to humans, despite the toxicity of their venom.

Poisonous part
The extremely toxic venom is a neurotoxin that affects the muscles and paralyzes the nervous sys-

tem, causing the release of the protein myoglobin, which stains the urine red, damages the kidneys, and affects the heart.

Symptoms

Unlike the bite of many other poisonous sea creatures, the bite of a sea snake seems like a harmless pinprick. Because symptoms appear very slowly—between 20 minutes and eight hours—the victim often does not connect the snakebite with subsequent symptoms. First, the victim feels weakness and then pain in the skeletal muscles. Victims notice numbness and thickening of the tongue and mouth, blurred vision, and difficulty in swallowing. Weakness increases, the eyelids droop, the jaws stiffen, and the pulse weakens and becomes irregular. Sometimes, nausea and vomiting are present. In cases of severe poisoning, symptoms worsen and cyanosis appears, followed by breathing problems and convulsions. Death may come in a few hours to a few days.

Treatment

Antivenin is available; the snake should be captured and identified to rule out the bite of a harmless water snake. Cortisone or epinephrine is sometimes given to prevent anaphylaxis, and fluids and electrolyte levels are monitored. If a person has not been severely bitten, recovery is rapid.

See also COBRA, KING; SNAKES, POISONOUS.

sea urchin (Diadema setosum; Toxpneustes elegans; Asthenosoma jimoni)   Of all the sea urchins, the sting from the long-spined variety *(D. setosum)* is the most poisonous. Red sea urchins *T. elegans* and *A. jimoni* are less venomous. Sea urchins are commonly found in warm waters around rocks or wrecks, where they can sting swimmers or divers even through shoes and gloves. They are rounded, about the size of a golf or tennis ball, with sharp spines radiating outward.

Poisonous part

Sea urchins have venomous spines with poisoned tips, and three pronged biting teeth that are extremely tenacious.

Symptoms

Although death is rare, the sting of the sea urchin penetrates soft tissue, causing an immediate severe stinging or throbbing pain, which may stay at the site of the wound or spread throughout the body and last for several hours or days. There may be redness and swelling at the site of the sting, and the area may become numb, followed by muscle weakness and possible paralysis.

Treatment

Contact medical help immediately. Remove spines; if the brittle tips break off and are not absorbed in two days, surgery may be required to remove them. Flush the wound with fresh- or salt water, and then soak the affected area in hot water or put hot compresses on it. The water should be very hot (122°F) so that the heat will deactivate the poison. Continue applying hot water for 30 minutes to an hour. Have the victim lie still with the stung part immobile and lower than the heart. Tie a flat strip of cloth snugly around a stung arm or leg two to four inches above the sting, loose enough to allow a pulse farther out on the limb. Check periodically and loosen if necessary, but do not remove it. If swelling reaches the band, tie another band two to four inches higher up and remove the first one. There may be a purple stain on the skin around the wound, which is merely a pigment of the spine and not dangerous.

sea wasp (Chironex fleckeri; Chiropsalmus quadrigatus)   One of the most venomous of the jellyfish, the sea wasp lives in warm water from Queensland northward to Malaya but also in cooler waters as far north as the central Atlantic seaboard; the Australian species is the most dangerous. Their tentacles may grow as long as 200 feet, although contact with only 20 feet of tentacle will be fatal. Sea wasps can be found close to shore, sometimes in only a few feet of water.

A moderate sting from a sea wasp can be fatal in a few minutes. The sea wasp is considered to be one of the most deadly organisms in the world, and in Australia alone it has caused more than 50 deaths in 20 years. In fact, the venom is so toxic that in laboratory experiments a solution diluted

10,000 times still killed the animal before the syringe could be extracted.

The only protection against the sting of sea wasp is the wearing of tights, which the wasps cannot penetrate; all life-saving teams in Queensland are required to wear them for this reason.

Poisonous part

The sea wasp's tentacles cluster at the corners of its body, and the stinging capsules within each contain a minute amount of one of the most deadly venoms ever discovered. The live nematocysts that contain the poison can live for months on the beach, if occasionally moistened with seawater, and are capable of injecting the poison; even nematocysts that have been dried on the beach for several weeks maintain potency.

Symptoms

The sting of the sea wasp can be fatal within seconds. In general, there are painful swellings and purple-brown wheals at the site of the sting, which later necrose. Pain is said to be excruciating and can cause the victim to become distraught and irrational. Symptoms include muscular spasms, breathing problems, rapid and weak pulse, pulmonary edema, shock, and respiratory failure followed almost always by death, within 30 seconds to three hours; in general, death occurs within 15 minutes. Even the mildest sting is not pleasant, with acute burning pain and a wheal that lasts for months.

Treatment

There is not usually time to administer first aid or an antidote, although a sea wasp antivenin is available in Australia. Stings from the sea wasp do not occur in the United States.

See also JELLYFISH.

Seconal   See BARBITURATES.

selective serotonin reuptake inhibitors (SSRIs)

This class of antidepressants was first introduced in 1987 with the marketing of fluoxetine (Prozac). Experts believe that selective serotonin reuptake inhibitors (SSRIs) help relieve depression by blocking the reabsorption (reuptake) of a brain chemical called serotonin, which is associated with depression, behavior, and mood. SSRIs allow more serotonin to remain in the brain, which in turn improves mood.

SSRIs are available in extended-release or controlled-release form, which provides the medication throughout a day or for a week at a time with a single dose. The SSRIs approved by the Food and Drug Administration to treat depression include citalopram (Celexa), escitalopram (Lexapro), fluoxetine (Prozac), fluvoxamine (Luvox), paroxetine (Paxil), and sertraline (Zoloft). Some of these drugs are also used to treat conditions other than depression.

Compared with other classes of antidepressants, SSRIs are generally less likely to have adverse interactions with other medications, and they are less dangerous if taken as an overdose.

Symptoms

An overdose of SSRIs rarely results in fatalities but in some cases causes a life-threatening condition called serotonin syndrome, in which dangerously high levels of serotonin accumulate in the brain. This syndrome can also occur when SSRIs are taken with other medications or supplements that have an influence on serotonin levels, such as monoamine oxidase inhibitors and St. John's wort. Signs and symptoms of serotonin syndrome include confusion, restlessness, hallucinations, extreme agitation, fluctuations in blood pressure, increased heart rate, nausea and vomiting, fever, seizures, and coma.

In some cases, antidepressants may be associated with worsening symptoms of depression or suicidal behavior or thoughts. These symptoms tend to appear early in treatment or when dosages are changed.

Treatment

If gastric lavage and/or charcoal are to be given, the airway must be clear. Gastric lavage is usually not necessary but may be performed within 60 minutes of suspected ingestion. Activated charcoal can be administered if indicated. Seizures and muscular rigidity are best managed with benzodiazepines.

selenium A metallic element found normally in the soil, selenium is necessary for human health but is toxic in large amounts, although few cases of selenium poisoning in humans have been reported. Selenium poisoning is more of a problem for farm animals and birds, although it can be a problem for farm families with wells polluted by runoff from selenium-rich agricultural soil.

Selenium is used in a wide variety of products because of its ability to produce electricity when light is shined on it; it is widely used in photoelectric cells, light meters, photocopying machines, and other electrical components. It is also used to create the red color in warning lights, traffic lights, and brake lights.

A well-balanced diet is the best way to obtain selenium; about two-thirds of dietary selenium comes from meat, fish, and dairy products, which provide enough selenium to satisfy daily requirements but not enough to be toxic.

Chronic poisoning may occur from numerous exposures during the manufacture of the wide range of products that use this element.

Symptoms
Chronic poisoning symptoms include pallor, garlicky odor to the breath, metallic taste, gastrointestinal disturbances, irritation of the nose, conjunctivitis, skin problems, drowsiness, and chest constriction.

Treatment
Removal from the environment and a selenium-free diet.

shellfish poisoning Shellfish are highly susceptible to bacterial and viral contamination because they live close to the shore, where pollution tends to be worst. Cooking usually destroys the microbes that infect shellfish—but eating raw clams, oysters, and other shellfish is linked to nearly 1,000 cases of hepatitis alone each year.

While shellfish by themselves are not poisonous, they can become contaminated by bacteria and other organisms from their environment and pass them on to humans when the shellfish is eaten. Oysters, clams, and mussels are particularly prone to becoming contaminated because of their meta-bolic system, which pumps water across the gills to isolate plankton for their food. This system makes them vulnerable to bacteria, viruses, or other contaminants in the water. Lobsters and other crustacean shellfish only rarely become contaminated.

In mussels, toxins are concentrated in the digestive glands, and toxicity is usually lost within weeks. But the Alaskan butter clam can remain toxic for up to two years after accumulating the toxin. However, the part of the mollusk that humans generally eat—the white meat, without the digestive glands—stores fairly small amounts of toxin.

Seafood contaminated with toxins may look and taste normal, but normal cooking methods don't affect the toxin. State shellfish screening programs test shellfish for the presence of these toxins and monitor the safety of shellfish harvest beds. However, people who catch their own shellfish from unapproved beds are at risk for a variety of toxic infections.

The toxins may be produced as fish spoil (as in scombrotoxin) or as the by-products of toxic plankton (paralytic shellfish poisoning), or they may naturally be present in the fish itself (tetrodotoxin).

Some types of plankton produce a toxin (saxitoxin) that is eaten by shellfish along the North American coasts. These plankton multiply rapidly during the warm summer months; because their color is pink or red, this phenomenon has come to be called "red tide." When people eat shellfish contaminated with the toxin, they can become very sick or die. It's not possible to build up immunity by becoming exposed to sublethal doses, and in some cases, the substance is so toxic that even one contaminated shellfish can be fatal if eaten. This is why clams, oysters, and mussels are not sold during months without an *r* (the summer months—May, June, July, and August).

Shellfish poisoning caused by these toxic plankton comes in four forms: neurotoxic shellfish poisoning (NSP), diarrheic shellfish poisoning (DSP), amnesic shellfish poisoning (ASP), and paralytic shellfish poisoning (PSP). Each has quite different etiology, symptoms and prognosis for recovery, but of the three, PSP is by far the most serious. All types are caused by 20 different toxins related to saxitoxin. The true incidence of these shellfish poisonings is not known, because so many cases are believed not to be reported.

Treatment

There is no known antidote to saxitoxin. As in any treatment of curarelike poisoning, administration of prostigmine may be effective, together with artificial respiration and oxygen as needed.

See also CIGUATERA; DINOFLAGELLATE; FISH CONTAMINATION; PARALYTIC SHELLFISH POISONING.

shigellosis Shigellosis is caused by four different species of *Shigella* bacteria common in developing countries where lack of sewage treatment is linked to contaminated food and water. It is less common in the United States but still causes about 300,000 cases each year. Shigellosis is very common among AIDS patients, and cases are most serious among them and among the very young and old. A person gets sick after ingesting bacteria, and only a few organisms can cause illness. A person is infectious from the time the diarrhea appears until the bacteria is no longer in the stool (about a month).

Shigellosis is found in milk and dairy products, poultry, mixed salads (tuna, potato, shrimp, macaroni, and chicken), and raw vegetables, but it can develop in any moist food that isn't thoroughly cooked. The bacteria multiply rapidly at room temperature.

Symptoms

Between eight hours to a week after eating tainted food or beverages, symptoms of nausea and vomiting, diarrhea, stomach cramps, weakness, vision problems, headache, and swallowing problems appear. Children or those with weakened immune systems may have more serious diarrhea.

Diagnosis

A culture of the stool will reveal the infection.

Treatment

Most people recover on their own, but some may need fluids to offset dehydration. Antibiotics will help stop the diarrhea, although *Shigella* is becoming resistant to some drugs. Antidiarrhea medications should not be taken.

Prevention

Confirmed cases must be reported to the local health department, which will begin an investigation and control measures in order to prevent large-scale outbreaks. Although several vaccines have been tested, none has yet been licensed. The most important way to prevent the spread of this disease is to carefully wash your hands after using the toilet.

sick building syndrome A condition in which people who occupy a building—most often either a place of employment or a home—experience acute health and comfort effects that appear to be associated with the time they spend in the building, but no specific cause or illness can be identified. The adverse effects may be limited to a particular room or area of the building or be widespread throughout the building. Symptoms may include headache, eye, nose, or throat irritation, dry cough, dry or itchy skin, dizziness, nausea, difficulty in concentrating, fatigue, and sensitivity to odors. Most people who suffer with this syndrome report that they get relief from their symptoms once they have been away from the building for some time. If the syndrome is associated with a place of employment, people often feel better over the weekend and then get symptoms again at the beginning of the work week.

Causes of or contributing factors to sick building syndrome may include improper or inadequate ventilation. When national energy conservation measures were initiated as a result of the 1973 oil embargo, the amount of outdoor air provided for ventilation in buildings was reduced from 15 cubic feet per minute (cfm) to five cfm per building occupant. This reduction in air ventilation rates was not adequate to maintain the health and comfort of the building occupants. Another factor in sick building syndrome is ineffective heating, ventilating, and air-conditioning systems.

Chemical contaminants from either indoor or outdoor sources may also be a cause of or contributing factor in sick building syndrome. Indoor air pollution sources may include adhesives, carpeting, copy machines, manufactured wood products, tobacco smoke, and cleaning supplies that may emit volatile organic compounds (VOCs), including formaldehyde. Tobacco smoke contributes VOCs, other toxic compounds, and particulate matter. Combustion products such as carbon monoxide, nitrogen dioxide, and respirable particles can come from unvented stoves, fireplaces, and heaters. Outdoor sources of chemical contaminants that can enter buildings include motor vehicle exhaust and pollutants from plumbing vents and sewer lines.

Biological contaminants, such as bacteria, pollen, viruses, and molds may breed in stagnant water that can accumulate in humidifiers, drain pans, and ducts, or where water has collected on carpeting, insulation, or ceiling tiles. Physical symptoms associated with biological contamination include cough, fever, chills, muscle aches, allergic reactions, and chest tightness. Legionnaire's disease and Pontiac fever are two similar conditions that are caused by a biological contaminant, the bacterium *Legionella pneumophila*. According to the Centers for Disease Control and Prevention, between 8,000 and 18,000 people are hospitalized each year with Legionnaire's disease, and it is believed the actual number is much greater because many cases are not diagnosed or reported.

The most serious of the indoor air pollutants is carbon monoxide, which, according to the Consumer Product Safety Commission, causes more than 200 deaths a year. Dangerous levels of the odorless gas may be caused by automobile exhaust and improperly installed or vented appliances. The CPSC now recommends that all homes be equipped with carbon monoxide detectors (similar to smoke alarms) that will sound a warning when the gas reaches dangerous levels.

See also CARBON MONOXIDE.

sidewinder *(Crotalus cerastes)*   Also known as the horned rattler, this is one of three rattlesnakes from the family Viperidae known for its quick sideways motion across the shifting desert floor. Its odd, sideways motion leaves a distinct trail of parallel J-shaped marks.

The sidewinder has a distinctive look, with a prominent triangular, hornlike projection over each eye. The snake is found in arid deserts with mesquite-crowned sand hills throughout the south-western United States and northeastern Mexico. It is most often encountered as it crosses roads at night in the spring; during the day, it usually hides in burrows or bushes.

Symptoms

Symptoms appear within 15 minutes and include excessive thirst, nausea, vomiting, shock, paralysis, respiratory problems, anemia, necrosis, kidney problems, and sometimes death. The bite of a rattlesnake is painful. Indications of a serious bite include swelling above the elbows or knees within two hours, hemorrhages, numbness at the puncture site, tingling around the mouth, yellow vision, vomiting, and violent spasms.

Treatment

Antivenin is available.

See also MASSASAUGA; PIT VIPERS; RATTLESNAKE, CANEBRAKE; RATTLESNAKE, CASCABEL; RATTLESNAKE, EASTERN DIAMONDBACK; RATTLESNAKE, MEXICAN WEST COAST, RATTLESNAKE, RED DIAMONDBACK; RATTLESNAKES; RATTLESNAKE, TIMBER; RATTLESNAKE, WESTERN DIAMONDBACK; SNAKES, POISONOUS; VIPER, GABOON; VIPER, JUMPING; VIPER, MALAYAN PIT; VIPER, RUSSEL'S; VIPER, SAWSCALED; VIPER, WAGLER'S PIT; VIPERS; WATER MOCCASIN; WUTU.

silver nitrate   This astringent is used primarily to prevent a serious form of conjunctivitis in newborns and may also be used on burns and dressings. It dissolves readily in water and is fatal when ingested either in its salt form or as a liquid.

Symptoms

Immediately upon ingestion, silver nitrate causes pain and burning in the mouth, blackened skin, mucous membranes, throat and abdomen, vomiting and diarrhea, collapse, shock, convulsions, coma, and death. Repeated doses over a long period of time will cause a permanent blue-black color in the skin.

Treatment

Treatment for poisoning should begin immediately after ingestion by washing out the stomach repeatedly with 1 percent sodium chloride (salt) solution.

After this lavage, administer a purgative, such as 30 grams of sodium sulphate in 250 milliliters of water, which should remain in the stomach. Demulcents such as milk or egg white can be given with pethidine or morphine if necessary for pain. Pay close attention to fluid balance and kidney function.

sleeping pills　The term "sleeping pills" is a broad one, encompassing a wide variety of drugs from different classes, all of which are used to treat insomnia. These drugs may include benzodiazepines, nonbenzodiazepine sedative hypnotics, barbiturates, antidepressants, and antihistamines (found in most over-the-counter sleep aids).

According to a 2005 National Institutes of Health conference statement, the antidepressant trazodone is the most commonly prescribed drug for treatment of insomnia in the Untied States, even though trazodone has not been officially approved by the Food and Drug Administration (FDA) for treatment of insomnia. Drugs that have been approved by the FDA for insomnia include the benzodiazepines estazolam (ProSom), temezepam (Restoril), flurazepam (Dalmane), and quazepam (Doral); nonbenzodiazepines zaleplon (Sonata), zolpidem (Ambien), and eszopiclone (Lunesta); ramelteon (Rozerem); and triazolam (Halcion). Some of the drugs are designed to help you fall asleep; others help you stay asleep.

The rule of thumb with sleeping pills is to take the least amount needed to get relief and to taper off of them quickly to avoid getting addicted to them. People who use sleeping pills regularly over time often develop tolerance and usually need more and more of the drug to achieve the desired effect.

Use of alcohol in combination with sleeping pills multiplies the effects. Other drugs, including those used to treat heart disease, diabetes, depression, and duodenal ulcers, may have an adverse impact on sleeping pills.

Symptoms

These depend on the type of drug taken, but typically include slurred speech, lack of coordination, unsteady gait, euphoria or depression, impaired attention or memory. Heart and/or lung failure are also possible.

Treatment

Initiate immediate gastric lavage where appropriate along with general symptomatic measures. Intravenous fluids should be administered as needed. Vital signs should be monitored and treated as appropriate.

See also BARBITURATES; BENZODIAZEPINES; DALMANE; ETHYL ALCOHOL.

slug bait　See METALDEHYDE.

smooth-scaled snake *(Parademansia microlepidotus)*　The most venomous land snake in the world, according to the *Guinness Book of World Records,* this snake is found in southwestern Queensland and northeastern South Australia and Tasmania. Until 1976, it was thought to be a Western form of the taipan, but its venom is actually quite different. The smooth-scaled snake grows to up to six feet, six inches long, and its venom has been measured at 0.00385 ounces after milking—enough to kill 125,000 mice.

Symptoms

Pain and swelling within 30 minutes, dilated pupils, and low blood pressure followed by muscle weakness and paralysis of breathing muscles.

Treatment

Antivenin is available.

See also SNAKES, POISONOUS; TAIPAN.

snakes, poisonous　There are about 3,000 species of snakes in the world, but only about 10 percent of them are poisonous. Venomous snakes come in all sizes, from the tiny desert vipers to the king cobra, growing up to 16 feet long; a king cobra, when angered, can rear up and stand as tall as a person. While there are many old folk methods to quickly determine if a snake is poisonous, such as counting the rows of scales, there is no practical way to tell the poisonous from the harmless.

According to World Health Organization statistics, about 50,000 people throughout the world die from snakebites each year—mostly in India;

about 8,000 victims are treated each year in the United States. The highest death rate from snakebite in the United States is reported from Arizona, Florida, Georgia, Texas, and Alabama, in that order. According to the *Guinness Book of World Records,* Burma has the highest mortality rate—15.4 deaths per 100,000 population each year.

There are only four varieties of snakes in the United States that are poisonous—the rattlesnake, copperhead, water moccasin, and coral snake, but they are widely distributed throughout the country. The water moccasin is distributed over the Southwest, the Gulf states, and the Mississippi valley as far north as southern Illinois. Of all poisonous snakes, the copperhead is probably more commonly found throughout the country, especially in North and South Carolina, West Virginia, Pennsylvania, Missouri, Oklahoma, Arkansas, and Illinois. Rattlesnakes are found throughout the continental United States.

The coral snake is usually associated with the southern United States. Of the 115 species in this country, only about 20 are dangerous, including 16 species of rattlesnakes. Generally, only the eastern and western diamondback, canebrake, timber, and Mojave rattlers (and a few subspecies) could be considered life threatening. Of these, diamondbacks are considered to be the most dangerous, because of their large size, the length of their fangs, the large quantity of venom and the nature of their venom.

Rattlers account for about 65 percent of the venomous snakebites that occur in this country each year, and for nearly all of the nine to 15 deaths. A smaller fraction of bites comes from copperheads, fewer still from cottonmouths, and only three or four bites a year from coral snakes. Many snakebite victims are children or members of religious sects that handle deadly snakes.

Poisonous part

Scientists have identified more than 100 proteins in rattlesnake venom, including deadly neurotoxic compounds that dissolve cells and damage blood vessels. Heart and kidney complications often follow. Most snakebite fatalities occur 18 to 32 hours after a bite, but death can occur within 60 minutes or after several days. Some snakes (such as cobras) lay eggs, while others (such as vipers) give birth to live young. Newly born venomous snakes are just as dangerous as their parents and can often be far more aggressive than the old folks; baby cobras, in particular, are vicious and will strike even while they are emerging from their eggs.

Symptoms

Fang marks and possibly teeth marks may be visible. Symptoms include an immediate, burning pain that spreads rapidly (especially with a pit viper's bite), and sudden swelling beginning soon after the bite in the bite area and then spreading throughout the body. (This is especially true for bites on the arm or leg.) Systemic symptoms include shock, nausea, weakness, and numbness; muscles may twitch and skin may tingle. There are a number of factors that influence the severity of a snakebite: the amount of venom injected; the size and species of the individual snake; the age, size, health, and sensitivity of the victim; the types of clothing worn; and the position and number of bites inflicted. If an hour passes after a snakebite and no symptoms appear, chances are not enough venom was injected and the danger is slight.

Treatment

Despite the long history of snakebites and their treatment, the problem of how to deal with snakebites remains controversial: ice or no ice? Tourniquet or constriction band? Cut and suck or not? More than 200 different first aid procedures for snakebite have been recommended by various experts.

The emphasis on treating a snakebite should be placed on getting prompt medical care, and first aid should never be considered to be a substitute for antivenin. Rapid treatment with an antivenin can help a snakebite victim regardless of whether or not the bite would have been fatal. Without antivenin treatment, hospital stays for venomous snake bites last about twice as long. The venom of all snakes in the Crotalidae family (rattlesnakes, copperheads, and water moccasins) contains similar poisons, and all can be treated with antivenin. A bite from the eastern coral snake requires a separate antivenin, and there is no antivenin for the western coral snake.

In addition, there are different types of venom, and it is useless to treat a victim with an antivenin for viper bites if the injury was caused by a cobra. And venom even differs among specimens from different areas, even within the same species; for example, antivenin from an Indian member of a particular species will not be very helpful against bites of Thai cobras of the species.

Here's what to do if someone is bitten by a venomous snake.

- Apply a pressure bandage over the bite site and on as much of the affected limb as possible.
- Immobilize the affected limb, using a splint if possible.
- Both pressure and immobilization are required.
- Reassure patient and arrange transport to nearest hospital without delay.
- Advise hospital of the impending arrival; maintain contact with hospital while transporting the patient.
- If paralysis occurs rapidly and breathing becomes labored or ceases, try mouth-to-mouth resuscitation.
- If blood pressure falls (patient feels faint or loses consciousness) elevate legs.
- Keep airway clear of secretions at all times.

And here's what NOT to do if bitten by a venomous snake.

- Do not try to kill or catch the snake for identification
- Do not wash the bite site (surface venom residues can be used in venom detection kits).
- Do not release the pressure bandage (hospital staff will decide when this is appropriate).
- Do not use cold/ice pack.
- Do not give the patient any beverages or food.
- Do not use any medication.
- Do not apply tight, narrow constricting bands.
- Do not use any form of electrical shock treatment.

Cutting into a snakebite is controversial. If you are trained, have the right equipment and are far from medical help, you can incise a snakebite. Treat

for shock and be prepared to give artificial respiration if breathing stops, if you are trained in CPR. Have someone phone ahead to alert the hospital, identifying the type of snake if possible (or take the dead snake with you).

Precautions
When moving through a snake-infested area, hikers should watch the path and never put feet or hands where they can't be seen. If walking through tall grass or bushes, poke the clumps with a stick to warn snakes. Do not reach above your head or put hands into crevices. Since about half of all snake strikes are below the knee, wear heavy, leather, high-top shoes or boots and loose-fitting long pants, with cuffs reaching over the tops of the shoes. When camping, avoid areas near rocks, logs, burrows, or caves. Always wear heavy gloves when cleaning up debris—especially logs or old lumber, and use a crowbar to move them.

Snakes are more dangerous during early spring; they've been storing venom and the poison glands are full. If a snake is spotted, back away from it for at least two to three feet. Snakes can strike about half their body length (and most are less than five feet long).

See also ADDER; ADDER, COMMON; ADDER, PUFF; BLACK SNAKE, AUSTRALIAN; BOOMSLANG; BROWN SNAKE; BUSHMASTER; CORAL SNAKE; CORAL SNAKE, ARIZONA; CORAL SNAKE, EASTERN; HABU, OKINAWA; KRAIT, BLUE; MAMBAS; MASSASAUGA; PIT VIPERS; RATTLESNAKE, CASCABEL; RATTLESNAKE, EASTERN DIAMONDBACK; RATTLESNAKE, MEXICAN WEST COAST, RATTLESNAKE, RED DIAMONDBACK; RATTLESNAKE, TIMBER; RATTLESNAKE, WESTERN DIAMONDBACK; RATTLESNAKES; SIDEWINDER; SMOOTH-SCALED SNAKE; VIPER, GABOON; VIPER, JUMPING; VIPER, MALAYAN PIT; VIPER, RUSSEL'S; VIPER, SAWSCALED; WATER MOCCASIN; WUTU.

sodium bicarbonate This buffering agent is used in the treatment of poisoning by methanol, ethylene glycol, or salicylate. It counteracts metabolic acidosis and enhances the elimination of salicylate or phenobarbital. It also helps to treat heart problems resulting from overdoses of cyclic antidepressants and some antiarrhythmic drugs. Used in gastric lavage solution, it can be helpful in the treatment of excessive iron ingestion.

sodium carbonate   See ALKALINE CORROSIVES.

sodium fluoroacetate   See COMPOUND 1080.

sodium hydroxide   See LYE.

sodium hypochlorite   The most common form of the active ingredient in bleach.
    See also ALKALINE CORROSIVES.

sodium phosphate   See ALKALINE CORROSIVES.

solanine   See POTATO.

solvent abuse   Certain volatile liquids give off intoxicating fumes that, when sniffed, produce an effect similar to getting "high" on drugs or alcohol. Glue sniffing is the most common form of solvent abuse, but many other substances are used (especially those containing toluene or acetone).
    The solvent is usually sniffed from a plastic bag containing the solvent, although sometimes aerosols are sprayed into the nose or mouth. The practice is often a group activity that usually lasts only for a few months at a time. However, solitary abuse is much more serious and may last for a much longer period of time.

Symptoms
Inhaling solvent fumes may cause hallucinations; chronic abuse may cause headache, vomiting, stupor, confusion, and coma. Death may occur as the result of a direct toxic effect on the heart, from a fall, choking on vomit, or asphyxiation due to the clinging bag around the nose and mouth. Other, long-term effects include damage to the membrane lining of the nose and throat, the kidneys, the liver, and the nervous system. The signs of solvent abuse

include intoxicated behavior, flushed face, mouth ulcers, solvent smell, and personality changes.

Treatment
Maintain airway, administer supplemental oxygen, and monitor blood gases and chest X-rays. Treat symptoms of coughing and coma and bronchospasm if they occur. Avoid the use of epinephrine because of the risk of aggravating arrhythmias.
    See also TRICHLOROETHANE; TRICHLOROETHYLENE.

South American rattlesnake   See RATTLESNAKE, CASCABEL.

spathiphyllum *(Spathiphyllum)*   Also known as the peace plant, this is an extremely common indoor potted plant popular as a commercial indoor landscape plant because of its limited light requirements. These plants, which can reach about two feet in height, produce a single white or greenish flower with a white spadix resembling a small ear of corn.

Poisonous part
All parts of this plant are toxic and contain water-insoluble raphides of calcium oxalate.

Symptoms
Upon ingestion, burning, swelling, and pain of the lips, mouth, tongue, and pharynx; because of this immediate pain, large amounts of this plant are not usually eaten. Contact dermatitis may be caused by the root juices.

Treatment
Cool liquids, including milk, held in the mouth and analgesics may ease the pain.
    See also OXALATES.

spiders, poisonous   Although most of the more than 50,000 species of spiders found in the United States actually possess poison glands connected to their fangs, only a very few are capable of piercing human skin. Those that can include the black widow *(Latrodectus)*, the brown recluse spider *(Loxosceles)*, the jumping spider *(Phidippus)*, and the tarantula (a common name given to many large spiders).

In general, most spider attacks occur when someone disturbs a spider's nest while working outdoors or making house repairs.

See also BLACK WIDOW SPIDER; BROWN RECLUSE SPIDER; TARANTULA.

spindle tree *(Euonymus europaeus)* This small tree has branches close to the ground and thin gray bark, looking very similar to its close cousin burning bush *(E. atropurpureus)*, except that its flowers are yellow-green. Introduced from Europe, this tree spread from cultivation in Massachusetts to Wisconsin and south.

Poisonous part

The leaves, seeds, and bark of this tree contain the cardiac glycoside evomonoside, similar to digitalis; a group of alkaloids, including evonine, that have not been evaluated; and a protein that inhibits protein synthesis in intact cells.

Symptoms

Within 10 to 12 hours, ingestion results in symptoms similar to those of meningitis: watery, bloody diarrhea; colic; vomiting; fever and convulsions; and liver damage that can be fatal within eight hours.

Treatment

Recommendation for treatment is difficult, since the underlying toxin is unknown. Replace fluids and electrolytes.

See also CARDIAC GLYCOSIDES.

spurge nettle *(Cnidolscolus stimulosus)* A perennial herb that is native to southeastern North America and also found in Europe and Asia. Spurge nettle, which is also known as "tread-softly," is covered with stinging hairs. It inflicts a painful sting on contact with the skin and can be poisonous to some people.

Poisonous part

Its toxin includes toxalbumins and cathartic oils. It can also cause skin reactions.

Symptoms

Contact produces instant, intense stinging and itching because of an irritating substance injected into the skin by the plant's stinging hairs, and causes a skin rash that disappears in about 30 minutes. A dull purple stain on the skin may linger for several weeks.

Treatment

Symptomatic.

squill *(Scilla)* **[Other names: Cuban lily, hyacinth-of-Peru, sea onion, star hyacinth.]** This hyacinth look-alike is found as a hardy perennial in the north temperate zones to southern Canada. It is often grown for its attractive blue, purple, or white flowers.

Poisonous part

The whole squill plant is poisonous and contains digitalislike glycosides.

Symptoms

There is a variable latency period between ingestion and symptoms, depending on the amount of the plant eaten. When they appear, symptoms include pain in the mouth, lips, tongue, and throat, nausea and vomiting, abdominal pain, cramps and diarrhea, hyperkalemia, and heart disturbances.

Treatment

Gastric lavage followed by the administration of activated charcoal and saline cathartics. Monitoring of potassium levels and electrocardiogram should be performed. In the event of heart problems: administration of atropine for conduction defects; phenytoin for rhythm disturbances.

See also DIGITALIS.

staphylococcus enterotoxin One of the most common types of food poisoning in the United States, affecting almost everyone at least once. Although the bacteria are easily destroyed by high heat during cooking, they also produce a heat-resistant toxin. It is believed that only a few strains of staphylococci produce enterotoxins, which may occur in a wide variety of foods (such as milk, cheese, ice cream, cream-filled bakery goods, dried beef, sausage, or chicken gravy). Poisoning with this type of bacteria most often occurs after eating food that has been kept warm for several hours before being served. In addition, food may be contaminated from infected food handlers.

Staphylococcus enterotoxin may be suspected when there has been only a brief interval between eating suspected tainted food and the onset of symptoms. It can be confimed by bacteriological examination for the presence of staphylococci; enterotoxin may also be produced by staphylococci in persons treated with broad-spectrum antibiotics.

The best way to prevent this type of food poisoning is to refrigerate perishable foods adequately. While heat does destroy the bacteria, it does not destroy the enterotoxin.

Symptoms

Symptoms usually appear within three hours of eating the tainted food; the incubation period depends on the amount of food eaten and the susceptibility of the consumer. (The aged, immunocompromised, and the very young are the most vulnerable.) Symptoms begin with salivation, followed by nausea, vomiting, abdominal cramps, prostration, and diarrhea; in severe poisoning, victims experience marked prostration together with vomiting, diarrhea, and sometimes, shock. Symptoms usually fade after five to six hours, although a few fatal cases have been reported among vulnerable populations.

Treatment

Significant loss of fluids and disruption of electrolyte balance may require parenteral administration of fluids and electrolytes; treatment for shock may be required following significant loss of fluids.

star of Bethlehem (Ornithogalum umbellatum; "wonder flower"—O. thyrosides) [Other names: African wonder flower, chincherinchee, dove's dung, nap at noon, summer snowflake, wonder flower.]   Found in warm climates, the flower of the Bible has creamy white, starlike flowers on upright slender stems that may reach two feet in height, and long, narrow leaves with onionlike bulbs. Found primarily in the Middle East, both species are also kept indoors and sold by florists as a cut flower. O. umbellatum has been naturalized in the southeastern United States, in Mississippi, Missouri, Kansas, and eastward.

Poisonous part

All parts of the star of Bethlehem plant are toxic, especially the onionlike bulb; the poisons are convallatoxin and convalloside (the same as lily of the valley) plus cardiac glycosides.

Symptoms

Immediately after ingestion, symptoms begin: shortness of breath, irritation of the mouth and throat, nausea, vomiting, abdominal pain, diarrhea, and respiratory problems. Fatalities have been reported from ingesting this plant.

Treatment

Gastric lavage and treatment of symptoms, followed by the administration of activated charcoal and saline cathartics. Electrocardiogram and potassium levels should be monitored repeatedly.

See also CARDIAC GLYCOSIDES; LILY OF THE VALLEY.

star-potato vine (Solanum seaforthianum)   Sometimes called the Brazilian nightshade, this South American plant is also cultivated in warmer areas in Florida and Hawaii. It is a member of a very large genus with 1,700 species, most of which have not been evaluated toxicologically.

Poisonous part

Human poisoning is usually attributed to immature fruit, which contains the toxin solanine glycoalkaloid.

Symptoms

While there is little danger of fatal poisoning in adults, children may ingest a fatal amount of this plant. Symptoms appear several hours after ingestion and include gastric irritation, scratchy throat, fever, and diarrhea (solanine poisoning is often confused with bacterial gastroenteritis).

Treatment

The same general supportive care that would be given in gastroenteritis cases; fluid replacement may be required.

Stelazine (trifluroperazine) This is one of the psychometric drugs used to treat psychotic anxiety and agitated depression. It is available as a tablet, liquid, or injection and works by depressing the central nervous system.

Symptoms

Within 20 minutes after an overdose, Stelazine causes agitation, convulsions, fever, low blood pressure, coma, and cardiac arrest.

Treatment

Do not induce vomiting; perform gastric lavage and administer Cogentin; treat other symptoms as they appear.

See also ANTIDEPRESSANTS.

stingray (*Urobatis halleri, Dasyatis longus,* etc.)
More than 1,500 cases of stingray attacks are reported in the United States each year, usually caused when a swimmer inadvertently steps on a stingray buried in the mud or sand. The *Dasyatis* stingrays are particularly noted for burying themselves in the mud or sand. When trod upon, the stingray flings its tail up and forward, burying the stinger in the victim's foot.

A stingray will never attack humans—fleeing if approached—unless it perceives itself under attack. When threatened, it can whip its tail around until it finds its attacker. It is possible to drive away stingrays by shuffling the feet in murky water.

Stingrays are found throughout the world and include the diamond, butterfly, European, eagle, California, and South American freshwater stingray. All large varieties found in freshwater are dangerous. Many stingrays do not travel far from their own area, seeming to display a sense of territory.

Poisonous part

The fearsome whiplike tail of the stingray is longer than its body, and near the base of its tail it has one, two, or three flattened barbed spines with small, sharp teeth connected to a poison sac; the barbs point backward, making it difficult to remove the barb after penetration. The tail is coated with venomous slime that can cause serious injury or even death to humans. Often, the entire stinger is left embedded in the wound, and pulling it out may further damage surrounding skin. When the spine stabs into the skin, it tears the sheath around the spine, which releases the venom, producing a violent reaction in the skin tissue. Some varieties of stingrays can inflict such a deep wound that they can transmit the tetanus bacilli, causing tetanus in their victims. The stingray venom is one of the most powerful vasoconstrictors among all the animal toxins and is markedly unstable. It has caused coronary vessel and resultant heart damage in animal experiments.

Symptoms

While death is rare, the sting of the stingray causes an immediate severe stinging or throbbing pain, which may stay at the site of the wound or spread throughout the body and last for several hours or days. Most stingray wounds are found on the ankle or foot and may be more of a laceration than a wound. There may be redness and swelling at the site of the sting, and the area may become numb, followed by dizziness, weakness, cramps, sweating, and falling blood pressure. Fatalities have been reported when the barb enters the chest or abdomen, but they are rare.

Treatment

There is no known antidote. Contact medical help immediately; flush the wound with salt water and then soak the affected area in hot water for one hour. The water should be very hot (122°F), so that the heat will deactivate the poison and also ease pain. Pain medication may be administered, and lacerations are surgically closed. Generally, victims recover within 48 hours, although hospitalization may be needed for those with persistent symptoms of chest pain, irregular pulse, or hypotension. Victims who have been stung on the chest or abdomen may require exploratory surgery. Tetanus shots and antibiotics are also necessary.

stonefish *(Synanceja horrida)* One of the world's most virulent animals, this large, unattractive fish gets its name from its resemblance to a piece of dead coral. It is found in coral reefs and mud flats in the Indo-Pacific and the waters around China, the Philippines, and Australia. Closely related to the scorpion fish and several other poisonous fish of the Scorpaenidae family, the stonefish has well-developed jagged spines and venom glands along its back that can penetrate a flipper or thin canvas shoe. This rough covering allows it to envelope itself in slime, coral debris and algae, camouflaging itself and increasing its chances of being stepped on. Stonefish are most often found in the Australian waters, where they have reportedly killed swimmers within hours of being stepped on.

Poisonous part

Symptoms are due primarily to stonustoxin, which produces immediate and extreme pain that spreads to the trunk of the body. Other systemic effects are due to potent myotoxins that act directly on all types of muscles. Death results from respiratory failure and usually occurs within hours.

Symptoms

The sting from the back fin spines of the stonefish is extremely painful, causing swelling, discoloration, loss of consciousness, and paralysis. The pain can be so severe that it may cause the victim to scream in agony. Victims who survive the first 24 hours usually will not die.

Treatment

Stonefish antivenin is available but difficult to find in remote areas. Otherwise, treatment is symptomatic and supportive. Irrigation and bleeding of the wound (to remove venom) should be followed by cleansing. Immerse the wound in hot water for one hour to deactivate the venom; administration of tetanus antitoxin and antibiotics is advised. Some researchers recommend the administration of emetine hydrochloride to alleviate pain and neutralize stonefish venom. Emetine is injected directly into the wound after the administration of a local anesthetic. Stonefish antivenin may also be used in other scorpion fish stings.

See also SCORPION FISH.

Streunex See BENZENE HEXACHLORIDE.

strychnine This bitter-tasting, colorless, crystalline powder is an extremely deadly chemical found in the seeds of a species of tropical plants called *Strychnos*. Strychnine is normally used as a rat poison; its bitter taste and scarcity on store shelves, however, make poisoning from this substance a rare occurrence. Still, when it occurs, strychnine poisoning causes some of the most dramatic symptoms of any toxic substance; its explosive convulsions are responsible for its frequent use in literature and film. A victim can be poisoned by strychnine either by swallowing it, by absorbing it through the skin, by eye contact, or by inhaling the dust. In the past it was used therapeutically as a tonic and general stimulant. Strychnine is found naturally in some seeds and plants, principally the tropical nux-vomica tree.

Symptoms

Strychnine attacks the central nervous system within 10 to 20 minutes, causing all the muscles to contract simultaneously, beginning with the victim's neck and face, and can be fatal if untreated. Arms and legs begin to spasm next, and the spasms become worse and worse until the victim's back arches almost continuously. The slightest sound or movement will bring on a fresh spate of spasms, and the strychnine victim dies from asphyxiation or exhaustion as a result of the spasms. Rigor mortis begins immediately, freezing the body in a spasm with the eyes wide open. The effects of strychnine are almost identical to those of tetanus.

Treatment

If treatment is begun before symptoms appear or after spasms have been controlled, physicians can pump the stomach and administer activated charcoal. Primary emphasis in treatment is to maintain breathing and to control spasms with a slow intravenous drip of succinylcholine or Valium (DIAZEPAM). The victim may also be placed on a ventilator. The victim should be kept quiet during spasms, since any noise or light will worsen the symptoms. With prompt medical attention, victims will recover within 24 hours.

See also NUX-VOMICA; RAT POISON.

succinylcholine See NEUROMUSCULAR BLOCKING AGENTS.

sulfites Any of several sulfur-based preservatives added to food to retard spoilage and discoloration. Sulfites are added to food to prevent browning of freshly cut fruits and vegetables when exposed to air, to control the growth of bacteria and molds, to prevent the breakdown of various oils that would lead to "off" flavors and to whiten potatoes.

It is impossible to tell by inspection or smell whether or not a food contains sulfites, but they are used in a wide variety of foods. Those that have some of the highest levels include dried fruits, dehydrated vegetables, and wine. Other foods that may contain sulfites are baked goods and mixes, alcoholic and nonalcoholic beverages, coffee and tea, condiments and relishes, dairy product substitutes, fresh and prepared fish and shellfish, fresh and processed fruits and fruit juices, fresh and processed vegetables and vegetable juices, gelatins, grain products, gravies and sauces, jams and jellies, nuts and their products, snack foods, soups and mixes, sugar and sweet sauces, toppings, and syrups. This does not mean, however, that all foods within these categories necessarily contain sulfites.

Sulfites are also used to preserve some prescription medications and drugs that are given intravenously; sensitive patients may react to either of these applications. Wine always contains sulfites because the yeasts that ferment the grapes unavoidably produce them.

All packaged foods now require labels that indicate the presence of sulfites, even if they are naturally present in detectable quantities. The chemical's GRAS (generally recognized as safe) rating was removed by the Food and Drug Administration in 1987. Foods sold in bulk, or served in restaurants, are not allowed to contain detectable levels of sulfites. (See Appendix A for a home kit.)

Symptoms

Sensitive individuals (especially asthmatics) experience a range of symptoms usually involving the respiratory system, ranging from mild to severe—even life threatening. These symptoms include narrowing of the airways, wheezing, breathing problems, nausea, stomach cramps, diarrhea, hives, itching, swelling, tingling, flushing, low blood pressure, blue tinge to the skin, shock, and loss of consciousness. It is estimated that as many as 10 percent of asthmatics may be sensitive to sulfites—especially those who take steroids for their condition. In addition, nonasthmatics can experience reactions as well. Chronic exposure to sulfites has not been shown to cause side effects or cancer.

Treatment

Supportive and symptomatic.

superantigens Proteins that cause food poisoning and toxic shock by whipping the immune system into a destructive frenzy. Normally, when a person's immune system encounters a virus, only about one in 10,000 of the disease-fighting T lymphocytes react. These lymphocytes target the alien virus or protein, called an "antigen," and kill it. But some of these antigens, called superantigens, arouse not just a few lymphocytes but as many as one in every five, which can launch an autoimmune attack and actually hurt the individual they should protect. And sometimes, superantigens can trigger the death of the lymphocytes, punching holes in the body's immune system.

surgeonfish A fish of tropical waters that is poisonous at certain times of the year because of contamination with poisonous dinoflagellates (plankton) often found in red tide. In addition, its sting causes severe pain.

Symptoms

The sting of the surgeonfish causes an immediate severe stinging or throbbing pain, which may stay at the site of the wound or spread throughout the body and last for several hours or days. There may be redness and swelling at the site of the sting, and the area may become numb. Death is rare.

Treatment

Contact medical help immediately; flush the wound with fresh- or salt water, and then soak the affected area in hot water or put hot compresses on it. The water should be very hot (122°F) in order to deactivate the poison. Continue applying hot water for 30 minutes to an hour.

See also DINOFLAGELLATE; FISH CONTAMINATION.

sushi   The popular Japanese dish made of raw fish that can cause a type of food poisoning. Raw fish may be tainted with a parasitic worm, *Anisakis simplex,* that infests small crustaceans on which many kinds of fish feed.

Symptoms

Gastrointestinal distress with abdominal pain, nausea, and vomiting.

Treatment

Symptomatic.

sweeteners, artificial   Synthetic compounds created to sweeten food, beverages, and medications and which provide no calories. The six artificial sweeteners currently approved by the Food and Drug Administration (FDA) include acesulfame potassium (Sunett), aspartame (Equal), D-Tagatose (Sugaree), neotame, saccharin (Sweet 'N Low), and sucralose (Splenda). These artificial sweeteners are 200 to 13,000 times sweeter than natural sugar. Sodium and calcium cyclamates were removed from the list of substances recognized as safe in food and beverages in October 1969 because of their carcinogenic effect on animals.

Although the United States originally banned saccharin on March 9, 1977, because it causes bladder cancer in laboratory animals, it was later determined that the mechanism responsible for the development of cancer did not apply to humans but only to rats. Therefore saccharin was allowed to re-enter the market in 2000. It can be found in many packaged foods and nearly all toothpastes in the United States. Aspartame was approved in 1981 as a general sweetener. It was followed by acesulfame potassium, which was approved for specific foods in 1988 and for general purposes in 2002; sucralose, which received tabletop sweetener approval in 1998 and general purpose approval in 1999; neotame, approved for general purposes in 2002; and D-tagatose, as a food additive in 2003.

Symptoms

Ingestion of very large amounts can produce symptoms that include vomiting, diarrhea, abdominal pain, frothing at the mouth, muscle spasms, convulsions, and stupor.

Treatment

If large doses of saccharin were ingested, perform gastric lavage or induce vomiting followed by the administration of a saline cathartic; aspartame overdose requires only supportive symptomatic treatment.

swimming pool disinfectants   Almost all of these products, used for keeping in-ground swimming pools free of contaminants, can be fire hazards and can cause gastric complaints if ingested. Most contain more than 70 percent calcium hypochlorite (70 percent available chlorine), which is a strong oxidant; exposure to high heat or contact with a range of household materials (such as mineral oils, kerosene, turpentine, lubricants, tobacco, etc.) can be a fire hazard.

Symptoms

Ingestion causes severe gastric symptoms; skin contact can result in a local dermatitis. Inhaling the fumes from decomposition is very irritating to eyes and lungs.

Treatment

If ingested, perform gastric lavage or induce vomiting. If eyes or skin have been contaminated, wash thoroughly with tap water immediately.

synthetic organic insecticides   Compounds include chlorobenzene derivatives such as DDT (dichlorodiphenyltrichloroethane), banned since 1973; TDE (tetrachlorodiphenylethane); DFDT (difluorodiphenyltrichloroethane); dimite dichlorodiphenylethanol; DMC (dichorodiphenyl methyl carbinol); methoxychlor; neotrane; ovotran; dilan. Also, indane derivatives, including chlordane (banned 1976); heptachlor (banned 1976); aldrin (banned 1974); dieldrin (banned 1974); endrin; kepone (chlordecone). Also, lindane (cyclohexane hexachloride) and toxaphene (chlorinated camphene). Finally, the phosphate esters, which include chlorothion; diazinon; DFP (diisopropyl-fluorophosphate); EPN; leptophos; malathion; metacide; OMPA (octamethylpyrophosphoramide); para-oxon; parathion; potosan; systox; TEPP (tetraethyl pyrophosphate); and thio-TEPP.

See also BOTANIC INSECTICIDES; INSECTICIDES; ORGANOPHOSPHATE INSECTICIDES.

Tagamet See CIMETIDINE.

taipan *(Oxyuranus scutellatus)* One of the world's deadliest snakes, the taipan is the largest cobra found in Australia and can grow to almost 13 feet. Brown on its back with a yellow underbelly, the nonhooded snake has extremely long fangs whose venom is so poisonous that it is fatal in a few moments. However, the number of fatalities is not too high, since the species is rare and lives in fairly undisturbed parts of northeast Australia.

Until 1976, the smooth-scaled, or fierce, snake *(Parademansia microlepidotus)* was considered to be a Western form of the taipan, but its venom is significantly different from that of the latter.

Symptoms

Within 15 to 30 minutes symptoms appear: pain and swelling, a drop in blood pressure and confusion, slurring of speech, dilation of the pupils, strabismus (eye irregularities), drooping of the upper eyelids, and muscle weakness. The respiratory muscles are affected last, and respiratory muscle paralysis is the most common cause of death.

Treatment

Antiserum is available.

See also ADDER, DEATH; ANTIVENIN; BROWN SNAKE; COBRA; COBRA, SPITTING; COPPERHEAD, AUSTRALIAN; CORAL SNAKE; SNAKES, POISONOUS; TIGER SNAKE.

tansy *(Tanacetum vulgare)* This common perennial herb was once a popular plant in a witch's arsenal during the Middle Ages. It gets its name from the Greek word *athanasia,* meaning "immortality"—it was the main ingredient in a potion designed to give immortality to Ganymede, a handsome Greek boy who became the eternal cupbearer for Zeus. Tansy may have gotten its reputation for immortal powers because its flowers do not easily wilt or because it was often placed in coffins as an insect repellent.

Today it is considered to be a weed in many places throughout the eastern United States and Pacific Northwest, growing wild in pastures and fields, along roadsides and in waste areas. Introduced into America from the Old World, it has pretty, flat yellow or white flowers that bloom from July through September; they are often used decoratively and look very much like yarrow. The plant grows to three feet, with dark green, fernlike leaves, and spreads in an ever-widening mass through underground runners. When crushed, its flowers and leaves smell faintly of pine.

Native to Europe, tansy has been naturalized in North America from Nova Scotia and Ontario to Minnesota, Missouri, and North Carolina, as well as in Oregon and Nevada.

The bitter oil of tansy has been used homeopathically to bring on menstruation, as an abortifacient by the American Indians and also as a treatment against intestinal worms.

Poisonous part

The leaves, flowers, and stem contain the toxic oil tanacetin. Poisoning often occurs after drinking too much tea or taking too much oil for medicinal reasons. The leaves also contain thujone in amounts that vary from plant to plant; thujone is a relatively toxic substance also found in wormwood.

Symptoms

Touching the plant can cause dermatitis. Within several hours after ingestion, symptoms appear, including frothing at the mouth, rapid and weak pulse, kidney problems, violent spasms, and convulsions followed by death.

Treatment

Perform gastric lavage and give symptomatic treatment.

See also HERBS, UNSAFE.

tarantula A common name given to many large, hairy spiders. The sight of one of these monsters might be enough to induce hysteria, but in fact tarantulas are fairly harmless. They are usually found in the Southwest, although they are also present in many other areas in the United States. While tarantulas do have venom, it is very mild and almost never causes a problem in humans, although sometimes an allergic response can occur. Captive tarantulas seldom try to bite. More and more popular in this country as pets, they are also sometimes used by jewelry stores to patrol window displays.

In the early days of the Old West, tarantulas were deeply feared, and their bite was believed to be fatal; it was thought that the only cure was whiskey, or "tarantula justice." True tarantulas (*Lycosa narbonensis*) originated in Europe, where they also have an unfounded reputation for being lethal. In fact, the superstition about the danger of a tarantula's bite originated in the Dark Ages when fears arose about the wolf spider (*Lycosa tarantula*).

During the Middle Ages in the town of Taranto, Italy, people claiming to have been bitten by this spider were seized with a dancing frenzy, born of the idea that the bite would be fatal if the victim did not dance hard and long enough to sweat the poison out of the system. The dance and the music to which it was performed were called "tarantellas" after the spider. The whole episode evolved into a popular fad involving a mass delusion—that these spiders bit people intentionally and that the venom was fatal.

In truth, the European spider is no more venomous and no more likely to bite than its American wolf spider relative. Still, historians are not sure what started the outbreak of biting and dancing.

One theory suggests that the dances, which were community affairs rather than individual performances, were actually pagan religious festivals masquerading as medical procedures to fool the clergy.

Symptoms

Although tarantulas rarely cause serious poisonings, their bite produces a painful skin reaction, with itching, swelling, redness and, on rare occasions, soreness and fever for several days. The pain from the bite results from the puncture wound of the fangs, not from any toxin, which is comparatively mild and intended to paralyze animals smaller than the tarantula itself. Of course, it is still possible to sustain an allergic reaction, in much the same way that some people are overly sensitive to a bee sting. Even more common is an allergy to tarantula hairs, which can cause a rash on some people. These hairs are used by the spider as a defense; when irritated, the tarantulas comb the hairs off their abdomens with their hind legs and throw them at the enemy. These flying hairs can actually divert an attack of a lizard or mouse if they land in the attacker's nose or eyes.

Treatment

Wash the wound and treat if infection occurs; give tetanus shot if necessary.

See also SPIDERS, POISONOUS.

taxine A plant alkaloid found in the common yew (*Taxus*) that can cause irregular or slow heartbeat and heart failure, and respiratory problems or failure. Ingestion of taxine can lead quickly to coma and death.

See also ALKALOIDS; YEW.

tear gas The most commonly used tear gases are chloroacetophenone (CN), ethylbromoacetate, bromoacetone, bromomethylethylketone, and ortho-chlorobenzylidene malononitril (CS). Tear gases can cause extreme irritation and swelling of the mucous membranes of the nose and eyes if discharged into the face and can even cause a temporary blindness.

It is usually expelled as a vapor that condenses to liquid droplets that are intensely irritating.

Symptoms

Exposure causes severe tearing and sneezing, chest tightness, coughing, nausea, and vomiting.

Treatment

Remove victim to fresh air—separate from other sufferers—face into the wind with eyes open, and have him or her breathe deeply. Tear gas should be washed off the skin with soap and water; eyes should be washed with saline or water. Thoroughly decontaminate the victim, including clothing, by washing with soap and water.

TEPP (tetraethylpyrophosphate) A highly toxic insecticide derived from phosphoric acid, TEPP is a colorless liquid with an agreeable odor that can be inhaled, absorbed through unbroken skin, or ingested. It is poisonous in all cases.

Symptoms

This central nervous system poison causes symptoms to appear within 15 minutes to four hours, including vision problems, headache, loss of depth perception, cramps, sweating, chest pain, cyanosis, anorexia, vomiting and diarrhea, paralysis, convulsions, low blood pressure, and death. Skin absorption irreversibly inhibits nerve signals.

Treatment

Administration of extremely large doses of atropine, plus treatment of symptoms.

See also ORGANOPHOSPHATE INSECTICIDES.

teratogen Any toxic substance (such as aspirin and caffeine) that can cause birth defects; teratogenicity is the ability to cause birth defects.

tetrachloroethane This industrial solvent is the most toxic of all the chlorinated hydrocarbons. It causes prolonged narcosis, liver damage, and severe toxic hepatitis, with acute yellow atrophy of the liver.

Symptoms

Contact causes irritation of the eyes, skin, and mucous membranes; inhalation causes cough, salivation, perspiration, confusion, vertigo and intoxication, with headache, excitement, weakness, nausea and vomiting, weak pulse, and stupor. Ingestion causes severe gastrointestinal irritation with abdominal cramps, diarrhea, and bloody stool. There may be kidney and liver damage.

Treatment

Remove victim from exposure immediately and maintain breathing. Induce vomiting or perform gastric lavage if ingested, and follow with a saline cathartic. For skin or eye contact, wash with water (using soap for skin) and remove contaminated clothing. Hemodialysis for kidney problems may reverse damage.

See also CHLORINATED HYDROCARBON PESTICIDES.

tetrodotoxin Toxin produced in the skin of pufferfish, California newts, sunfish, porcupine fish and some South American frogs that is similar to saxitoxin and interferes with the transfer of salt and neuronal transmission in muscles. Three cases of tetrodotoxin poisoning occurred among California chefs who shared contaminated fugu (pufferfish) brought from Japan by a coworker as a prepackaged, ready-to-eat product in 1996. None of the victims ate very much (only between ¼ to 1½ oz.), and symptoms began between three and 20 minutes after eating the fugu.

The chef who brought the fugu from Japan failed to declare this item through customs. The remaining fugu was obtained for toxin analysis at the Food and Drug Administration (FDA). Although individuals cannot bring fugu into the United States, the FDA has permitted fugu to be imported and served in Japanese restaurants by certified fugu chefs on special occasions. A cooperative agreement with the Japanese Ministry of Health and Welfare ensures fugu is properly processed and certified safe for consumption before export by the government of Japan.

If cleaned and dressed properly, the fugu flesh or musculature is edible and considered a delicacy by some people in Japan, who may pay the equivalent of $400 or more for one meal. Despite careful preparation, fugu remains a common cause of fatal food poisoning in Japan, accounting for approximately 50 deaths annually.

The order Tetraodontoidea includes ocean sunfishes, porcupine fishes and fugu, which are among the most poisonous of all marine creatures. These species inhabit the shallow waters of the temperate and tropical zones and can be exported from China, Japan, Mexico, the Philippines, and Taiwan. The liver, gonads, intestines, and skin of these fish contain tetrodotoxin, a powerful neurotoxin that can be fatal in about 60 percent of those who eat it. Other animals (such as the California newt and the eastern salamander) also possess tetrodotoxin in lethal quantities.

Symptoms

Paresthesias begin 10 to 45 minutes after ingestion, usually as tingling of the tongue and inner surface of the mouth. Other common symptoms include vomiting, lightheadedness, dizziness, feelings of doom, and weakness. An ascending paralysis develops, and death can occur within six to 24 hours, secondary to respiratory muscle paralysis. Other signs include salivation, muscle twitching, chest pain, and convulsions. Severe poisoning is indicated by low blood pressure, slow heartbeat, depressed corneal reflexes, and fixed dilated pupils.

Diagnosis

Tetrodotoxin poisoning is based on clinical symptoms and a history of ingestion.

Treatment

There is no antidote to tetrodotoxin, and there is great controversy over the relative benefits of the administration of atropine, edrophonium, or pyridostigmine. Otherwise, treatment is supportive. Replace fluid and electrolytes; induce vomiting or perform gastric lavage if ingestion occurred within the preceding hour.

See also FISH CONTAMINATION; PUFFERFISH; SAXITOXIN.

thallium This soft metal is a minor constituent in ores and is commonly found in flue dusts; thallium salts are used in industry and chemical analysis, including the manufacture of optical lenses, photoelectric cells, and costume jewelry.

As a rodenticide, it is a tasteless, odorless inorganic chemical pesticide banned for household use in the United States since 1965. However, poison control centers still report cases of thallium poisoning, primarily from old products still found on home and store shelves. Before it was banned for such use, thallium was contained in a wide range of pesticide products designed to control roaches, ants, silverfish, water bugs, moles, mice, and rats. Poisoning most often occurs by accidentally ingesting rat or ant bait; chronic poisoning can also occur from skin absorption.

The minimum lethal dose of thallium salts is between 12 and 15 milligrams per kilogram, although its toxicity varies depending on the compound. There are reports of fatalities following adult ingestion of as little as 200 mg, and only one ounce of a 1 percent concentration can kill a 55-pound child.

Symptoms

Thallium acts by breaking down all cells in the body, especially hair follicles and the central nervous system. From one to three weeks after ingestion, hair begins to fall out, followed by pain in the extremities, fever, conjunctivitis, abdominal pain and nausea, bloody diarrhea, lethargy, tremors, convulsions, and cyanosis. In severe poisonings, pulmonary edema and pneumonia may be followed by death from respiratory failure. There may also be organic brain damage, causing personality changes, anxiety or depression, and even psychotic behavior.

Treatment

There is no recommended specific treatment in the United States. Prussian blue is believed to enhance removal of thallium from tissues and increases kidney and fecal elimination, but it is not available for use in the United States. Activated charcoal is probably just as good at enhancing fecal elimination. Induce vomiting or perform gastric lavage, followed by the administration of activated charcoal for at least five days with potassium chloride, plus symptomatic treatment. For skin contamination, all thallium should be washed off the skin with soap and water.

See also RAT POISON.

theophylline This potent bronchodilator has been widely used in the treatment of asthma and to prevent attacks of apnea (cessation of breathing) in premature infants for the past 70 years. The drug is also used to treat heart failure, since it stimulates heart rate. It is used less frequently today because newer drugs with fewer side effects are now available. Most common brands include Theo-Dur and Slo-Phyllin. Other brands include Theo-24, Uniphyl, and Uni-dor.

Poisoning by theophylline may either be chronic or acute, with different symptoms in each case.

Symptoms

Poisoning by an acute single dose is usually the result of a suicide attempt or accidental child poisoning, although it may be caused by an accidental therapeutic overdose. In these cases, symptoms include vomiting, tremors, anxiety, and rapid heartbeat, with high blood sugar and metabolic acidosis. With severe overdose, there may be irregular heartbeat and seizures that may not appear until 12 or 16 hours following ingestion.

Chronic poisoning occurs when excessive doses are given over at least a 24-hour period, or when another drug interferes with its metabolism. Victims of chronic poisoning are usually the very old and the very young. Symptoms include vomiting and rapid heart rate without accompanying metabolic effects. Seizures are common in higher doses.

Treatment

Treat symptoms and monitor vital signs and electrocardiogram. Give activated charcoal repeatedly.

thermometers Despite frequent calls to poison control centers by desperate parents whose child has broken a thermometer and swallowed the mercury, this type of accident actually represents very little danger. Ingestion of the free metal from the thermometer does no harm, since in this state mercury is not absorbed from the gastrointestinal tract. Still, parents may wish to rinse the child's mouth with water.

Provided that the child has not cut the lip from the glass, has no embedded glass in the mouth or throat, and can freely breathe and swallow, the glass should not pose a threat to the child's health, either.

Likewise, outdoor thermometers (which contain only small amounts of xylene, toluene, alcohol, or other chemicals) are harmless.

It is important to clean up mercury spills. A filter tip from a cigarette may be helpful. After the mercury is removed, wash the area with a phosphate detergent.

See also MERCURY.

thiamine (vitamin B$_1$) This B-complex vitamin is used as part of the treatment in persons poisoned with ethylene glycol.

Thorazine (chlorpromazine) This synthetic chemical is derived from phenothiazine and is used primarily to treat manic-depression, although it can also be used to treat hiccups, tetanus, and severe behavior problems in children and adults. It is available as a tablet, syrup, suppository or injection. In April 2005, the Food and Drug Administration notified healthcare professionals that patients with dementia-related psychosis treated with atypical antipsychotic drugs are at an increased risk of death. Since that notification was issued, the FDA reviewed additional information that indicates the risk is also associated with conventional antipsychotics. Antipsychotics are not indicated for the treatment of dementia-related psychosis. Therefore, Thorazine packaging must now include a statement of this increased risk in a boxed warning and in the warnings section of the labeling.

Combining Thorazine with barbiturates, narcotics, or alcohol can be dangerous.

Symptoms

When taken in large doses, Thorazine can cause drowsiness, fainting, low blood pressure, fast heartbeat, tremor, dizziness, electrocardiogram changes, convulsions, and coma. Since Thorazine suppresses the cough reflex, a person can aspirate vomitus while under the influence of this drug. Thorazine has also been linked to "phenothiazine sudden death" among psychiatric patients who take the drug in large doses. Patients who are receiving an overdose will also often exhibit balance problems, slobbering, stuttering, restlessness, hand tremors, and contraction of the face and neck muscles.

Treatment

Perform gastric lavage; treat symptoms, and give fluids to offset severe low blood pressure.

See also ANTIDEPRESSANTS.

thrombolytics   See ANTICOAGULANTS.

tiger snake (Notechis scutatus)   Considered to be the most dangerous snake of southern Australia, this relatively small member of the cobra family has no hood and is colored with yellow and brown bands. It is commonly found in wet areas of Australia and Tasmania. The snake is only about four feet long, and when about to strike, it flattens its head and appears to jump.

Symptoms

Beginning 15 to 30 minutes after a bite, symptoms include pain, swelling, falling blood pressure and convulsions, and, quite often, death, which is caused by respiratory failure. Symptoms resemble poisoning from the deadly nightshade alkaloids. The respiratory muscles are affected last, and respiratory muscle paralysis is the most common cause of death.

Treatment

The specific antivenin should be used.

See also ANTIVENIN; COBRA; SNAKES, POISONOUS.

TNT   See TRINITROLUENE.

toad, bufo   Under stress, all toads of this genus secrete venom contained in glands behind their eyes at the base of the skull. There are many different species of *Bufo* found throughout the world; the biggest one is the marine toad *(Bufo marinus)*, which can grow bigger than a dinner plate. The marine toad originated in South America but has been introduced all over the world because of its penchant for eating rodents and insects. In the United States it is found in southern Florida, where dogs may occasionally bite one. While technically capable of killing a small dog who eats a toad, the bufo has such a terrible taste that dogs immediately spit it out; no cases of canine deaths from bufo poisoning have been reported.

Poisonous part

Toads of the *Bufo* genus have venom containing bufonin, bufogin, and bufotalin compounds (called bufotoxin), whose action is similar to that of digitalis.

Symptoms

Untreated skin contact may cause a generalized skin irritation.

Treatment

Upon skin contact, immediately wash with water and soap. Eye contact may be extremely painful; affected eyes should be washed out with copious amounts of water or saline solution.

tobacco (Nicotiana)   A member of the nightshade family, tobacco is responsible for one of the most widespread narcotic habits in the world and has been used by the Central and South American Indians since prehistoric times. It was popularized in Europe by the French ambassador Jean Nicot de Villemain, who introduced Catherine de Médicis to tobacco chewing.

The plant may be an annual or perennial; if perennial, it usually grows into a large shrub or small tree. Its tubular flowers may be white, yellow, or red, and its fruit contains tiny seeds. *N. tabacum* is the most common species used for smoking tobacco; several species are grown in the United States.

Poisonous part

The whole plant is poisonous, although the most dangerous poisoning results from eating the large, fresh leaves in a salad, using infusions for enemas or absorbing the alkaloid through the skin during harvest. Other ways of obtaining the nicotine are also dangerous, in descending order: chewing without spitting; inhaling the smoke; chewing and spitting; inhaling as snuff; and smoking without inhaling.

In addition, the smoke of tobacco neutralizes 500 milligrams of vitamin C in the body for every pack of cigarettes smoked. Although the specific toxin varies depending on the species, all include nicotine and related alkaloids, including anabasine; nicotine is so potent it is sometimes used as an insecticide. Tobacco is also a botanical cousin to the heart regulator digitalis.

Symptoms
Ingestion can produce anxiety, irritability, confusion, halting speech, dizziness, sleepiness, stupor, nausea, vomiting, appetite loss, tinnitus (ringing in the ears), cough, trembling, heart palpitations, and irregular pulse. Reports in the literature include one death of a child from blowing soap bubbles through a tobacco pipe and another from accidentally swallowing snuff.

Treatment
Gastric lavage followed by administration of activated charcoal.

See also NICOTINE; NICOTINE GUM; NICOTINE PATCH.

toilet cleaners See ALKALINE CORROSIVES.

toxalbumins See PHYTOTOXINS.

toxaphene The chemical name of this synthetic organic pesticide is chlorinated camphene, which can be used as a spray, a wettable powder, or a dust to combat a range of insects, ticks, and mites. This tasteless, pleasant-smelling insecticide is fat soluble but does not dissolve in water.

Symptoms
When accidentally ingested or absorbed into the skin, toxaphene can cause symptoms similar to those caused by DDT, including a range of neurological symptoms and convulsions. Lethal doses result in a series of convulsions followed by anoxia (absence of oxygen supply to tissue) and respiratory failure. While there have been no adverse reports of chronic, low-level cases of poisoning, toxaphene is carcinogenic in animals. Fatal dose is estimated to be five grams per 70 kilograms.

Treatment
Gastric lavage followed by saline, cathartics. Early administration of barbiturates to prevent convulsions. Following the onset of convulsions, administration of faster-acting intravenous barbiturates (even to the point of sedation).

See also DDT; SYNTHETIC ORGANIC INSECTICIDES.

toxin A poisonous substance, especially a protein that is produced by some bacteria, animals, insects, and plants; a toxin is less complex than a poison or a venom but not as identifiable as a chemical compound. Occasionally, bacterial toxins are subdivided into endotoxins (released from dead bacteria), exotoxins (released from living bacteria), and enterotoxins (intestinal inflammators). Sometimes, the term "toxin" is restricted to poisons spontaneously produced by a living organism ("biotoxin"). Toxins produced by fungi are called mycotoxins; higher plants produce phytotoxins, and animal toxins are called zootoxins.

While some biotoxins seem to have little benefit to the organism that produces them, they may be involved in some unknown way in metabolism. However, many other biotoxins are noticeably helpful to their organism, primarily by inhibiting predators—especially insects.

toxoid A bacterial toxin that has been deactivated by either heat or chemicals, which removes its toxicity but maintains its ability to stimulate antibody production by the immune system. Certain types of toxoids are used in immunizations against specific diseases, such as diphtheria or tetanus.

See also EXOTOXIN.

toxoplasmosis This disease is caused by the parasite *Toxoplasma gondii,* which is transmitted to humans via undercooked meat or by coming in contact with contaminated animal feces (such as when cleaning a cat's litter box). It's most serious in pregnant women: 7 percent of exposed fetuses have minor abnormalities, and 3 percent have severe damage. Highest risk occurs if the mother has been infected during the first six months of pregnancy.

It is found in undercooked beef, mutton, or lamb from an infected animal; unpasteurized milk from an infected goat; or water contaminated with cat feces. Humans aren't infectious to each other.

Symptoms

Symptoms appear between five and 20 days after exposure. Clinical signs are usually mild, with a slight swelling of lymph nodes with a low-grade fever, fatigue, sore throat, or slight body rash. High risk individuals may experience severe symptoms involving multiple organs.

Diagnosis

Blood tests reveal the parasite.

Treatment

Severe cases are treated with sulfanamides and pyrimethamine; healthy nonpregnant young adults don't need to be treated.

Complications

In infants born to infected mothers, complications include eye problems, water on the brain, jaundice, vomiting, fever, convulsions, or mental retardation. High-risk individuals may have fatal pneumonia or heart infection.

Prevention

High-risk people should avoid eating raw or undercooked meat, and pregnant women should avoid contact with a cat's litter box.

tranquilizers See ANTIANXIETY DRUGS.

trichinellosis A type of potentially fatal food poisoning caused by the larvae of a parasitic worm (*Trichinella spiralis*) that enters the body and pen-

etrates the muscles. Trichinellosis was once very common and usually caused by eating undercooked pork. However, the number of cases per year has been declining because of legislation that prohibits feeding raw meat garbage to hogs and with increased public awareness of the dangers of eating raw or undercooked pork products. During 1997–2001, an average of 12 cases per year were reported. Routine inspection of carcasses for trichinella organisms is not done in the United States because the disease is on the decline, and irradiation of pork carcasses can eradicate the larvae. Today, more cases are associated with eating raw or undercooked wild game meats than with pork.

Symptoms

Symptoms, including diarrhea, nausea, fever, sore muscles, and swollen eyelids, appear between one and seven weeks after eating contaminated food. These symptoms are followed by pain and bleeding in the eyes, thirst, chills, sweating, and weakness. Symptoms may last for months. Partial immunity may follow an infection.

Diagnosis

Blood tests can confirm the infection by detecting antibodies to the larvae or by a muscle biopsy that reveals the larvae themselves.

Treatment

Mebendazole is an effective treatment; failure to treat the infection could be fatal. Bed rest is recommended to prevent relapse.

Complications

In severe cases, there may be heart and neurological problems that can progress to fatal heart failure, either in the first two weeks after infection, or between the fourth and eighth week.

Prevention

All pork products and wild game should be cooked completely (at least 170°F) for 35 minutes per pound. Pork should be a gray color on the inside, with no visible pink. Storing infected meat in a freezer with a temperature no higher than -13°F for 10 days also will kill the parasite. Pork or pork products should never be eaten raw, and even smoked or salted meat may still have organisms. Pork should not be ground in the same grinder as other meats, and afterward the grinder should be cleaned well.

trichloroethane Also known as methyl chloroform, this common household solvent is found as an ingredient in a wide range of products, including fabric cleaners, spot removers, insecticides, and paint removers. Together with trichloroethylene, it is used in most typewriter correction fluids, a form in which it can be abused by those who sniff it for its euphoric effects. It is available in two forms: 1,1,2 and (more commonly) 1,1,1-. A colorless, heavy liquid, it is considered by the National Institute of Occupational Safety and Health (NIOSH) to be a possible carcinogen. There is potential for abuse in those who have access to the substance and sniff the vapors.

Because of several deaths resulting from intentionally sniffing typewriter correction fluid, manufacturers have added oil of mustard as a deterrent, in both Liquid Paper and Liquid Paper Thinner (which contains more trichloroethane than the correctional fluid).

Symptoms

Trichloroethane is a central nervous system depressant, but it also affects the heart, liver, and kidneys and can reach toxic levels as a result of inhalation, skin contact, or ingestion. It has a rapid anesthetic action and was used for this purpose prior to the 1960s, until safer agents were developed. Symptoms depend on the concentration and type of exposure but generally include headache, eye irritation, vertigo, sleepiness, visual disturbances, nausea, stupor, unconsciousness, and coma. In extreme cases, inhaling these fumes can be fatal. Skin contact causes severe swelling followed by sloughing of the skin.

Ingestion causes symptoms including burning mouth, nausea, vomiting, abdominal pain, and heart irregularities. Chronic abuse by sniffing produces weight loss, nausea, fatigue, visual problems, dermatitis, and jaundice. The lethal dose in humans is reportedly between 0.5 and 5 milliliters per kilogram.

Treatment

Move victim to a well-ventilated area and remove contaminated clothing; management is mainly supportive. Oxygen and artificial respiration should be used in the event of respiratory failure. Give supplemental oxygen and treat hydrocarbon aspiration pneumonitis if it occurs. Treat seizures, coma, and arrhythmias if they occur, but do not use epinephrine because of a risk of inducing or worsening cardiac arrhythmias. There is no specific antidote. If ingested, do NOT induce vomiting; perform gastric lavage if the patient is seen within an hour of ingestion or has taken a large overdose. This is followed by the administration of activated charcoal and a cathartic.

See also TRICHLOROETHYLENE.

trichloroethylene This common household solvent is used as an inhalation anesthetic, a metal degreaser, a solvent for oils and greases, and a paint remover. Together with trichloroethane, it is used in most typewriter correction fluids, a form in which it can be abused by those who sniff it for its euphoric effects. A colorless, heavy liquid, it was formerly popular as an anesthetic during labor prior to 1965. There is potential for abuse in those who have access to the substance and sniff the vapors.

Symptoms

Trichloroethylene is a central nervous system depressant, but it also affects the heart, liver, and kidneys. Symptoms depend on the concentration and type of exposure but generally include headache, eye irritation, vertigo, sleepiness, visual disturbances, nausea, stupor, unconsciousness, and coma. In extreme cases, inhaling these fumes can be fatal.

Skin contact causes severe erythema followed by sloughing of the skin. Ingestion causes symptoms including burning mouth, nausea, vomiting, abdominal pain, and heart irregularities. Chronic abuse by sniffing produces weight loss, nausea, fatigue, visual problems, dermatitis, and jaundice.

Treatment

Move victim to a well-ventilated area and remove contaminated clothing; management is mainly supportive. Oxygen and artificial respiration should be used in the event of respiratory failure. If ingested, perform gastric lavage followed by the administration of a saline cathartic.

See also TRICHLOROETHANE.

trihexyphenidyl (Artane)   An anticholinergic drug used together with other drugs to relieve the symptoms of Parkinson's disease (rigidity and tremors); it is also used to treat symptoms of excessive use of Haldol (haloperidol) and Thorazine. These symptoms (unsteady gait, slobbering, slurring words, shuffling feet) are similar to those of Parkinson's disease.

trinitrotoluene (TNT)   This solid, colorless to pale yellow explosive blows up when heated to 240°F (or when shocked); it becomes even more explosive when combined with oxidizers. Prolonged skin contact will cause a type of skin rash; inhalation and ingestion of TNT are far more toxic.

Until industry tightened safety practices in the 1950s, TNT exposure was responsible for fatal cases of aplastic anemia and toxic hepatitis.

Symptoms

The principal symptom of inhalation of TNT dust or vapor is jaundice of the skin, nails, and hair. Other symptoms include sneezing, coughing, sore throat, yellow stain on skin, hair or nails, rash, blue color, pallor, nausea, anorexia, anemia, kidney failure, delirium, convulsions, and coma. Chronic poisoning causes stomach disorders with heart irregularities and kidney failure. Fatal toxic dose is between one and two grams.

Treatment

Ingested TNT should be removed by induced vomiting or gastric lavage, followed by the administration of a cathartic. For skin contamination, thoroughly wash with soap and water. Soap with 10 percent potassium sulfite will turn red in contact with TNT and can be used to determine thorough cleansing. Observe victim for possible liver damage.

tropical rattlesnake   See RATTLESNAKE, CASCABEL.

trumpet plant (*Solandra*)   Also known as chalice vine, this climbing woody vine has large, showy yellow trumpet-shaped flowers with fleshy berries. It is found in tropical America and Mexico and is cultivated outdoors in Florida, the West Indies, and Hawaii.

Poisonous part

All parts of the plant are toxic, including the nectar, and contain atropine alkaloids.

Symptoms

Following ingestion, symptoms include dry mouth, fast heartbeat, dry, hot flushed skin, fever, and blurred vision. Children are particularly prone to excitement, headache, delirium, and hallucinations.

Treatment

If poisoning is severe enough to cause high fever or delirium, administer slow intravenous drip of physostigmine until symptoms disappear; repeated administration may be required.

See also ATROPINE.

trunkfish (*Lactoria cornutus*)   A fish of tropical oceans that is poisonous at certain times of the year because of feeding on poisonous plankton. Symptoms may develop quickly or slowly and involve tingling sensations in the lips and mouth followed by numbness, nausea, vomiting, abdominal cramps, weakness, paralysis, convulsions, skin rash, coma, and death in about 12 percent of cases.

See also CIGUATERA; DINOFLAGELLATE; FISH CONTAMINATION.

tularemia   Every state except Hawaii has reported cases of tularemia, which is also known as rabbit fever. It is caused by the bacterium *Francisella tularensis,* which is typically found in rabbits, hares, and rodents. About 200 cases per year are reported in the United States, but more may go unreported. The vast majority of cases occur in rural areas, usually in the south central and western states, and are caused by the bites of flies and ticks, handling infected animals, eating or drinking contaminated food or water, or by inhaling airborne bacteria. The bacteria can stay alive in soil or water for several weeks. The disease is not known to spread from person to person.

Franciscella tularensis is very infectious, however: as few as 10 to 50 organisms can cause disease. This fact makes it a potential biological weapon. If the bacteria were used as a weapon, the attack would be airborne, because exposure to the organisms by inhalation causes severe respiratory illness, including life-threatening pneumonia and systemic infection.

Symptoms

Symptoms typically occur within three to five days from time of infection, but the range can be from one to 14 days. If the bacteria are inhaled, symptoms can include sudden onset of fever, chills, headache, muscle aches, joint pain, dry cough, and progressive weakness. The infection can then progress to severe respiratory illness, including life-threatening pneumonia. Signs and symptoms that can occur from other sources (e.g., bites, handling infected animals, contaminated food and water) include skin ulcers, inflamed eyes, sore throat, diarrhea, mouth sores, swollen lymph glands, and pneumonia.

Treatment

Tularemia can be fatal if the infected individual is not treated with the appropriate antibiotics. Treatment is usually prescribed for 10 to 14 days. Oral antibiotics may include those in the tetracycline class (e.g., doxycycline) or fluoroquinolone class (e.g., ciprofloxacin). Injected antibiotics may include streptomycin or gentamicin. A vaccine for tularemia is currently under review by the Food and Drug Administration.

Prevention

To prevent infection by *F. tularensis,* use insect repellent on your skin and treat clothing with repellent containing permethrin. Wash your hands often with soap and warm water, especially if you have handled animal carcasses. Consult a veterinarian if you notice any change in the behavior of your pets, especially rabbits, hares, and rodents.

tuna, bluefin   One of a group of scombroid fishes (including mackerel, swordfish, and others) that contain a chemical in the flesh called histidine. When these fish are allowed to stand at room temperature for several hours, histidine interacts with bacteria to form a histaminelike substance called saurine. Scombroid fish are more susceptible to the development of saurine poison than most other kinds of fish. All of the species that are potentially toxic live in temperate or tropical waters, especially around California and Hawaii; even commercially canned tuna can become toxic, although the most common fish responsible is mahimahi.

Scombroid poisoning can be prevented simply by adequately refrigerating fish.

Symptoms

Symptoms of saurine poisoning resemble those of a severe allergy: Soon after eating the affected fish (which is said to have a sharp, pungent taste), the victim begins to experience headache, throbbing blood vessels in the neck, nausea, vomiting, burning throat, massive welts, and itching. Recovery occurs after eight to 12 hours.

Treatment

Gastric lavage; administration of antihistamines or the histamine blocker cimetidine (Tagamet).

See also FISH CONTAMINATION; SCROMBROID POISONING.

tuna, skipjack (Euthynnus pelamis)   One of a group of scombroid fishes (including mackerel, swordfish, and allies) that contain a chemical in the flesh called histidine. When these fish are allowed to stand at room temperature for several hours, histidine forms a histaminelike substance called saurine. Scombroid fish are more susceptible to the development of saurine poison than most other kinds of fish.

See also FISH CONTAMINATION; SCROMBROID POISONING; TUNA, BLUEFIN.

turbantop (Gyromitra esculenta)   Also called false morel *(G. infula),* this mushroom varies in toxicity from variety to variety and individual to individual. Those found in North America are almost all poisonous, but a few of the European varieties are extremely tasty and harmless. The turbantop is brown with a thick, hollow stem.

Poisonous part

The poisonous compound is monomethylhydrazine (mmh), found in all *Gyromitra* mushrooms. It destroys the red blood cells and affects the kidneys and central nervous system. Some of the toxins in these mushrooms may be removed by drying, boiling, rinsing, and reboiling.

Symptoms

Symptoms begin between two hours and a day after ingestion and can include severe liver damage, vomiting, diarrhea, jaundice, convulsions, destruction of red blood cells, and coma. Fatality rate from liver failure ranges from 15 to 40 percent. Toxicity in humans varies from one individual to the next. Overall fatality rate is about 15 percent.

Treatment

Give pyridoxine for seizures; treat methemoglobinemia with methylene blue.

See also *GYROMITRA;* MUSHROOM POISONING; MUSHROOM TOXINS.

turpentine This common household solvent is used as a thinner for paint, varnish, and lacquer. A volatile oil, turpentine is derived from sapwood of cone-bearing trees like pines and firs and has been used medically as a skin irritant. Still, it is not usually fatal, since its fumes make it too painful to swallow or inhale for any appreciable length of time.

Symptoms

Breathing these solvent fumes can cause headache, eye irritation, dizziness, visual disturbances, nausea, unconsciousness, and convulsions. With skin contact, it causes local irritation and immediate reddening. Ingestion can result in abdominal pain, nausea, vomiting, diarrhea, urinary prob-

lems, unconsciousness, shallow breathing, and convulsions. In extreme cases, kidney failure and pulmonary edema can be fatal.

Treatment

Avoid vomiting. Gastric lavage followed by the administration of demulcents, such as milk. For skin contamination, wash thoroughly with soap and water.

See also PETROLEUM DISTILLATES; VOLATILE OILS.

2,4-D [Trade names: Agrotect, Lawn-Keep, Rider, Super D Weedone, Weed-B-Gon, Weedone.] This herbicide was introduced in 1946 as the first hormonelike weed killer and has grown to become the most extensively used herbicide in the world. In 1985, agriculture and forestry applications in the United States accounted for nearly 40 million pounds of 2,4-D. As an herbicide, it is fairly selective; it is toxic to many broad-leaved plants but does not affect grasses (such as cereal crops, ornamental lawns, or pastures). It works by interfering with normal plant growth processes, and it is also used to control ripening of fruit and root development.

This corrosive white powder is widely used in agriculture to control weeds in corn, wheat, sorghum, oats, barley, and sugarcane, with considerable chance for widespread exposure. It is available as an aerial or ground spray, or by direct injection into plants.

Studies suggest that normal exposure levels of 2,4-D for agricultural and forestry workers and animals such as deer, rabbits, and fish are considerably lower than those levels producing toxic effects. Protective clothing should be worn when applying the herbicide. It is uncertain to what extent the public is exposed, but it is possible that some residue remains on food; therefore, experts suggest washing all fresh produce.

Symptoms

When ingested in large doses, 2,4-D cause gastrointestinal irritation, spasms of the heart and central nervous system depression. It is also a skin and eye irritant, and prolonged inhalation causes coughing, dizziness, and temporary loss of coordination. Prolonged exposure to low levels can produce a variety of responses ranging from a reversible loss of coordination to stomach ulcers—and sometimes death.

A review by the International Agency for Cancer Research concluded there were insufficient data to assess the carcinogenicity of 2,4-D.

Treatment

Induce vomiting or perform gastric lavage, followed by the administration of activated charcoal and a saline cathartic. Quinidine may be necessary if ventricular fibrillation occurs. Chronic exposure can produce aplastic anemia.

universal antidote   Although milk is most popularly considered to be the universal antidote, there is really no such thing, according to most toxicologists. Milk is actually used to dilute poison, not combat its effects, and it is only useful with some toxic substances. Another so-called universal antidote—two parts activated charcoal, one part milk of magnesia, and one part strong tea solution—is also ineffective, despite its popularity in the press. According to toxicology experts, the use of activated charcoal alone would be much more effective, and some evidence suggests that the addition of milk of magnesia and tea actually interferes with the absorptive activity of the charcoal.

Salt water, which at one time was considered to be a universal antidote because of its ability to absorb poison in the stomach, can be harmful and actually cause cardiac arrest. Because many antidotes are dangerous in and of themselves, no treatment should be considered before talking with a physician or poison control center. Using an antidote depends on the type and amount of substance ingested, and how much time has passed between ingestion and treatment.

See also CHARCOAL, ACTIVATED.

urushiol   A resin contained in the sap of poison oak, poison ivy, and poison sumac that causes contact dermatitis in seven out of 10 Americans who come in contact with it. About five out of 10 Americans are extremely sensitive to urushiol.

See also POISON IVY; POISON OAK; POISON SUMAC.

Vacor (PNU, or 2 percent N-3-pyridylmethy-N'p-nitrophenylurea) This yellow or green rat killer causes irreversible insulin-dependent diabetes and autonomic nervous system injury. Fatal poisonings are usually the result of suicide, since ingestion of a small amount will not usually be fatal. Vacor was banned for household sale in 1979, but it is still found in some homes and is available to professional exterminators.

Ingestion of one packet of Vacor (39 grams) has caused acute toxicity.

Symptoms
Because Vacor destroys the insulin-producing cells in the pancreas, symptoms include twitching, low blood pressure, thirst, diabetes, nausea and vomiting, abdominal and chest pain, weakness, blurred vision, lethargy, impaired mental function, delirium, collapse, coma, and respiratory failure ending in death.

Treatment
Administer nicotinamide within 30 minutes, followed by symptomatic treatment; although its success has not been proven in humans, its use can prevent PNU-induced diabetes in rats. Induce vomiting or perform gastric lavage, followed by the administration of activated charcoal and a cathartic. Treat coma and give intravenous fluids for low blood pressure; chronic therapy includes a high-salt diet and fluorocortisone. Treat diabetes as usual.

See also NICOTINAMIDE; RAT POISON.

Valium See DIAZEPAM.

valproic acid An anticonvulsant, valproic acid is a prescription medication that is used alone or with other medications to treat certain types of seizures, mania in people who have bipolar disorder, and to prevent migraine headaches. It is available as Depakene and Depakote, and under the generic names divalproex sodium and valproate sodium. It works by increasing the amount of gamma-aminobutyric acid (GABA), a natural substance found in the brain.

Use of valproic acid is associated with an increased risk of suicidal behavior, which can occur as early as one week after starting the medication. It is also linked to liver failure resulting in death. On rare occasions use of valproic acid also may cause life-threatening pancreatitis (inflammation of the pancreas). Since the mid-1990s there has been a steady increase in the number of reported overdoses and deaths, with the majority occurring in people older than 19 years. A likely reason for this increase is that valproic acid is being used more and more as a mood stabilizer as opposed to its primary use as an anticonvulsant.

Symptoms
Overdose can cause irregular heartbeat, weak pulse, shallow breathing, sleepiness, and coma. Symptoms of suicidal behavior include anxiety, agitation, hostility, mania, withdrawing from family and friends, new or worsening depression, and preoccupation with death and dying. If you suddenly stop taking valproic acid, you may experience severe, prolonged, and possibly life-threatening seizures.

Treatment
Naloxone can reverse the central nervous system depressant effects of a valproic acid overdose. This drug should be used with caution, however, because it could also reverse the antiepileptic benefits of valproic acid. Because valproic acid is

absorbed very rapidly, gastric lavage is usually of limited value.

venin de crapaud   An ancient poison popular throughout Europe during the 15th century, it was made by feeding arsenic to toads and distilling the juices from their bodies after they died.

See also ARSENIC.

Vibrio parahaemolyticus   Poisoning caused by eating fish or shellfish contaminated with the *Vibrio parahaemolyticus* bacteria. Sporadic outbreaks of this type of gastroenteritis have appeared in the United States, and it is very common in Japan, where large outbreaks often occur. The illness appears when the bacteria attach themselves to a person's small intestine and secrete an as-yet-unidentified toxin.

Anyone who eats raw, improperly cooked contaminated fish and shellfish is at risk, especially during the warmer months. Improper refrigeration of contaminated seafood allows the bacteria to grow, increasing the chance of infection.

Symptoms
Between four and 96 hours after ingestion, infected diners may experience diarrhea, abdominal cramps, nausea and vomiting, headache, fever, and chills.

Diagnosis
This organism can be cultured from a person's stool.

Treatment
In most cases, the infection will clear up by itself. Only a few cases require hospitalization and treatment with antibiotics. The illness is usually mild, although some people may need to be hospitalized.

Prevention
Seafoods should be completely cooked for at least 15 minutes at 160°F.

See also FISH CONTAMINATION; *VIBRIO VULNIFICUS*.

Vibrio vulnificus   This rare bacteria was first recognized to cause an unusually severe syndrome of foodborne illness, called "primary septicemia" (blood poisoning), that can seriously affect people with an underlying disease. Those at high risk for infection with serious consequences include people with liver disease, iron disorder (hemochromatosis), diabetes, cancer, HIV infection or AIDS, and long-term steroid use (such as chronic asthma patients). However, when eaten by healthy people, *Vibrio* causes only minor stomach discomfort.

Between 1988 and 2006, the Centers for Disease Control and Prevention (CDC) received reports of more than 900 infections caused by *V. vulnificus* from the Gulf Coast states alone, which is where the majority of cases occur. The CDC then collaborated with Alabama, Florida, Louisiana, Mississippi, and Texas to monitor the number of cases of the infection in the Gulf Coast area, and therefore cases of *V. vulnificus* and other *Vibrio* species are nationally notifiable.

Vibrio is found in raw or undercooked contaminated seafood such as oysters, clams, and crabs harvested in warm water, especially the Gulf of Mexico.

Symptoms
Healthy patients become ill between 12 hours and a week after eating raw contaminated seafood with gastrointestinal complaints. Among certain people—cancer patients, diabetics, the elderly, and those with weak immune systems—the risk of serious illness rises sharply; the fatality rate is more than 50 percent.

Treatment
If you suspect *V. vulnificus* infection of a wound, antibiotic treatment should be initiated immediately. Doxycycline plus cephalosporin is usually recommended. Severe cases may require limb amputation.

Complications
Blood clotting problems can occur.

Prevention
People at high risk should avoid raw seafood.

See also FISH CONTAMINATION; *VIBRIO PARAHAEMOLYTICUS*.

viper, gaboon *(Bitis gabonica)* This close relative of the puff adder is found in African rain forests and remnant forest and thickets, although it is not arboreal. One of the largest and heaviest Old World vipers, it is usually placid but capable of lightning strikes and is considered to be one of the most dangerous snakes.

The gaboon viper is easily concealed by its colors: purple, crimson, rose, pale blue, silver, yellow russet, and black, arranged in complex geometrical patterns. It has the longest fangs of any snake in the world (almost two inches) and has enough venom to kill 200 people. Yet it is so placid that small children can pick one up by the tail and carry it.

Symptoms

A bite from the gaboon viper may pass unnoticed until the pain begins—and when it may be too late to administer antivenin. Although less toxic than that of its puff adder cousin, gaboon viper venom can still be fatal. Without treatment, victims begin bleeding from the gums, nose and eyes and experience chills, fever, sweating, falling blood pressure, convulsions, and death. In cases of a severe bite, the victim will also experience swelling above the elbows or knees within two hours.

Treatment

Antivenin is available.

See also MASSASAUGA; PIT VIPERS; RATTLESNAKE; CANEBRAKE; RATTLESNAKE, CASCABEL; RATTLESNAKE, EASTERN DIAMONDBACK; RATTLESNAKE, MEXICAN WEST COAST, RATTLESNAKE, RED DIAMONDBACK; RATTLESNAKE, TIMBER; RATTLESNAKE, WESTERN DIAMONDBACK; RATTLESNAKES; SIDEWINDER; SNAKES, POISONOUS; VIPER, JUMPING; VIPER, MALAYAN PIT; VIPER, RUSSEL'S; VIPER, SAWSCALED; VIPER, WAGLER'S PIT; WATER MOCCASIN; WUTU.

viper, horned See SIDEWINDER.

viper, jumping *(Bothrops)* Also known as the tommygoff, this aggressive relative of the fer-de-lance is found throughout Central and South America. Brown or gray with diamond-shaped crosswise marks, it can grow to about two feet long and can strike with such force that it can lift itself off the ground. Its venom is not as dangerous as that of others in the fer-de-lance group.

Symptoms

Because the venom interferes with the coagulation of the blood, it hemorrhages into muscles and the nervous system and results in bleeding from the gums, nose, mouth, and rectum. It is possible to assess the seriousness of the bite by checking the level of swelling or hemorrhages that appear above the elbows or knees two hours after the bite. After a person is bitten, the area above the bite quickly swells and turns purple. The victim vomits blood, perspires, and collapses within an hour, with blood flowing from the nose and eyes, followed by unconsciousness and death if no antivenin is administered. In fact, absent antivenin, death from cardiorespiratory failure is unavoidable.

Treatment

Antivenin is available.

See also MASSASAUGA; PIT VIPERS; RATTLESNAKE; CANEBRAKE; RATTLESNAKE, CASCABEL; RATTLESNAKE, EASTERN DIAMONDBACK; RATTLESNAKE, MEXICAN WEST COAST, RATTLESNAKE, RED DIAMONDBACK; RATTLESNAKE, TIMBER; RATTLESNAKE, WESTERN DIAMONDBACK; RATTLESNAKES; SIDEWINDER; SNAKES, POISONOUS; VIPER, GABOON; VIPER, MALAYAN PIT; VIPER, RUSSEL'S; VIPER, SAWSCALED; VIPER, WAGLER'S PIT; VIPERS; WATER MOCCASIN; WUTU.

viper, Malayan pit *(Agkistrodon rhodostoma)* Found in forests, plantations, and other cultivated areas, this snake (also known as the Malayan moccasin) is often quick to strike. Its long, tubular fangs are located in a maxillary bone than can be rotated 90 degrees, effectively swinging the fangs from a vertical to a horizontal position. The head is triangular with large scales, and the small eyes have vertical pupils; its snout is pointed and upturned, and the sturdy body is reddish brown with a series of dark brown crossbands that narrow along the back's midline. A light stripe extends from the eye to the nape of neck, and there is a wide light-colored band on the lip.

This snake is normally found in forested areas, where it stays coiled up under rocks or dense vegetation; at twilight it hunts for food. Fairly aggressive, when molested it assumes a threatening posture, curling up its body and vibrating the tip of its tail.

Symptoms

Those who have been bitten by vipers show much the same symptoms as victims of cobra bites, plus bleeding from the gums, chills, and fever. It is possible to assess the seriousness of the bite by checking the level of swelling or hemorrhages that appear above the elbows or knees two hours after the bite. After a person is bitten, the area above the bite quickly swells and turns purple. The victim vomits blood, perspires, and collapses within an hour, with blood flowing from the nose and eyes, followed by unconsciousness and death if no antivenin is administered. In fact, absent antivenin, death from cardiorespiratory failure is unavoidable.

Treatment

Antivenin is available.

viper, Palestine *(Vipera palestinae)* This member of the viper family is a considerable threat in the Middle East and causes more cases of snakebite in Palestine than any other venomous snake.

See also MASSASAUGA; PIT VIPERS; RATTLESNAKE; CANEBRAKE; RATTLESNAKE, CASCABEL; RATTLESNAKE, EASTERN DIAMONDBACK; RATTLESNAKE, MEXICAN WEST COAST; RATTLESNAKE, RED DIAMONDBACK; RATTLESNAKE, TIMBER; RATTLESNAKE, WESTERN DIAMONDBACK; RATTLESNAKES; SIDEWINDER; SNAKES, POISONOUS; VIPER, GABOON; VIPER, JUMPING; VIPER, RUSSEL'S; VIPER, SAWSCALED; VIPER, WAGLER'S PIT; VIPERS; WATER MOCCASIN; WUTU.

viper, Russell's *(Vipera russelli)* Also called the tic polonga or daboia, the Russell's viper is found in both forests and open occupied areas from the Himalayas and southern China to Sri Lanka and Indonesia. This snake is very aggressive and is one of the most deadly in the world. Growing up to 5 feet long, it has rows of reddish brown spots circled by black and white lines, with a wide head and a square snout.

Aggressive and assertive, it is normally found on margins of woods and forests, brushy fields, mountain meadows, cultivated lands, and thickets near villages, usually on the ground—but it is also capable of climbing fences to find prey.

This viper is active mainly at twilight and during the night, coiling up under stones and brushy places during the day. It is generally lazy and slow, but when irritated it becomes aggressive, hissing loudly and striking with force and speed.

Symptoms

Those who have been bitten by vipers show much the same symptoms as victims of cobra bites, plus bleeding from the gums, chills, and fever. It is possible to assess the seriousness of the bite by checking the level of swelling or hemorrhages that appear above the elbows or knees two hours after the bite. After a person is bitten, the area above the bite quickly swells and turns purple. The victim vomits blood, perspires, and collapses within an hour, with blood flowing from the nose and eyes, followed by unconsciousness and death if no antivenin is administered. In fact, absent antivenin, death from cardiorespiratory failure is unavoidable.

Treatment

Antivenin is available.

See also MASSASAUGA; PIT VIPERS; RATTLESNAKE; CANEBRAKE; RATTLESNAKE, CASCABEL; RATTLESNAKE, EASTERN DIAMONDBACK; RATTLESNAKE, MEXICAN WEST COAST, RATTLESNAKE, RED DIAMONDBACK; RATTLESNAKE, TIMBER; RATTLESNAKE, WESTERN DIAMONDBACK; RATTLESNAKES; SIDEWINDER; SNAKES, POISONOUS; VIPER, GABOON; VIPER, JUMPING; VIPER, MALAYAN PIT; VIPER, SAWSCALED; VIPER, WAGLER'S PIT; VIPERS; WATER MOCCASIN; WUTU.

viper, sawscaled *(Echis carinatus)* The most venomous of the Viperidae vipers, the sawscaled viper is found in semidesert and dry, arid regions in the Afro-Asian deserts, India, and Sri Lanka. This alert and vicious snake is known for its irritability and aggressiveness; its bite is usually fatal. A small snake no longer than two feet, it has a gray sandy color with rows of white spots and zigzag lines.

Active at night, this snake is easily disguised and can be very dangerous in a land were most of the people don't wear shoes. Even a newborn snake can kill a person and will bite with very little provocation. When disturbed, this snake moves itself into an S shape, rubbing its scales together to produce a hissing sound. It moves in a peculiar sidewise motion known as sidewinding.

While there is a solid market for the sale of these snakes, the 200,000 animals brought to the United States over a period of six years have done little to decimate the population.

Symptoms

The venom of the sawscaled viper is unusually toxic; it causes both internal and external hemorrhages and is fatal within 12 to 16 days after the bite. Those who have been bitten by vipers show much the same symptoms as victims of cobra bites, plus bleeding from the gums, chills, and fever. It is possible to assess the seriousness of the bite by checking the level of swelling or hemorrhages that appear above the elbows or knees two hours after the bite. After a person is bitten, the area above the bite quickly swells and turns purple. The victim vomits blood, perspires, and collapses within an hour, with blood flowing from the nose and eyes, followed by unconsciousness and death if no antivenin is administered. In fact, absent antivenin, death from cardiorespiratory failure is unavoidable.

Treatment

Antivenin is available.

See also MASSASAUGA; PIT VIPERS; RATTLESNAKE; CANEBRAKE; RATTLESNAKE, CASCABEL; RATTLESNAKE, EASTERN DIAMONDBACK; RATTLESNAKE, MEXICAN WEST COAST, RATTLESNAKE, RED DIAMONDBACK; RATTLESNAKE, TIMBER; RATTLESNAKE, WESTERN AND DIAMONDBACK; RATTLESNAKES; SIDEWINDER; SNAKES, POISONOUS; VIPER, GABOON; VIPER, JUMPING; VIPER, MALAYAN PIT; VIPER, RUSSELL'S; VIPER, WAGLER'S PIT; VIPERS; WATER MOCCASIN; WUTU.

viper, Wagler's pit *(Trimeresurus Wagleri)* A species of snake found in Asia and one of a group collectively known as fer-de-lance. The venom of this snake remains almost completely poisonous even after being in a sterilizer. It causes extremely fast collapse and death, without local swelling.

Symptoms

With a bite from this viper, blood cannot coagulate and hemorrhages into muscles and the central nervous system. There is local pain, bleeding from the bite, gums, nose, mouth, and rectum. Those who have been bitten by vipers show much the same symptoms as victims of cobra bites, plus bleeding from the gums, chills, and fever. It is possible to assess the seriousness of the bite by checking the level of swelling or hemorrhages that appear above the elbows or knees two hours after the bite. After a person is bitten, the area above the bite quickly swells and turns purple. The victim vomits blood, perspires, and collapses within an hour, with blood flowing from the nose and eyes, followed by unconsciousness and death if no antivenin is administered. In fact, absent antivenin, death from cardiorespiratory failure is unavoidable.

Treatment

Antivenin is available.

See also MASSASAUGA; PIT VIPERS; RATTLESNAKE, CANEBRAKE; RATTLESNAKE, CASCABEL; RATTLESNAKE, EASTERN DIAMONDBACK; RATTLESNAKE, MEXICAN WEST COAST, RATTLESNAKE, RED DIAMONDBACK; RATTLESNAKE, TIMBER; RATTLESNAKE, WESTERN DIAMONDBACK; RATTLESNAKES; SIDEWINDER; SNAKES, POISONOUS; VIPER, GABOON; VIPER, JUMPING; VIPER, MALAYAN PIT; VIPER, RUSSELL'S; VIPER, SAWSCALED; VIPERS; WATER MOCCASIN; WUTU.

vipers *(Viperidae)* This major family of poisonous snakes includes some 160 species found in most parts of the world; they possess the most efficient way of injecting venom of all snakes. The Viperidae family consists primarily of two subfamilies: the pit vipers (Crotalinae), found throughout the Americas and southeastern Asia, numbering about 120 species; and the Viperinae, numbering 39 species, including the European adder, the sawscaled viper, and the puff adder found throughout Europe, Africa, and Asia.

In general, vipers share many of the same characteristics; for example, the head is triangular or spade shaped, distinct from the body. Because they are so different from other groups, the vipers are the most easily identified of all poisonous snakes. Their long, tubular fangs are located in a maxillary bone that can be rotated 90 degrees, effectively swinging the fangs from a vertical to a horizontal position.

The true vipers (Viperinae) differ from the pit vipers in internal anatomy, and they also lack the temperature-sensitive pit organs. The pit vipers (Crotalinae) are characterized by a unique sense organ on each side of the head between the nostril and the eye. As the snake moves its head, it can ascertain the direction of objects by sensing heat; if the object is directly in front of the snake, the heat radiation will enter both the left and right pit organs at the same time, which indicates distance as well as direction.

The bites of even the smallest European vipers are always potentially dangerous. The Russell's viper (one of the largest members of the subfamily) is one of the deadliest snakes in the world.

Symptoms

Those who have been bitten by vipers show much the same symptoms as victims of cobra bites, plus bleeding from the gums, chills, and fever. It is possible to assess the seriousness of the bite by checking the level of swelling or hemorrhages that appear above the elbows or knees two hours after the bite. After a person is bitten, the area above the bite quickly swells and turns purple. The victim vomits blood, perspires, and collapses within an hour, with blood flowing from the nose and eyes, followed by unconsciousness and death if no antivenin is administered. In fact, absent antivenin, death from cardiorespiratory failure is unavoidable.

Treatment

Antivenin is available.

See also MASSASAUGA; PIT VIPERS; RATTLESNAKE, CANEBRAKE; RATTLESNAKE, CASCABEL; RATTLESNAKE, EASTERN DIAMONDBACK; RATTLESNAKE, MEXICAN WEST COAST, RATTLESNAKE, RED DIAMONDBACK; RATTLESNAKE, TIMBER; RATTLESNAKE, WESTERN DIAMONDBACK; RATTLESNAKES; SIDEWINDER; SNAKES, POISONOUS; VIPER, GABOON; VIPER, JUMPING; VIPER, MALAYAN PIT; VIPER, RUSSELL'S; VIPER, SAWSCALED; VIPER, WAGLER'S PIT; WATER MOCCASIN; WUTU.

vitamins　Vitamin supplementation is increasingly common in the United States, with people choosing both individual vitamins and multivitamin formulations with or without minerals. In fact, multivitamin supplements are typically the most popular type of dietary supplement reported in surveys and studies. According to the National Health and Nutrition Examination Survey (NHANES), 52 percent of adults said they took a dietary supplement in the past month, and 35 percent reported regular use of a multivitamin-multimineral supplement. The NHANES III data note overall dietary supplement use of 40 percent.

Although many Americans take vitamin supplements according to directions from their healthcare providers or product labeling, some take megadoses of vitamins, which can be toxic. This is true whether a vitamin is "natural" or "synthetic." A natural vitamin is one that has been extracted from a substance found in nature (e.g., vitamins A and D are extracted from cod liver oil, vitamin E from wheat germ oil). Because extraction processes are expensive, most vitamins are manufactured (synthetic) by drug companies.

According to the U.S. Pharmacopeia there is no proof that natural vitamins are better than synthetic ones, with the exception of vitamin E, while some other sources include beta-carotene on the list. Natural beta-carotene is derived from algae, and it contains many carotenes that the synthetic form does not possess. For all other vitamins, the synthetic and natural forms function equally well.

Vitamins are either water soluble or fat (oil) soluble. Water soluble vitamins dissolve easily in water, are passed out of the body in the urine, and usually don't cause toxicity. Among the water-soluble vitamins are the B vitamins (thiamine, riboflavin, niacin, pantotheate, pyridoxine, cobalamin, folate, biotin), and vitamin C; vitamins A, D, E, and K are fat-soluble and are not so easily excreted from the body. Because fat-soluble vitamins accumulate in the body, megadoses of them are more likely to cause toxicity than megadoses of water-soluble vitamins.

For more than 50 years, Americans turned to the RDA (Recommended Daily Allowance) to tell them the safe, correct dosage of vitamins they should take. The RDAs underwent changes over the years, with one of the most significant being the steps taken by the Food and Drug Administration (FDA) in 1990 when it announced that it would average the RDAs for all age groups, resulting in new figures that were lower and reportedly a better reflection of a typical American's vitamin needs.

Then in 1997 the Food and Nutrition Board of the National Academy of Sciences decided to change how nutritionists and nutrition scientists evaluated the diets of healthy people. Thus they revised the RDAs and created a new way to evaluate nutrient values and new dietary reference values, designed not only to prevent nutrient deficiencies, but also to reduce the risk of chronic diseases such as osteoporosis, cardiovascular disease, and cancer. This new system is called the Dietary Reference Intakes (DRIs), of which there are four types of DRI reference values:

- Estimated Average Requirement (EAR): daily nutrient intake value estimated to meet the requirement of 50 percent of healthy individuals in a specific gender and life stage
- Recommended Dietary Allowance (RDA): average daily dietary intake level sufficient to meet the nutrient requirement of 97–98 percent of healthy individuals in a specific gender and life stage
- Adequate Intake (AI): used when an RDA cannot be determined, it is based on observed or experimentally determined estimates of nutrient intake by groups of healthy people, presumed to be adequate
- Tolerable Upper Intake Level (UL): the highest level of daily nutrient intake that is likely to pose no risk of adverse health effects for nearly all individuals in the general population.

According to the American Association of Poison Control Centers' Toxic Exposure Surveillance System, 62,446 exposures to different types of vitamins were reported to poison control centers across the United States in 2005. Of those exposures, 48,604 occurred in children younger than age six years. Overall, there were 73 major adverse outcomes and one death associated with these reported incidents.

vitamin A Excessive use of vitamin A (either as a daily supplement or as an acne treatment) can cause liver and kidney problems. Megadoses of this vitamin have also been used (more than 50,000 International Units (IU) daily for months) to treat children with learning disabilities or as an "anticancer" treatment for adults. Reports indicate that doses over 40,000 International Units per day for several months have resulted in hypervitaminosis A in adults; acute ingestion of more than 12,000 International Units per kilogram may lead to stomach problems. Other studies suggest that doses in excess of 25,000 International Units (five times the recommended daily allowance) can lead to liver damage, hair loss, blurred vision, and headaches.

Symptoms

In children, symptoms of vitamin A toxicity include irritability, anorexia, skin problems, swollen legs and forearms, hair loss, bleeding lips, severe headache, and a craving for butter. Massive doses of vitamin A may also increase pressure within the skull. Symptoms in adults are much the same, only not so serious. In adults, changes in menstruation and skin pigmentation have been reported.

Treatment

Withdrawal from the vitamin. According to experts, treating vitamin A overdose with vitamin E is controversial. Steroids may relieve intracranial pressure in children. The symptoms will disappear in a few weeks after the megadoses have stopped. Recent studies also suggest that elevated levels of vitamin A may increase bone resorption and promote development of osteoporosis.

vitamin B₆ (pyridoxine) This B-complex vitamin is used to manage seizures caused by poisoning by the Gyromitra mushrooms, hydrazine (rocket fuel), or isoniazid. It is also given as part of the therapy for ethylene glycol poisoning.

vitamin D   Vitamin D is essential for the formation of strong bones and has been added to milk since the 1930s as a way to reduce the incidence of rickets. Toxicity with vitamins D_3 or D_4 is rare and would require between 5,000 and 10,000 International Units (IU) daily for several months, although some sensitive people experience symptoms at lower doses. In daily doses of 50,000 International Units (125 times the U.S. RDA) this vitamin can cause the buildup of calcium deposits in the blood that can interfere with the functioning of muscles, including the heart. Sunbathing, which stimulates the body's production of vitamin D, will not create an overdose, however.

A spate of vitamin D poisonings were linked to accidental overdoses in milk fortification at one dairy in Boston, in dosages ranging up to 232,565 International Units. Normally, milk contains 400 International Units of vitamin D per quart. In testing across the country, milk and formula were found to rarely contain the amount of vitamin D as stated on the label; most dairies, however, add too little rather than too much.

Symptoms
Anorexia, nausea, vomiting, fatigue, weakness, headache, diarrhea, and weight loss. Kidney problems, excess calcium in the blood (hypercalcemia) and osteoporosis may also occur. Megadoses of vitamin D during pregnancy are implicated in a variety of fetal abnormalities, including mental retardation and supravalvular aortic stenosis. In severe cases, overdoses of vitamin D can cause irreversible kidney and cardiovascular damage.

Treatment
Withdrawal from the vitamin. The excess levels of calcium in the blood may continue for a few weeks, which may require a restriction in the amount of calcium intake, plenty of fluids, and the administration of glucocorticoids. Vitamin D can also be removed with dialysis.

vitamin E   Acute poisoning with vitamin E is rare, although chronic use of extreme megadoses of this vitamin (more than 600 International Units per day) could cause headaches, dizziness, fatigue, stomach problems, swollen lips, and muscle weakness.

vitamin K (phytonadione)   This vitamin is used to reverse the excessive anticoagulation following overdose of coumarin and indanedione derivatives and is also used in the treatment of salicylate poisoning.

water soluble vitamins   Probably the most popular vitamin to be taken in very large doses is vitamin C, which very rarely causes toxic symptoms beyond stomach irritation and diarrhea after very large doses. However, it can result in scurvy in those who abruptly discontinue taking megadoses, and there have been reports that chewable tablets have eroded teeth if taken daily for more than three years. Earlier reports of vitamin C causing kidney stones is unsupported by research.

Thiamine (vitamin B_1) toxicity has been reported in doses of five milligrams per day for about a month and can cause headaches, irritability, sleeplessness, tachycardia, and weakness.

Toxicity with vitamin B_6 has been reported in doses of two per day for four months, or more quickly at higher doses, causing symptoms including unsteadiness and numb hands and feet. Symptoms disappear after stopping the vitamin; also, some reports indicate that numbness lingers for up to six months.

Niacin in doses of 2,000 International Units (more than 100 times the RDA) may help lower cholesterol, but people who take this much should watch for possible symptoms of jaundice and liver damage.

volatile oils   Also known as essential oils, these are colorless liquids that evaporate quickly and are often used as skin irritants; many have reputations as abortifacients. One of the best-known essential oils is camphor, found in many over-the-counter products including Campho-Phenique, Vicks Vaporub, camphorated oil, and Mentholatum. Topical application of these products leads to inflammation

VOLATILE OILS

Birch oil	Contains 98% methyl salicylate
Camphor oil	FDA banned in 1980 as liniment; causes fetal deaths
Clove oil	Contains 80–90% eugenol
Cinnamon oil	Can burn skin after prolonged contact; potent antigen and smoked as a hallucinogen
Eugenol	Phenol derived from clove oil
Eucalyptus oil	Contains 70% eucalyptol; toxic
Gualacol	Nontoxic
Lavender oil	Contains coumarin
Menthol	Alcohol derived from various mint oils; toxic
Myristica oil	Nutmeg oil, used as a hallucinogen
Pennyroyal oil	Can be fatal
Peppermint oil	Contains 50% menthol; toxic
Thymol	Antiseptic
Turpentine oil	Toxic
Wintergreen oil	Contains methyl salicylate, toxic

followed by a feeling of comfort, but if ingested they can be fatal.

Plants that contain volatile oils include nutmeg, pine, absinthe, pennyroyal, juniper, savin, rue, citronella, sassafras, hemlock, anise, cinnamon, pepper, clove, rape, tansy, eucalyptus, turpentine, and menthol.

Symptoms

Acute ingestion of 15 milliliters of a volatile oil can be fatal, since it irritates all tissues, damages the kidneys, and causes swelling in the lungs, brain, and lining of the stomach. Symptoms include nausea, vomiting, diarrhea, unconsciousness, shallow breathing, and convulsions. Inhaling the volatile oils causes dizziness, rapid and shallow breathing, rapid heartbeat, unconsciousness, or convulsions. Further, volatile oils in amounts large enough to cause an abortion are also large enough to cause irreversible kidney and liver damage.

Treatment

There are no specific antidotes. Administer liquid petrolatum or castor oil and then perform gastric lavage, followed immediately by the administration of activated charcoal. Give milk or mineral oil to ease stomach irritation, give plenty of fluids and keep the victim warm and quiet. Convulsions can be controlled with diazepam or barbiturates.

See also CAMPHOR.

vomiting Emesis, or vomiting, is the violent expulsion of the contents of the stomach. It is so traumatic, in fact, that the stomach nearly turns itself inside out, forcing itself into the lower area of the esophagus. Vomiting is a symptom of an underlying disease or medical condition and not a specific illness.

When vomiting is associated with poisoning, whether the poisoned patient vomits on his or her own or after vomiting has been induced, follow these steps:

- If possible have the person vomit into a bucket or sink so you can bring some of the vomited material to the hospital. This can help the doctor identify the poison involved.

- Make sure the person doesn't inhale the vomited material into the lungs. To prevent this, hold small children face down over your knees while they vomit. A larger person should bend way over or lie down with head hanging off the side of a bed. The chin should be held lower than the level of the hips.

- If the poison has spilled on the person's clothing, skin, or eyes, remove the clothing and flush the skin or eyes with water.

- Monitor vital signs if possible.

- If the person stops breathing, perform CPR (cardiopulmonary resuscitation).

- Treat for shock: Keep the victim quiet and lying down, with head tilted to one side. Raise the feet unless breathing problems or pain result. Loosen clothing and cover the victim with a blanket to conserve body heat. Keep the victim calm. Moisten the lips, but don't give any liquids or sedatives. If the person becomes nauseated, roll him or her to the side so the victim can't inhale the vomit. Call 911 or get the victim to the hospital as soon as possible.

warfarin A derivative of the blood thinner coumarin, warfarin is used to interfere with the body's ability to clot blood. Many other drugs interact with warfarin, strengthening its action. Warfarin is also used as a rat poison.

Symptoms

An overdose seriously interferes with clotting ability, so a victim could bleed to death from a cut. Other symptoms include a sudden hemorrhage of the larynx, trachea, or lungs, bringing up bright red blood and a salty taste into the mouth; bloody stools; hemorrhages and widespread bruising; skin rash; fever; and vomiting. Kidney and liver damage are often fatal, and repeated daily doses of anticoagulants have led to death, even two weeks after the drug has been discontinued.

Treatment

Bed rest together with the administration of mephenytoin; therapy with vitamin K improves blood clotting within 48 hours.

See also ANTICOAGULANTS; RAT POISON.

water arum (*Calla palustris* L.) [Other names: female water dragon, water dragon, wild calla.] This small, water-loving plant has heart-shaped leaves on 10-inch stems, with thick clusters of red berries, and grows in swampy areas in parts of Canada, Colorado, Texas, and Florida.

Poisonous part

The whole plant—especially the root—is toxic and contains calcium oxalate raphides.

Symptoms

Chewing any part of this plant almost immediately causes burning of the lips, mouth, tongue, and throat; therefore, large amounts of the poison are rarely swallowed. Contact dermatitis is also common.

Treatment

Pain and swelling fade by themselves; keeping cold liquids or demulcents (such as milk) in the mouth may ease the pain. The oxalates are insoluble and do not cause systemic poisoning.

See also OXALATES.

water dropwort *(Oenanthe crocata)* [Other names: dead men's fingers, hemlock water dropwort.] This European perennial has been accidentally naturalized into marshy areas in Washington, D.C.; it grows to five feet tall with a bundle of long, thin roots containing latex, which turns to orange when exposed to air. Its white flowers appear in ball clusters. Its cousin, *O. sarmentosa*, grows on the west coast from southwest Alaska to central California and is not toxic.

Poisonous part

The entire plant is toxic, especially the roots, which contain an unsaturated aliphatic compound called oenanthotoxin, closely related to the poisons contained in water hemlocks.

Symptoms

After ingesting the root, the victim experiences salivation followed within minutes by convulsions.

Treatment

Assist breathing; convulsions respond to intravenous diazepam.

See also HEMLOCK, WATER.

water lily See DEATH CAMAS.

water moccasin *(Agkistrodon piscivorus)* This aquatic pit viper (also known as "cottonmouth" because of the color of the inside of its mouth) is found throughout the southeastern United States and is particularly dangerous because it won't move away if disturbed. It does give a warning before striking, however; when bothered, it stands its ground and repeatedly opens its mouth wide, showing the white interior of its mouth. Unlike other water snakes, the water moccasin swims with its head well out of the water, and its eyes are not visible from directly above.

Usually more than three feet long, with a heavy body and broad head, it has a black, olive, or brown body with dark crossbands. Young snakes have strong pattern colors and bright, yellow-tipped tails.

The water moccasin is never far from water and is found in swamps, lakes, rivers, irrigation ditches, canals, rice fields, and clear, rocky mountain streams of the southeastern United States, from Virginia to the upper Florida Keys, west to Illinois, southern Missouri, Oklahoma, and Texas. There is also an isolated population in north central Missouri.

While this snake may be seen sunning itself during the day, it is more often active at night, when it preys on frogs, fishes, other snakes, and birds. The water moccasin is one of the very few snakes that feeds on carrion; in the wild, it has been seen eating fish heads and entrails thrown away by fishermen.

The shoes of the North American Indians—called moccasins—got their name from the skins of the water moccasins, from which they were made.

Symptoms

The bite of the water moccasin is far more venomous than that of the copperhead and can be fatal. Its venom dissolves whatever tissue it touches, and the victim dies from bleeding to death within the body's tissues. The wound site darkens and oozes fluid while swelling spreads, with an extensive hemorrhage beneath the wound area and hemorrhages in the heart, lungs, and other organs. Symptoms may begin within 10 minutes and alternate between hyperactivity and quietness, culminating in death because the veins that carry blood to and from the heart have been destroyed.

Treatment

Antivenin is available.

See also MASSASAUGA; PIT VIPERS; RATTLESNAKE, CANEBRAKE; RATTLESNAKE, CASCABEL; RATTLESNAKE, EASTERN DIAMONDBACK; RATTLESNAKE, MEXICAN WEST COAST, RATTLESNAKE, RED DIAMONDBACK; RATTLESNAKE, TIMBER; RATTLESNAKE, WESTERN DIAMONDBACK; RATTLESNAKES; SIDEWINDER; SNAKES, POISONOUS; VIPER, GABOON; VIPER, JUMPING; VIPER, MALAYAN PIT; VIPER, RUSSEL'S; VIPER, SAWSCALED; VIPER, WAGLER'S PIT; VIPERS; WUTU.

Weedol See PARAQUAT.

weever fish *(Trachinus)* While most fish are not particularly poisonous, the weever is another matter. Found in the British Isles and continental Europe as far south as Morocco, it lives in water up to 160 feet deep, although it is most at home in less than 20 feet of water with clean sand on the bottom.

Weevers are particularly abundant in the Mediterranean Sea, where it is possible to find several varieties, including the spotted weever *(Trachinus araneus)* and the greater weever *(T. draco),* which is sold for food throughout Europe.

The fish lies buried just below the sand's surface, where it can sting anyone who steps on it with its first dorsal fin and the spines on the gill covers. Weevers hunt at night, catching and eating small crustaceans and fish, but they do not use their poisonous spines for anything other than defense.

Symptoms

While death is rare, the sting from the back fin spines of the weaver fish causes an immediate severe stinging or throbbing pain, which may stay at the site of the wound or spread throughout the body and last for several hours or days. Pain can be so severe that the victim loses consciousness. There may be redness and swelling at the site of the sting, and the area may become numb.

Treatment

There is no known antidote. Contact medical help immediately; flush the wound with fresh- or salt water and then soak the affected area in hot water or put hot compresses on it. The water should be very hot (122°F), so that the heat will deactivate the poison. Continue applying hot water for 30 minutes to an hour. Folk wisdom also advocates applying urine to the sting site.

white snakeroot *(Eupatorium rugosum or Ageratine altissima)*   This eastern North American herb causes "milk sickness," which occurs after consuming dairy products from livestock poisoned by the plant. The milk of cows that feed on the plant becomes poisoned by tremetol, an unstable alcohol that occurs together with an incomplete resin acid.

Milk sickness was common in the United States from North Carolina to the Midwest until the late 19th century, when milk processing methods improved. In fact, it spread like wildfire throughout the western pioneers in the early 19th century; Abraham Lincoln's mother Nancy Hanks Lincoln died of the disease when he was only seven. In Dubois County, Indiana, at that time, the death toll was as high as one out of every two people.

Although physicians often confused the illness with other diseases and had little time to publicize information about the strange new symptoms, settlers realized that the sickness seemed to be associated with drinking milk from cows with "trembles," a disease they got by grazing on woodland plants. Soon, they had narrowed their suspicions to poison ivy and white snakeroot, and in 1821 the Tennessee legislature required fencing around certain forested areas to "prevent animals from eating an unknown vegetable, thereby imparting to their milk and flesh qualities highly deleterious."

The mystery was finally solved by two women: Anna Pierce, an Illinois doctor who had taken midwife and nursing courses at a time when women were not accepted in medical school, and a fugitive Shawnee woman. When milk sickness arrived in Anna Pierce's town, killing her mother and sister-in-law and sickening her father, Pierce made a series of critical observations about the disease and campaigned to prevent drinking milk during the summer.

Then she befriended a Shawnee woman known as Aunt Shawnee, a fugitive from an area of forced relocations of Native Americans. Aunt Shawnee showed Anna the white snakeroot, explaining that it caused both trembles and milk sickness and was used by the Shawnee as a treatment for snakebite. When Pierce fed snakeroot to a calf, it developed trembles; in 1928, scientists isolated tremetol, an alcohol similar to rotenone, from the white snakeroot; in 1987, scientists discovered that the constituents of snakeroot are not in themselves toxic but are converted to toxic substances by the body's own metabolic processes.

White snakeroot belongs to the family of medicinally active plants including joe-pye weed (used to cool fevers), boneset (similar to aspirin), and dog fennel (used to treat insect bites). It thrives in deep, rich, loamy soil that is often found in woods, and its toxicity varies from region to region, being least dangerous in the East and the South.

Today snakeroot only occasionally kills livestock, and milk sickness is almost nonexistent because of the improvement of eastern pastures, clearing of woodlots and the mixing of milk from many cows in commercial dairy operations. It remains a possibility for those who drink milk or eat cheese from their own cows, or who buy dairy products directly from farmers whose cows browse in rich woods.

Symptoms

Anyone who consumes milk or other dairy products from cows that have eaten the plant will become weak, nauseated, constipated, prostrate, and delirious; between 10 and 25 percent of victims will die. There is a latency period ranging from several hours to several days. Milk sickness also causes a sickly sweet breath, a product of acidosis due to a buildup of lactic acid in the muscles, and thirst, with a burning sensation in the stomach.

Treatment

Treat liver damage and anuria; other treatment is symptomatic.

window cleaner   See ISOPROPYL ALCOHOL.

wintergreen, oil of   See SALICYLATES.

wintersweet *(Acokanthera oblongifolia)* This dense evergreen shrub is native of Africa, with large leathery leaves and fragrant flowers. The fruit resembles a reddish purple plum with two seeds. Wintersweet is often found as a hedge in California, Florida, and Hawaii and as a greenhouse plant.

Poisonous part

The fruit pulp is considered to be edible in some areas, although it contains small amounts of a cardiac glycoside similar to ouabain; the seeds contain the greatest amount, although the toxin is distributed throughout the plant (including the wood).

Symptoms

Mouth pain, nausea, vomiting, abdominal pain, cramps, diarrhea, and possible heart rhythm disturbances.

Treatment

Induce vomiting or perform gastric lavage, followed by the administration of activated charcoal and saline cathartics. Electrocardiogram and potassium levels should be monitored. Phenytoin or atropine may be required to treat seizures.

wonder flower *(Ornithogalum thyrsoides)* A lily plant of Old World origin, the wonder flower is a common garden plant with an oniony bulb and grasslike leaves, with white flowers borne in a cluster on an upright spike; seeds are contained in a capsule.

Poisonous part

All parts of the plant are poisonous, especially the bulb, and contain convallatoxin and convalloside, a digitalislike glycoside identical to those of the toxic lily of the valley.

Symptoms

Digitalis glycoside toxicity has a variable latency period depending on how much was ingested; symptoms include pain in the mouth, nausea, vomiting, abdominal pain, cramps, and diarrhea, with heart problems and rhythm disturbances.

Treatment

Perform gastric lavage or induce vomiting, followed by the administration of activated charcoal and saline cathartics. Monitor electrocardiogram and blood levels of potassium. Administration of atropine or phenytoin may be required to prevent seizures.

See also LILY OF THE VALLEY.

wood alcohol   See METHYL ALCOHOL.

wood preservative   See PETROLEUM DISTILLATES.

wutu *(Bothrops alternus)* A dangerous South American pit viper and cousin of the fer-de-lance.

Symptoms

With a bite from this viper, blood cannot coagulate and hemorrhages into muscles and the nervous system. There is local pain, bleeding from the bite, gums, nose, mouth, and rectum. Shock and respiratory arrest are followed by death.

Treatment

Antivenin is available.

See also ADDER; MASSASAUGA; PIT VIPERS; RATTLESNAKE, CANEBRAKE; RATTLESNAKE, CASCABEL; RATTLESNAKE, EASTERN DIAMONDBACK; RATTLESNAKE, MEXICAN WEST COAST, RATTLESNAKE, RED DIAMONDBACK; RATTLESNAKE, TIMBER; RATTLESNAKE, WESTERN DIAMONDBACK; RATTLESNAKES; SIDEWINDER; SNAKES, POISONOUS; VIPER, GABOON; VIPER, JUMPING; VIPER, MALAYAN PIT; VIPER, RUSSEL'S; VIPER, SAWSCALED; VIPER, WAGLER'S PIT; WATER MOCCASIN; VIPERS.

Yersiniosis A type of food poisoning caused by the *Yersinia* bacteria. Most cases that occur in humans are caused by one species, *Y. enterocolitica.* Contamination usually is associated with pork products, as well as milk, oysters, fish, beef, lamb, and game. Yersiniosis is usually self-limiting and causes a mild-to-moderate infection. The Centers for Disease Control and Prevention estimates that 17,000 cases occur each year in the United States.

Symptoms
Between one to seven days after ingesting tainted food, the victim may experience acute diarrhea and fever, stomach pain that may be mistaken for appendicitis, and bloody diarrhea. Adults experience painful joints as well.

Treatment
Antibiotics are effective and should be taken up to seven days; serious illness may require hospitalization.

Complications
Internal infection and arthritis.

Prevention
Consumers should avoid eating raw pork or unpasteurized milk and maintain good kitchen cleaning standards.

yew *(Taxus)* The poisonous yews include the English yew *(T. baccata),* Pacific or western yew *(T. brevifolia),* American yew or ground hemlock *(T. canadensis),* and Japanese yew *(T. cuspidata).* Yew trees are found throughout the Northern Hemisphere and in ancient times were used as an aborti-facient—often with deadly consequences. Survival after yew poisoning is uncommon.

Yew trees are evergreen, with reddish brown scaly bark and needlelike leaves; the hard seeds are green or black. English yew grows in the southern United States; western yew is found from Alaska south along British Columbia's coast, to western Washington, Oregon, California, Idaho, and Montana. Canada yew is found in Pennsylvania, West Virginia to Iowa and north. Japanese yew is found throughout the northern temperate zone.

Poisonous part
All parts of this evergreen shrub except the red berries contain the poison taxine—especially the wood bark, leaves, and seeds. While the red berries are not poisonous, the small black seeds inside the berries may be toxic.

Symptoms
Symptoms appear after about an hour and include dizziness, dry mouth, nausea, vomiting, diarrhea, stomach pain, difficulty in breathing, muscle weakness, slow heartbeat, rash, and blue lips. Convulsions, shock and coma are followed by death from heart or respiratory failure. Chewing the needles can also cause an anaphylactic reaction. Ingestion of English or Japanese yew foliage may cause sudden death, as the alkaloid weakens and eventually stops the heart.

Treatment
Gastric lavage followed by activated charcoal; a temporary pacemaker may be necessary; oxygen given as needed. Epinephrine is given in the treatment of anaphylactic shock.

APPENDIXES

APPENDIX I
HOME TESTING KITS FOR TOXIC SUBSTANCES

Asbestos

Air Tech International
4112 Tulare Drive
Silver Spring, MD 20906
(240) 388-0030
http://www.air-techinternational.com/testkits.html

Professional House Doctors, Inc.
Healthy Home Test Kits
7110 Oliver Smith Drive
Des Moines, IA 50322
http://prohousedr.com/DIYTestKits.htm

Carbon Monoxide Detectors/Alarms

Air Tech International
4112 Tulare Drive
Silver Spring, MD 20906
(240) 388-0030
http://www.air-techinternational.com/testkits.html

First Alert
Purchase carbon monoxide detectors/alarms
online or locate a store near you
http://www.firstalert.com/carbon_monoxide_
alarms.php

Kidde
1016 Corporate Park Drive
Mebane, NC 27302
Consumer hotline: (800) 880-6788
Offers a line of carbon monoxide detectors and
alarms

Formaldehyde

Air Tech International
4112 Tulare Drive
Silver Spring, MD 20906
(240) 388-0030
http://www.air-techinternational.com/testkits.html

Professional House Doctors, Inc.
Healthy Home Test Kits
7110 Oliver Smith Drive
Des Moines, IA 50322
http://prohousedr.com/DIYTestKits.htm

Sylvane, Inc.
1495 Hembree Road, Suite 400
Roswell, GA 30076
http://www.sylvane.com/formaldehyde-test-kit.html

Heavy Metals and Minerals

Vivagen Health Products
PO Box 142998
Gainesville, FL 32614-2998
(800) 307-9232
http://www.vivagen.net/tests_distillers.htm
Test kits for heavy metals (in fluids or substances)
and minerals (in hair)

Lead

Health Goods
PO Box 6463
Manchester, NJ 03108-6463
(888) 878-2497
http://www.healthgoods.com/shopping/Home_
Test_Kits/Lead_Paint_Testing.asp
Offers several lead test kits

Professional House Doctors, Inc.
Healthy Home Test Kits
7110 Oliver Smith Drive
Des Moines, IA 50322
http://prohousedr.com/DIYTestKits.htm

Miscellaneous

Air Tech International
4112 Tulare Drive
Silver Spring, MD 20906
(240) 388-0030
http://www.air-techinternational.com/testkits.html
Provides test kits for pesticides in water

Test Medical Symptoms @ Home, Inc.
6633 Ashman Road
Maria Stein, OH 45860
(888) 595-3136 (Sales)
http://www.testsymptomsathome.com/index2.asp
Provides date rape tests and test kits for chlorine, fluoride, nerve agents, cyanide, etc.

Mold

Air Tech International
4112 Tulare Drive
Silver Spring, MD 20906
(240) 388-0030
http://www.air-techinternational.com/testkits.html

First Alert
Purchase home mold test kits online or locate a store near you
http://www.firstalert.com/safety_products_item.php?pid=58

First Environmental Services, Inc.
2604 Powers Avenue, Suite 2
Jacksonville, FL 32207
(800) 541-9457 (order)
(904) 823-1928 (information)
http://www.Envirotester.com
Provides tests for mold, bacteria, and yeasts

Home Health Science, Inc.
BioScience & Safety Products
12 Wilson Drive
Sparta, NJ 07871
(877) 276-8250 (technical help)
http://www.moldcheck.com

National Allergy Supply
1620-D Satellite Blvd
Duluth, GA 30097

(800) 522-1448
http://www.natlallergy.com/product.asp?pn=1315&bhcd2=1208126740

Toxic Mold Lab
20728 56th Avenue West
Lynnwood, WA 98036
(800) 351-9564
http://www.toxicmoldlab.com

Radon

Air Tech International
4112 Tulare Drive
Silver Spring, MD 20906
(240) 388-0030
http://www.air-techinternational.com/testkits.html

Health Goods
PO Box 6463
Manchester, NJ 03108-6463
(888) 878-2497
http://www.healthgoods.com/shopping/Home_Test_Kits/Radon_Testing.asp
Offers several radon testing and monitoring items

Professional House Doctors, Inc.
Healthy Home Test Kits
7110 Oliver Smith Drive
Des Moines, IA 50322
http://prohousedr.com/DIYTestKits.htm

Sulfites

Sulfitest Center Laboratories
35 Channel Drive
Port Washington, NY 11050
(800) 645-6335

Water Quality

Health Goods
PO Box 6463
Manchester, NJ 03108-6463
(888) 878-2497
http://www.healthgoods.com/shopping/Home_Test_Kits/Water_Quality_Testing.asp
Provides nearly a dozen different water quality test kits

APPENDIX II
HOTLINES

Arts Materials
Arts and Crafts Theater Safety
www.artscraftstheatersafety.org
ACTS is a nonprofit that provides health, safety, industrial hygiene, technical services, and safety publications to arts communities.

Air and Water Pollution Issues

Acid Rain
(202) 343-9620

Environmental Justice
(800) 962-6215

Indoor Air Quality Information Clearinghouse
(800) 438-4318

Safe Drinking Water Hotline
(800) 426-4791

Food Poisoning

USDA Meat and Poultry Hotline
(888) 674-6854 or email: mphotline.fsis@usda.gov

Lead and Radon

National Lead Information Center Hotline
(800) 434-5323

National Radon Hotline
(800) 767-7236

Pesticides and Poisons

National Pesticide Information Center
(800) 858-7378 6:30 A.M.–4:30 P.M. PT

National Poison Control Hotline
(800) 222-1222

Pet Poisoning

Animal Poison Control Center
(888) 426-4435
A $60 consultation fee may be applied to your credit card.

Toxic Chemicals

Superfund/EPCRA Hotline
(800) 424-9346 10 A.M.–3 P.M. Monday–Thursday
(800) 424-8802 to report oil or chemical spills
http://www.epa.gov/superfund/contacts/index.htm for more contacts
Answers questions about Superfund regulations, oil pollution prevention, and cleanup operations. It no longer handles solid waste questions.

APPENDIX III
NEWSLETTERS

Clean Water Report
7600A Leesburg Pike
West Bldg., Suite 300
Falls Church, VA 22043
For professionals. The Clean Water Report includes information on key actions from Congress, the courts, industry, states, and municipalities nationwide on hazardous waste, nuclear waste, solid waste, and more.

Food Chemical News
Agra Informa, Inc.
http://www.foodregulation.com/aius/home.
jsp?pagetitle=aiusfp&pubId=ag096
Weekly issue online and in print on the latest on food policy and regulations, foodborne pathogens and illness. By subscription.

Pesticide and Toxic Chemical News
Agra Informa, Inc.
http://www.foodregulation.com/aius/home.
jsp?pagetitle=aiusfp&pubId= ag100
Weekly issue online and in print on regulation, legislation, and litigation of pesticides and toxic substances. By subscription.

Poison Antidote
Utah Poison Control Center
585 Komas Drive
Salt Lake City, UT 84108
http://uuhsc.utah.edu/poison/publiced/antidote/
Quarterly newsletter for parents, health-care providers, daycare providers, health educators, and others

Poison Online
5340 Fryling Road, Suite 101
Erie, PA 16510
http://www.pollutiononline.com/content/member
ship/register.asp?TypeofPage=register
Information on gas detection, emissions, dust control, industry news, pollution control, and more. Delivered via e-mail twice weekly.

Poison Prevention Newsletter
SUNY Upstate Medical University
750 E. Adams Street
Syracuse, NY 13210
www.upstate.edu/poison/pdf/pp_newsletter/2008/
march_08.pdf
Monthly newsletter for consumers; available online

APPENDIX IV
ORGANIZATIONS

Academy of Toxicological Sciences
1821 Michael Faraday Drive, Suite 300
Reston, VA 20190
(703) 438-3103
Recognizes and certifies currently active toxicologists who have demonstrated certain levels of knowledge and experience in toxicology

American Academy of Clinical Toxicology
777 East Park Drive
Harrisburg, PA 17105
(717) 558-7847
Nonprofit dedicated to the advancement of research, education, prevention, and treatment of diseases caused by chemicals, drugs, and toxins

American Academy of Environmental Medicine
6505 E. Central Avenue #296
Wichita, KS 67206
(316) 684-5500
Provides information on the interactions between humans and the environment and the effects on health

American Academy of Veterinary and Comparative Toxicology
Murray State University in Kentucky
715 North Drive, PO Box 2000
Hopkinsville, KY 42240
(270) 886-3959
Fosters and encourages education, training, and research in veterinary toxicology. Publishes *Veterinary and Human Toxicology* quarterly.

American Association of Poison Control Centers
515 King Street, Suite 510
Alexandria, VA 22314

(703) 894-1858
http://www.aapcc.org
Provides a forum for poison centers and interested individuals to promote the reduction of morbidity and mortality from poisoning through professional and public education and research.

American College of Toxicology
9650 Rockville Pike
Bethesda, MD 20814
(301) 634-7840
http://www.actox.org
Its purpose is to educate and lead toxicology professionals in the exchange of information on the current status of safety assessment and the application of new developments in the field.

Animal Poison Control Center
American Society for the Prevention of Cruelty to Animals
424 E. 92nd Street
New York, NY 10128-6804
(888) 426-4435
http://www.aspca.org/site/PageServer?pagename=pro_apcc
A 24-hour-a-day emergency center, staffed by veterinary health specialists, that provides information on pet poisons. A $60 consultation fee is charged.

Chemical Industry Institute of Toxicology
PO Box 12137
Research Triangle Park, NC 27709
(919) 558-1200
http://www.thehamner.org/institutes/ciit/
A nonprofit research institute whose mission is to develop better scientific understanding of how environmental chemicals impact human health

Center for Health, Environment and Justice

PO Box 6806

Falls Church, VA 22040

(703) 237-2249

http://www.chej.org

A nonprofit organization that provides information on how to manage chemical waste

Center for Research on Occupational and Environmental Toxicology (CROET)

3181 SW Sam Jackson Park Road, L606

Portland, OR 97239-3098

(800) 457-8627

http://www.ohsu.edu/croet/

Their mission is to promote health and prevent disease and disability in the workplace through research, outreach, and education.

National Inhalant Prevention Coalition (NIPC)

322A Thompson Street

Chattanooga, TN 37405

(800) 269-4237

http://www.inhalants.org/

NIPC is an inhalant referral and information clearinghouse; it develops informational materials, produces a quarterly newsletter, provides training, and leads an education and awareness campaign.

National Safety Council

1121 Spring Lake Drive

Itasca, IL 60143-3201

(630) 285-1121

http://www.nsc.org/issues/poison/

Information on poisons, medication overdoses, inhalants, hazardous household chemicals, etc.

National Pesticide Information Center

Oregon State University

333 Weniger Hall

Corvallis, OR 97331

(800) 858-7378

http://npic.orst.edu

Serves as a source of unbiased information on pesticide chemistry, toxicology, and environmental fate to industry, government, medical, and agricultural personnel, and the general public

Safe Kids Worldwide

1301 Pennsylvania Ave NW, Suite 1000

Washington, DC 20004

(202) 662-0600

http://www.safekids.org

Safe Kids Worldwide promotes changes in behaviors, laws, attitudes, and the environment to prevent accidental injury to children.

Toxicology Information Response Center (TIRC)

ORNL

1060 Commerce Park, MS 6480

Oak Ridge, TN 37830

(865) 576-1746

http://www.ornl.gov/sci/techresources/tirc/hmepg.shtml

TIRC is an information center that operates under the sponsorship of the National Library of Medicine and serves as an international center for toxicology and related information.

Governmental Organizations

Agency for Toxic Substances and Disease Registry (ATSDR)

1825 Century Boulevard

Atlanta, GA 30345

(800) 232-4636

http://www.atsdr.cdc.gov/

The ATSDR is a federal public health agency of the U.S. Department of Health and Human Services that provides health information to prevent harmful exposure and diseases related to toxic substances.

Centers for Disease Control and Prevention

1600 Clifton Road NE

Atlanta, GA 30333

(800) 311-3435

http://www.cdc.gov

The CDC develops programs to deal with environmental health problems, including those that involve environmental, chemical, and radiation emergencies.

Chemical Hazard Response Information System (CHRIS)

US Coast Guard

2100 Second Street SW

Washington, DC 20593
(202) 267-2200
http://www.chrismanual.org
CHRIS provides information during emergencies that involve the water transport of hazardous chemicals.

Consumer Product Safety Commission
4330 East-West Highway
Bethesda, MD 20814
(800) 638-2772
http://www.cps.gov
Among CPSC's many responsibilities is the review and tracking of chemicals that may pose a chronic hazard to consumers from their presence in consumer products.

Council on Environmental Quality
722 Jackson Place NW
Washington, DC 20503
(202) 395-5750
http://www.whitehouse.gov/ceq/
The Council coordinates federal environmental efforts and works with agencies and other White House offices to develop environmental policies and initiatives.

Department of Agriculture
1400 Independence Avenue SW
Washington, DC 20250
Contact http://www.usda.gov for a list of offices and agencies.
The USDA is involved in several areas of toxicology, including the Food Safety and Inspection Service, Animal and Plant Health Inspection Service, Food Quality Assurance Program, and Food and Nutrition Service.

Department of Energy
1000 Independence Avenue SW
Washington, DC 20585
(202) 586-4403
http://www.energy.gov/index.htm
Several offices within the Department of Energy are involved in toxicology-related research and risk reduction efforts, including Civilian Radioactive Waste Management, Environmental Management, and Health, Safety, and Security.

Department of the Interior
18th and C Street NW
Washington, DC 20240
http://www.doi.gov
This agency conducts a wide variety of activities and initiatives related to toxicology, including surveillance of pesticides and other environmental pollutants, and the Healthy Lands and Water for America initiatives.

Department of Transportation (DOT)
1200 New Jersey Avenue SE
Washington, DC 20590
(202) 366-4000
http://www.dot.gov
The DOT has an office of Hazardous Materials Safety that coordinates a national safety program for the safe transport of hazardous materials by air, water, highway, and rail.

Environmental Protection Agency (EPA)
1200 Pennsylvania Avenue NW
Washington, DC 20460
http://www.epa.gov
To contact your regional office: http://www.epa.gov/epahome/comments.htm#2
To access a list of EPA hotlines: http://www.epa.gov/epahome/hotline.htm
The EPA is the main federal agency responsible for identifying and controlling environmental pollutants, solid waste, pesticides, toxins, radiation, and energy.

Food and Drug Administration (FDA)
5600 Fishers Lane
Rockville, MD 20857
(301) 443-1240
http://www.fda.gov
Recalls and safety alerts: http://www.fda.gov/opacom/7alerts.html
The FDA is the primary consumer health protection agency of the federal government responsible for ensuring the safety of food, biologicals, and cosmetics. The Poisoning Surveillance and Epidemiology Branch assists poison control centers and stimulates research and development of antidotes.

National Center for Toxicological Research (NCTR)
3900 NCTR Road
Jefferson, AR 72079
(870) 543-7130
http://www.fda.gov/NCTR/
Conducts research to support and anticipate the FDA's regulatory needs

National Institute of Environmental Health Sciences
PO Box 12233
Research Triangle Park, NC 27709
(919) 541-3345
http://www.niehs.nih.gov/
The mission of the NIEHS is to reduce the burden of human illness and disability by understanding how the environment influences the development and progression of human disease.

National Institute of Neurological Disorders and Stroke
For health or medical questions and general information:
NIH Neurological Institute

PO Box 5801
Bethesda, MD 20824
(800) 352-9424
http://www.ninds.nih.gov/
Among its broad research interests are drug-induced adverse reactions and neurotoxic substances.

Toxicology and Environmental Health Information Program
National Library of Medicine, Specialized Information Services
Two Democracy Plaza, Suite 510
6707 Democracy Boulevard, MSC 5467
Bethesda, MD 20892-5467
(301) 496-1131
http://www.nlm.nih.gov/pubs/factsheets/tehipfs.html
TEHIP maintains a comprehensive toxicology and environmental health Web site that includes access to resources produced by TEHIP and other government entities. TEHIP is also responsible for the Toxicology Data Network, which is an integrated system of toxicology and environmental health databases.

APPENDIX V
POISON EDUCATION AND INFORMATION MATERIALS

Children and Poison Safety

American Association of Poison Control Centers
http://www.aapcc.org/games/games.htm
Online games for kids regarding poisons and prevention

Checklists for Healthy Child, Healthy World
http://healthychild.org/resources/checklist/
A comprehensive list of checklists, provided by the American Academy of Pediatrics. Some of the topics include "What To Do in a Pesticide Emergency," "Avoid Arsenic Exposure from CCA-Treated Wood," "Prevent Mold Exposure," "Reduce Gas Pollution in your Home," "Protecting Your Baby from Environmental Toxins During Pregnancy," and "Clean Carpets without Dangerous Chemicals."

Connecticut Poison Control Center
http://poisoncontrol.uchc.edu/education/index.htm
Education programs and poison prevention materials for pre-K through adult. Provides interactive programs, brochures, posters, and newsletter. Some are available for free download.

For Your Information—Pesticides and Child Safety
National Service Center for Environmental Publications
PO Box 42419
Cincinnati, OH 45242
(800) 490-9198
http://www.epa.gov/agriculture/achs.html
Brochure offers tips on safeguarding children from accidental pesticide poisonings or exposures. Free.

Healthy Child Healthy World
http://healthychild.org/main/categories/hazards
Videos, articles, and checklists on toxins that are in a child's world

Learn about Chemicals around Your House
http://www.epa.gov/kidshometour/
EPA Web site offered to children on household chemicals and pesticides

Mr. Yuk
http://www.mryuk.com.
Mr. Yuk was created by the Pittsburgh Poison Center at Children's Hospital of Pittsburgh to educate children and adults about poison prevention. Mr. Yuk stickers and additional poison prevention educational materials (e.g., games, posters, brochures, stickers) can be ordered online.

National Safe Kids Campaign
1301 Pennsylvania Avenue NW, Suite 1000
Washington, DC 20004
(202) 662-0600
http://www.usa.safekids.org/poison/
Offers poison prevention resources, including fact sheet, games, posters, brochures, and a children's booklet, Filbert Prevents a Poison

A Parent's Guide to Insect Repellents
http://patiented.aap.org/content.aspx?aid=5556
Available from the American Academy of Pediatrics online bookstore

Pittsburgh Poison Center at Children's Hospital of Pittsburgh
3705 Fifth Avenue
Pittsburgh, PA 15213-2583

Preschool Poison Prevention

http://www.first-school.ws/activities/firststeps/
    poisonsafety.htm

Lessons and activities geared toward preschool children

Protect Your Child From Poison

America Academy of Pediatrics

37925 Eagle Way

Chicago, IL 60678-1379

(888) 227-1770

http://patiented.aap.org/content.aspx?aid=5135.

A concise yet complete guide to preventing and treating childhood poisoning, including symptoms and treatment guidelines for poisons, poison center contact information, and more. Sold in packs of 100. Fee.

Quills Up—Stay Away! Poison Prevention Program

http://www.poison.org/prevent/preschool.asp

An educational program, designed for preschool children, that features Spike, the porcupine puppet. A project of the CDC/National Capital Poison Center. The program features a teacher's guide, video, and teaching materials.

Read the Label First! Protect Your Kids

National Service Center for Environmental Publications

PO Box 42419

Cincinnati, OH 45242

(800) 490-9198

http://www.epa.gov/ncepihom

Online brochure about protecting children from exposure to household cleaners and pesticides available at http://www.epa.gov/oppt/labeling/pubs/rtlf/kids.pdf

The SDA Kid's Corner

The Soap and Detergent Association

475 Park Avenue South

New York, NY 10016

http://www.cleaning101.com/sdakids/index.cfm

A children's Web site with information on safe use of soaps and detergents, hand washing, and safe disposal of cleaning products

First Aid for Poisoning

First Aid Fast

American National Red Cross

2025 E Street, NW

Washington, DC 20006

(800) 733-2767

An illustrated quick-reference guide that provides step-by-step guidance for poisonings, injuries, cardiac emergencies, and more. Sized to fit in a purse or briefcase; also available in Spanish. Available from your local American Red Cross office.

Food Safety

Thermy Food Safety Educational Materials

U.S. Department of Agriculture

http://www.fsis.usda.gov/food_safety_education/
    thermy/index.asp

Educational materials, including teachers' materials, games, coloring books, fact sheets, and more

USDA/Food Safety Information Center

Education and Training Materials Database

http://foodsafety.nal.usda.gov/fsic/fseddb/fseddb
    excerpts.php?Focus=Consumers

More than 80 educational and training items related to food safety, ranging from books, videos, booklets, and posters to curriculi

General

Chemical Encyclopedia

http://healthychild.org/resources/chemical/

An online encyclopedia of toxic chemicals, provided by the American Academy of Pediatrics

National Institute on Drug Abuse

National Institutes of Health

6001 Executive Boulevard, Room 5213

Bethesda, MD 20892-9561

http://www.nida.nih.gov/students.html

Provides educational materials on the effects of drugs on children

Poison Prevention Community Action Kit

National Safety Council

1025 Connecticut Avenue NW, #1200

Washington, DC 20036

http://www.nsc.org/issues/poison/index.htm

A three-ring binder that includes fact sheets, PowerPoint presentations, children's activities, and more. The information is available both in hard copy and on a CD-ROM. Single copies free.

What You Need to Know About the Safety of Art & Craft Materials

The Art and Creative Materials Institute, Inc.

PO Box 479

Hanson, MA 02341

(781) 293-4100

http://www.acminet.org

A 12-page booklet. Single copies are free; quantities upon request.

Household Poison Safety

Consumer Aerosol Products Council

99 Canal Center Plaza, Suite 310

Alexandria, VA 22314

(703) 683-1044

http://www.nocfcs.org/

Provides teaching materials, including Classroom Aerosol Adventure Teacher's Kit and Video, fact sheets, and science projects for kids about safe use of aerosols at home

Formaldehyde

National Safety Council, Environmental Health Center

1025 Connecticut Avenue NW, Suite 1200

Washington, DC 20036

http://www.nsc.org/EHC/indoor/formald.htm

Online fact page

Formaldehyde and Cancer: Questions and Answers

National Cancer Institute

NCI Public Inquiries Office

6116 Executive Boulevard, Room 3036A

Bethesda, MD 20892-8322

http://www.cancer.gov/cancertopics/factsheet/Risk/formaldehyde

Provides online facts on formaldehyde

The Inside Story: A Guide to Indoor Air Quality

Office of Radiation and Indoor Air (6609J)

Cosponsored with the Consumer Product Safety Commission

http://www.epa.gov/iaq/pubs/insidest.html

A comprehensive booklet (EPA 402-K-93-007) available for free download online U.S. EPA/Office of Air and Radiation

Poison Room by Room

National Safety Council

1121 Spring Lake Drive

Itasca, IL 60143-3201

(630) 285-1121

http://www.nsc.org/resources/issues/poisonpretips/room_by_room.aspx

Lead Poisoning

"Charlie Goes to Town"

Superintendent of Documents

U.S. Government Printing Office

Washington, DC 20402

Item #0431-I-01

EPA's Charlie chipmunk is dedicated to keeping children lead-free in this coloring book.

CLEARCorps/USA

1416 Sulphur Spring Road

Baltimore, MD 21227

(410) 247-3339

http://www.clearcorps.org/

Information on protecting children from lead poisoning. Offers comic/coloring book, quiz, brochures, fact sheets, all available online; also a DVD, "Jimmy's Getting Better."

Protect Your Family from Lead in Your Home

U.S. Department of Housing and Urban Development

451 Seventh Street SW, P-3206

Washington, DC 20410

(202) 755-1785

http://www.epa.gov/lead/pubs/leadpdfe.pdf

Comprehensive booklet from the EPA on lead, lead poisoning, how to remove lead paint, how to remodel a home that has lead paint, and more

Pesticides

Pesticide Outreach Material Catalog

http://www.healthyhousing.org/clearinghouse/docs/Article0323.pdf

A catalog provided by the EPA, offering more than 120 free publications, fact sheets, posters, activity books, and other educational materials

Poisonous Plants

Help Your Kids Outsmart Poison Ivy, Oak and Sumac at Camp

http://www.education.com/reference/article/Ref_Help_Your_Kids/
Article to help parents prepare children for safety at summer camp

Safe Medication Use

Medicines and You: A Guide for Older Adults

FDA/MEDYOU, PSC Personal Property Facility
16071 Industrial Drive
Gaithersburg, MD 20877
(800) 677-1116
http://www.cfhinfo.org
A 17-page educational guide that offers tips for talking to health-care professionals, ways seniors can lower medicine costs, facts about drug interactions, and a medicine record

Over-the-Counter Medicines: What's Right For You?

Consumer Healthcare Products Association, Communications
900 19th Street NW
Washington, DC 20006
http://www.chpa-info.org
Offers tips in both English and Spanish on how to read medication labels, avoid drug interactions, use over-the-counter drugs when pregnant or nursing, dosing, and more. Up to 100 copies free.

Prescription Medicine Information and Education Resources

National Council on Patient Information and Education
(301) 656-8565
ncpie@erols.com
http://www.talkaboutrx.org for an order form
Brochures available from the National Council on Patient Information and Education (NCPIE) are

designed to help consumers and their health-care providers better communicate about prescription medicines. They include:

- "Talk About Prescriptions." Month Planning Kit for Health Care Professionals and Communicators. A two-pocket folder includes fact sheets, the latest statistics detailing "Prescription Medicine Misuse," and a poster. $15 each.
- "The National Medication Checkup Kit for Health Care Professionals." Contains an advertising packet, posters, an evaluation form, and 25 consumer brochures explaining the value of having a medication checkup. Developed by NCPIE in cooperation with Glaxo Wellcome, Inc. $20 per kit.
- "Prescription Medicines and You: A Consumer Guide" (brochure)—A 16-page, large-type booklet developed jointly by NCPIE and the U.S. Agency for Health Care Policy and Research. Includes forms to help keep track of medicines, and questions to ask with each new prescription medicine. Available in six languages: English, Spanish, Chinese, Korean, Vietnamese, and Cambodian. $25 for 100 copies.
- "Medicine: Before You Take It, Talk About It" (brochure): $20 for 100 copies.
- "Get the Answers." Personal Medical Information Wallet Card—Available in English or Spanish. $15 for 100 cards.
- "Alcohol and Medicine: Ask Before You Mix" (brochure). $20 for 100 copies. "Buying Prescription Medicines Online: A Consumer Safety Guide" (brochure). $18.50 for 100 copies.

What You Should Know about Taking Medicines Safely

Pharmaceutical Research and Manufacturers of America
950 F Street, NW, Suite 300
Washington, DC 20004
(202) 835-3400
http://www.phrma.org/files/Health%20Literacy%20Brochure%2010.1.07.pdf
A 12-page booklet

APPENDIX VI
REGIONAL POISON CONTROL CENTERS

The U.S. National Poison Hotline phone number is (800) 222-1222. When you call this number you will be automatically and immediately linked to the poison center nearest you in the United States. A poison expert is available 24 hours a day, seven days a week. The following poison control centers are members of the American Association of Poison Control Centers and the U.S. Poison Control Center. The list was last updated in August 2006. For pet poisonings, dial 888-426-4435, the Animal Poison Control Center, 24 hours a day, seven days a week.

ALABAMA

Alabama Poison Center
2503 Phoenix Drive
Tuscaloosa, AL 35405
(800) 462-0800

Regional Poison Control Center
Children's Hospital
1600 7th Avenue South
Birmingham, AL 35233

ALASKA

Alaska Poison Control System
Community Health and EMS
Injury Surveillance and Prevention Program
PO Box 110616
Juneau, AK 99811-0616

ARIZONA

Arizona Poison & Drug Info Center
Arizona Health Sciences Center, Room 1156
1501 North Campbell Avenue
Tucson, AZ 85724
(800) 222-1222 (emergency phone)

Banner Poison Control Center
901 East Willetta Street
Phoenix, AZ 85006

Samaritan Regional Poison Center
Good Samaritan Regional Medical Center
1111 E. McDowell Road—Ancillary 1
Phoenix, AZ 85006

ARKANSAS

Arkansas Poison & Drug Info Center
College of Pharmacy
University of Arkansas for Medical Sciences
4301 W. Markham, Mail Slot 522-2
Little Rock, AR 72205

CALIFORNIA

California Poison Control System: Fresno/ Madera Division
Children's Hospital Central California
9300 Valley Children's Place, MB15
Madera, CA 93638-8762

California Poison Control System: Sacramento Division
UC Davis Medical Center
2315 Stockton Boulevard
Sacramento, CA 95817-2201

California Poison Control System: San Diego Division
University of California, San Diego Medical Center
200 West Arbor Drive
San Diego, CA 92103-8925

California Poison Control System: San Francisco Division
UCSF Box 1369
San Francisco, CA 94143-1369

COLORADO

Rocky Mountain Poison & Drug Center
1010 Yosemite Street, Suite 200
Mail Code 0180
Denver, CO 80230-6800

CONNECTICUT

Connecticut Poison Control Center
University of Connecticut Health Center
263 Farmington Avenue
Farmington, CT 06030-5365

DELAWARE

The Poison Control Center
34th and Civic Center Boulevard
Philadelphia, PA 19104-4303

DISTRICT OF COLUMBIA

National Capital Poison Center
3201 New Mexico Avenue, NW, Suite 310
Washington, DC 20016

FLORIDA

**Florida Poison Information
Center–Jacksonville**
655 West Eighth Street
Jacksonville, FL 32209

Florida Poison Information Center–Miami
University of Miami, Department of Pediatrics
PO Box 016960 (R-131)
Miami, FL 33101

Florida Poison Information Center–Tampa
Tampa General Hospital
PO Box 1289
Tampa, FL 33601

GEORGIA

Georgia Poison Center
CHOA at Hughes Spalding
Grady Health System
80 Jesse Hill Jr. Drive, SE
PO Box 26066
Atlanta, GA 30303-3050

HAWAII

Hawaii Poison Center
1319 Punahou Street
Honolulu, Hawaii 96826

IDAHO

Rocky Mountain Poison & Drug Center
777 Bannock Street
Mail Code 0180
Denver, CO 80204-4028

ILLINOIS

Illinois Poison Center
222 South Riverside Plaza, Suite 1900
Chicago, IL 60606

INDIANA

Indiana Poison Center
Methodist Hospital, Room AG373
Clarian Health Partners
I-65 at 21st Street
Indianapolis, IN 46206-1367

IOWA

Iowa Statewide Poison Control Center
Iowa Health System & University of Iowa
   Hospitals & Clinics
2910 Hamilton Boulevard Lower A
Sioux City, IA 51104

KANSAS

Mid-America Poison Center
University of Kansas Medical Center
3901 Rainbow Boulevard, Room B-400
Kansas City, KS 66160-7231

KENTUCKY

Kentucky Regional Poison Center
Medical Towers South, Suite 847
234 East Gray Street
Louisville, KY 40202

LOUISIANA

**Louisiana Drug & Poison Information
Center**
University of Louisiana at Monroe
College of Pharmacy, Sugar Hall
Monroe, Louisiana 71209-6430

Louisiana Poison Center
1455 Wilkinson Street
Shreveport, LA 71103

MAINE

Northern New England Poison Center
Maine Medical Center
22 Bramhall Street
Portland, ME 04102

MARYLAND

Maryland Poison Center
University of Maryland at Baltimore
20 North Pine Street, PH 772
Baltimore, MD 21201

National Capital Poison Center
3201 New Mexico Avenue, NW, Suite 310
Washington, DC 20016

MASSACHUSETTS

Regional Center for Poison Control and Prevention
Children's Hospital Boston
300 Longwood Avenue
Boston, MA 02115

MICHIGAN

Children's Hospital of Michigan
Regional Poison Control Center
4160 John R. Harper Professional Building, Suite 616
Detroit, MI 48201

DeVos Children's Hospital
Regional Poison Center
1300 Michigan NE, Suite 203
Grand Rapids, MI 49503

MINNESOTA

Hennepin County Medical Center
701 Park Avenue
Minneapolis, MN 55415

MISSISSIPPI

Mississippi Regional Poison Control Center
University of Mississippi Medical Center
2500 North State Street
Jackson, MS 39216

MISSOURI

Missouri Regional Poison Center
7980 Clayton Road, Suite 200
St. Louis, MO 63117

MONTANA

Rocky Mountain Poison & Drug Center
777 Bannock Street
Mail Code 0180
Denver, CO 80204-4028

NEBRASKA

The Poison Center
Children's Hospital
8200 Dodge Street
Omaha, NE 68114

NEVADA

Oregon Health Sciences University
3181 SW Sam Jackson Park Road, CB550
Portland, OR 97201

Rocky Mountain Poison & Drug Center
777 Bannock Street
Mail Code 0180
Denver, CO 80204-4028

NEW HAMPSHIRE

New Hampshire Poison Information Center
Dartmouth-Hitchcock Medical Center
One Medical Center Drive
Lebanon, NH 03756

Northern New England Poison Center
22 Bramhall Street
Portland, ME 04102

NEW JERSEY

New Jersey Poison Information & Education System
University of Medicine and Dentistry at New Jersey
65 Bergen Street
Newark, NJ 07101-3001

NEW MEXICO

New Mexico Poison & Drug Information Center
Health Science Center Library
Room 130
University of New Mexico
Albuquerque, NM 87131-1076

NEW YORK

Central New York Poison Center
750 East Adams Street
Syracuse, NY 13210

**The Finger Lakes Regional Poison & Drug
Information Center**
University of Rochester Medical Center
601 Elmwood Avenue, Box 321
Rochester, NY 14642

**Long Island Regional Poison & Drug
Information Center**
Winthrop University Hospital
259 First Street
Mineola, NY 11501

New York City Poison Control Center
NYC Bureau of Public Health Labs
455 First Avenue
Room 123, Box 81
New York, NY 10016

Western New York Poison Center
Children's Hospital of Buffalo
219 Bryant Street
Buffalo, NY 14222

NORTH CAROLINA

Carolinas Poison Center
Carolinas Medical Center
5000 Airport Center Parkway, Suite B
Charlotte, NC 28208

NORTH DAKOTA

Hennepin County Medical Center
701 Park Avenue
Minneapolis, MN 55415

North Dakota Poison Information Center
Meritcare Medical Center
720 4th Street North
Fargo, North Dakota 58122

OHIO

Central Ohio Poison Center
700 Children's Drive, Room L032
Columbus, OH 43205

**Cincinnati Drug & Poison Information
Center**
3333 Burnet Avenue
Vernon Place, Third Floor
Cincinnati, OH 45229-9004

Greater Cleveland Poison Center
11100 Euclid Avenue, MP 6007
Cleveland, OH 44106-6007

OKLAHOMA

Oklahoma Poison Control Center
Children's Hospital at OU Medical Center
940 NE 13th Street, Room 3510
Oklahoma City, OK 73104

OREGON

Oregon Poison Center
Oregon Health & Science University
3181 SW Sam Jackson Park Road, CB550
Portland, OR 97239

PENNSYLVANIA

Central Pennsylvania Poison Center
Pennsylvania State University
The Milton S. Hershey Medical Center
MC H043, PO Box 850
500 University Drive
Hershey, PA 17033-0850

Pittsburgh Poison Center
Children's Hospital of Pittsburgh
3705 Fifth Avenue
Pittsburgh, PA 15213

The Poison Control Center
The Children's Hospital of Philadelphia
34th and Civic Center Boulevard
CHOP North Suite 985
Philadelphia, PA 19104-4303

PUERTO RICO

Puerto Rico Poison Center
PO Box 367212
San Juan, PR

RHODE ISLAND

**Regional Center for Poison Control and
Prevention**
300 Longwood Avenue
Boston, MA 02115

SOUTH CAROLINA

Palmetto Poison Center
College of Pharmacy
University of South Carolina
Columbia, SC 29208

SOUTH DAKOTA

Hennepin County Medical Center
701 Park Avenue
Minneapolis, MN 55415

TENNESSEE

Middle Tennessee Poison Center
501 Oxford House
1161 21st Avenue South
Nashville, TN 37232-4632

Southern Poison Center
University of Tennessee
875 Monroe Avenue, Suite 104
Memphis, Tennessee 38163

TEXAS

Central Texas Poison Center
Scott and White Memorial Hospital
2401 South 31st Street
Temple, TX 76508

North Texas Poison Center
Parkland Memorial Hospital
5201 Harry Hines Boulevard
Dallas, TX 75235

South Texas Poison Center
University of Texas Medical Branch
3112 Trauma Center
901 Harborside Dive
Galveston, TX 77555-1175

South Texas Poison Center
University Texas Health Science Center, San
    Antonio
Department of Surgery
Mail Code 7849, 7703 Floyd Curl Drive
San Antonio, TX 78229-3900

Texas Panhandle Poison Center
Northwest Texas Hospital

1501 S. Coulter Drive
Amarillo, TX 79106

West Texas Regional Poison Center
Thomason Hospital
4815 Alameda Avenue
El Paso, TX 79905

UTAH

Utah Poison Control Center
410 Chipeta Way, Suite 230
Salt Lake City, UT 84108-1208

VERMONT

Northern New England Poison Center
22 Bramhall Street
Portland, ME 04102

Vermont Poison Center
Fletcher Allen Health Care
111 Colchester Avenue
Burlington, VT 05401

VIRGINIA

Blue Ridge Poison Center
University of Virginia Health System
1222 Jefferson Park Avenue
Charlottesville, VA 22903

National Capital Poison Center
3201 New Mexico Avenue NW, Suite 310
Washington, DC 20016

Virginia Poison Center
401 North 12th Street
PO Box 980522
Richmond, VA 23298-0522

WASHINGTON

Washington Poison Center
155 NE 100th Street, Suite 400
Seattle, WA 98125-8011

WEST VIRGINIA

West Virginia Poison Center
3110 MacCorkle Avenue, SE
Charleston, WV 25304

WISCONSIN

Wisconsin Poison Center
Children's Hospital of Wisconsin
PO Box 1997, Mail Station 677A
Milwaukee, WI 53201-1997

WYOMING

Nebraska Regional Poison Center
8200 Dodge Street
Omaha, NE 68114

APPENDIX VII
WEB SITES

American Association of Poison Control Centers
http://www.aapcc.org
Information on all aspects of poisoning

Tox Town
http://toxtown.nlm.nih.gov/
An interactive guide to commonly encountered toxic substances, your health, and the environment; provided by the National Library of Medicine/National Institutes of Health

Bites and Stings

Medline Plus, Insect Bites and Stings
http://www.nlm.nih.gov/medlineplus/ency/article/000033.htm

Pest Products, Bites and Stings
http://www.pestproducts.com/bitesandstings.htm
Comprehensive information on bites and stings

Snakes
http://www.fda.gov/Fdac/features/995_snakes.html

Carbon Monoxide Poisoning

Centers for Disease Control
http://www.cdc.gov/co/faqs.htm

Environmental Protection Agency
http://www.epa.gov/iaq/pubs/coftsht.html

Food Safety

Food Safety at Home, School, and When Eating Out
http://www.cfsan.fda.gov/~dms/cbook.html
An activity book for children to color, provided by the USDA

USDA Food Safety and Inspection Service
http://www.fsis.usda.gov/Factsheets/
Fact sheets on meat and poultry preparation, foodborne illnesses, safe food handling, etc.

Household Items

Children and Household Poisons
http://www.fda.gov/opacom/lowlit/poison.html
FDA site on how to protect your children from poisons

Household Hazardous Materials—A Guide for Citizens
http://training.fema.gov/emiweb/is/is55.asp
An interactive Web-based course

Household Products Database
http://www.nlm.nih.gov/pubs/factsheets/householdproducts.html
Provides information on the potential health effects of chemicals contained in more than 7,000 household products; provided by the National Library of Medicine/National Institutes of Health

Lead Poisoning Information
http://www.leadpro.com/facts.html
Information on the basics of lead poisoning; links

Medication Safety/Poisoning
http://poisoncontrol.uchc.edu/poisons/medications.htm

Poison and Drug Information Center
http://www.pharmacy.arizona.edu/outreach/poison/hazard.php
Provides poison and medication-related emergency treatment advice, referral assistance, poison prevention, and information on toxins and proper use of medications

Poison-Proof Your House

http://www.healthyhouseinstitute.
     com/a_680-Poison_Proof_Your_Home

Healthy House Institute provides information on how to poison-proof your house

Poison-Proof Your House, Room-by-Room

http://www.epa.gov/opp00001/factsheets/room
     byroom-checklist.htm

EPA site that provides a one-room-at-a-time checklist

Poison Plants

Poison Oak, Sumac, Ivy

http://www.medicinenet.com/poison_ivy/
     article.htm

Poisonous Plants

http://www.ansci.cornell.edu/plants/index.html

Cornell University's poisonous plants informational database

Poisonous Plants for Cats

http://www.cfainc.org/articles/plants.html

List provided by the Cat Fanciers Association

Poisonous Plants for Dogs

http://www.uexplore.com/health/poison
     plants.htm

List of plants poisonous to dogs

Poisonous Plants for Pets

http://www.aspca.org/site/PageServer?pagename=
     pro_apcc_common

Workplace Hazards

HazMap

http://hazmap.nlm.nih.gov/

An occupational toxicology database that provides information about the health effects of exposure to chemicals and biologicals in the workplace; provided by the National Library of Medicine/National Institutes of Health

GLOSSARY

abortifacient Substance that causes abortions.

acetylcholine A type of chemical messenger between nerves and muscles, as well as many other sites in the nervous system. The actions of acetylcholine are called "cholinergic."

acidosis A disturbance of the body's acid-base balance, in which there is a buildup or loss of alkali (base). An overdose of aspirin is a common cause of acidosis.

alkali Another name for "base," an alkali includes a variety of substances, some of which are corrosive. Examples of alkalis include caustic soda, lime, bicarbonate of soda and antacids.

alkaloid A group of nitrogen-containing substances isolated from plants for use as a drug. Morphine, codeine and nicotine are all examples of alkaloids.

alkalosis A disturbance of the body's acid-base balance, in which there is a buildup of alkali (base) or loss of acid. Metabolic alkalosis may occur in an antacid overdose or after severe vomiting.

antiarrhythmic drugs A class of drugs used to treat different types of irregular heartbeats.

antihistamines A group of drugs that blocks the effects of histamine (a chemical released during an allergic reaction).

bacteria Commonly known as "germs," these are a group of single-celled microbes that multiply by dividing in two, some of which cause disease.

bradycardia An abnormally slow heartbeat.

cathartic A drug given by mouth or suppository that stimulates movement of the bowels.

chelating agents Chemicals used to treat metal poisoning (such as with lead, arsenic, or mercury). They act by combining with the metal to form a less poisonous substance, which is then excreted.

cyanosis Bluish coloration of the skin and mucous membranes due to too much hemoglobin in the blood.

It's usually most noticeable in the nail beds and on lips or tongue.

dehydration The loss of essential bodily fluids and chemicals (especially electrolytes, sodium, and potassium).

edema The medical term for swelling.

endotracheal tube A narrow plastic tube threaded through the mouth or nose, into the windpipe (trachea). It is used to provide oxygen into the lungs if a patient isn't breathing well enough alone.

food poisoning Any illness that is caused by eating contaminated food or water.

gastric lavage Washing out the stomach with water in order to remove a poisonous substance.

gastroenteritis An inflammation of the intestinal tract and the stomach that often causes pain, bloating and gas, nausea or vomiting, and diarrhea.

hallucinogens Substances that are ingested to induce alterations of consciousness. They can be classified according to their chemical structure and the compound from which they are derived.

histamine A chemical released by cells that causes allergy symptoms.

hyperkalemia The presence of an abnormally high concentration of potassium in the blood (also called *hyperpotassemia*).

hypotension Low blood pressure.

hypothermia Low body temperature (below 95°F) that may lead to unconsciousness or death.

incubation period The time between exposure to a poison and the onset of symptoms.

leukopenia An abnormal decrease in the number of white blood cells.

metabolic acidosis An abnormal condition of too much acid in the blood and tissues caused by abnormal metabolism.

mycotoxins Toxins produced by fungi (mushrooms, molds, and yeasts).

nerve block The injection of a local anesthetic into or around a nerve to produce loss of sensation in a part of the body supplied by that nerve.

parasites Organisms that grow, feed, and are sheltered on or in a different organism (host) but contribute nothing to the survival of the host.

peritoneal dialysis A technique used to remove waste products from the blood and excess fluid from the body.

persistent organic pollutants Chemical substances that persist in the environment, accumulate through the food chain, and pose a risk of causing damage to human health and the environment.

plankton Tiny organisms (plants and animals) that float freely in water.

pneumonitis Inflammation of the lungs characterized by coughing, breathing problems, and sometimes wheezing.

protozoa Single-celled animals found in soil and water.

psychosomatic A term used to describe physical symptoms that appear to have been caused (or made worse) by psychological problems.

solvent An organic liquid (such as benzene or other volatile petroleum distillates) that when inhaled can cause intoxication, as well as membrane damage.

species A group of closely related organisms. For example, some members of the *Bacillus* species include *Bacillus cereus* and *Bacillus subtilis*. There can be subspecies, subtypes, and strains within a species.

spore A dormant state of bacteria that protects genetic and other materials needed for life. Spores are often highly resistant to high or low temperatures and dehydration.

tachycardia Rapid heartbeat.

toxin Poisons produced by some harmful bacteria.

vasodilator A group of drugs that act to widen the blood vessels.

vertigo An illusion that one's surroundings are moving or spinning.

virus Microbes that are smaller than bacteria and that need a host cell in order to reproduce.

xenoestrogens Substances foreign to the human body that directly or indirectly act like estrogens in the body.

zoonosis Any infectious disease that can be transmitted from other animals (wild or domestic) to humans, or from humans to animals.

REFERENCES

Abramowitz, Melissa. "Microscopic Monsters." *Fit* (March/April 1997): 80–82.

Adler, Tina. "Feeding microbes to get rid of nitrates." *Science News* 148 (July 15, 1995): 39.

Alavanja, M. C. R., et al. "Use of agricultural pesticides and prostate cancer risk in the Agricultural Health Study cohort." *American Journal of Epidemiology* 157 (2003): 800–814.

Alber, John I., and Alber, Delores M. *Baby-Safe Houseplants & Cut Flowers*. Highland, Ill.: Genus Books, 1991.

Allison, Malorye. "Not Just for Kids." *Harvard Health Letter* 17 (May 1992): 6–8.

Altekruse, S. F.; Cohen, M. L.; and Swerdlow, D. L. "Emerging Foodborne Diseases." In *Emerging Infections Diseases*. Washingon, D.C.: Centers for Disease Control, 1998.

AMAP (Arctic Monitoring and Assessment Programme). October 9–10, 2002 AMAP Progress Report to the Arctic Council Ministerial Meeting.

Anderson, I. "Should potassium permanganate be used in wound care?" *Nursing Times* 99, no. 31 (August 5–11, 2003): 61.

Anderson, Kathryn D.; Rouse, Thomas M.; and Randolph, Judson G. "A Controlled Trial of Corticosteroids in Children with Corrosive Injury of the Esophagus." *New England Journal of Medicine* 323 (September 6, 1990): 637–640.

Angle, C. R. "Is Ipecac Obsolete?" *Journal of Toxicology, Clinical Toxicology 29*, no. 4 (1991): 513–514.

Arena, J. M. "Plants That Poison." *Emergency Medicine* 21: 20–35.

———. *Poisoning: Toxicology, Symptoms, Treatment*. Springfield, Ill.: Charles C. Thomas, 1986.

Arnon, S. S., et al. "Human botulism immune globulin for the treatment of infant botulism." *New England Journal of Medicine* 354, no. 5 (2006): 462–471.

Auerbach, Paul S. "Marine Envenomations." *New England Journal of Medicine* 325 (August 15, 1991): 486–494.

Auger, J., et al. "Decline in semen quality among fertile men in Paris during the past 20 years." *New England Journal of Medicine* 332, no. 5 (February 1995): 281–285.

Balint, G. A., et al. "Ricin: The toxic protein of castor oil seeds." *Toxicology* 2 (1974): 77–102.

Ball, Susan. "Should patients with HIV boil their drinking water?" *AIDS Reader* 8, no. 1 (1998): 4–6.

Barlam, T. F., and McCloud, E. "Severe Gastrointestinal Illness Associated with Olestra Ingestion." *Journal of Pediatric Gastroenterology and Nutrition* 37, no. 1 (July 2003): 95–96.

Baroff, L. J., et al. "Relationship of Poison Control Contact and Injuries to Children." *Annals of Emergency Medicine* 21, no. 2 (February 1992): 153–157.

Barone, Michael. "Chances Are." *U.S. News & World Report*, July 1, 1991, p. 19.

Baskin, E. *The Poppy and Other Deadly Plants*. New York: Delacorte Press, 1967.

Beal, Clifford F. "Poison Bomb Alert: Chemical Weapons." *World Monitor: The Christian Science Monitor Monthly* 3 (September 1990): 62–67.

Behler, John L., and King, F. Wayne. *The Audubon Society Field Guide to North American Reptiles and Amphibians*. New York: Alfred A. Knopf, 1991.

Bellenir, Karen, and Dresser, Peter D., eds. *Food and Animal Borne Diseases Sourcebook,* vol. 7. Detroit, Mich.: Gale Research, 1995.

Besser, R. E.; Lett, S. M.; Weber, T.; et al. "An outbreak of diarrhea and hemolytic uremic syndrome from *E. coli 0157:H7* in fresh pressed apple cider." *Journal of the American Medical Association* 269 (1993): 2,217–2,220.

Beyer, Lisa. "Coping with Chemicals." *Time* 137 (February 25, 1991): 47–48.

Bidleman, T. F., et al. "Persistent Organic Pollutants: General Characteristics and Continental Pathways in North America. Draft Intermin Report to the Secretariat of the Commission for Environmental Cooperation." 1997.

Bittman, Mark. "How to Buy and Eat Fish." *New York Times' Good Health Magazine* 141 (April 26, 1992): S18.

Bosveld, Jane. "Food Poisoning: The Culprit Could Be in Your Kitchen." *McCall's* 119 (March 1992): 32.

Boyce, T. G.; Swerdlow, D. L.; and Griffin, P. M. "Escherichia coli O157:H7 and the hemolytic-uremic syndrome." *New England Journal of Medicine* 333 (1995): 364–368.

Bremness, Lesley. *Herbs*. London: Dorling Kindersley, for Readers Digest, 1990.

Brent, Jeffrey, et al. "Fomepizole for the Treatment of Ethylene Glycol Poisoning." *New England Journal of Medicine* 340, no. 11 (March 18, 1999): 832–838, 879–881.

Brouwer, A., et al. "Polychlorinated biphenyl (PCB)-Contaminated Fish Induces Vitamin A and Thyroid Hormone Deficiency in the Common Seal *(Phoca vitulina)*." *Aquatic Toxicology* 15: 99–106.

Browder, Sue. "Are You Allergic to the Modern World?" *Woman's Day* (April 1, 1992): 56, 102.

Burros, Marian. "An Ounce of Prevention in Food-Poisoning Season." *New York Times,* July 18, 1992, pp. N18, L13.

Calvino, J., et al. "Voluntary ingestion of Cortinarius mushrooms leading to chronic interstitial nephritis." *American Journal of Nephrology* 18, no. 6 (1998) 565–569.

Casarett, Louis J.; Amdur, Mary O.; and Klaassen, Curtis D., eds. *Casarett and Doull's Toxicology: The Basic Science of Poisons,* 5th ed. New York: McGraw-Hill, 1995.

Castleman, Michael. "Lead Again." *Sierra* 77 (July/August 1992): 25–26.

Centers for Disease Control and Prevention (CDC). *Addressing Emerging Infectious Disease Threats to Health: A Prevention Strategy for the United States.* Atlanta: U.S. DHHS, 1994.

———. "Facts about Cyclospora." CDC Media Relations. Available http://www.cdc.gov/od/oc/media/fact/cyclospo.htm, 1998.

———. "Facts about Norwalk virus," CDC Media Relations. Available http://www.cdc.gov/od/oc/media/fact/norwalkv.htm, 1998.

———. "Food & Water Borne Bacterial Diseases." Washington, D.C.: CDC Fax Information Service, 1996.

Chestnut, V. K. *Thirty Poisonous Plants of North America.* Seattle: Shorey, 1976.

Chollar, Susan. "The Poison Eaters: Some Cultivated Bacteria Are Finally Getting Down to Business, Gobbling Up Hazardous Pollutants." *Discover* 11 (April 1990): 76–79.

Christian, Donna. "Protecting Your Family from Food Poisoning." *Good Housekeeping* (April 1998): 68.

Chugh, S. N. "Incidence and Outcome of Aluminum Phosphide Poisoning in a Hospital Study." *Journal of the American Medical Association* 267 (February 5, 1992): 642.

Cloudsley-Thompson, John L. *Spiders and Scorpions.* New York: McGraw-Hill, 1980.

Cobb, Nathaniel, and Etzel, Ruth A. "Unintentional Carbon Monoxide-Related Deaths in the United States, 1979 through 1988." *Journal of the American Medical Association* 266 (August 7, 1991): 659–663.

Cobe, Patricia. "A Safer Chicken in Every Pot." *Ladies Home Journal* (February 1998): 146.

Colborn, T. et al. *Our Stolen Future.* New York: Dutton, 1996.

Conroy, S. "Magnesium as treatment for aconitine poisoning. Electronic letter." *Heart* (December 4, 2000). Also available online. URL: http://heart.bmj.com/cgi/eletters/84/4/e8#40.

Consumer Reports. "Poison Ivy Protection? (A Question of Health)." *Consumer Reports* 56 (June 1991): 424.

Cooper, Peter. *Poisoning by Drugs and Chemicals, Plants and Animals.* Chicago: Alchemist Publications, 1974.

Cottler, L. B., et al. "Ecstasy abuse and dependence among adolescents and young adults: Applicability and reliability of DSM-IV criteria." *Human Psychopharmacology* 16 (2001): 599–606.

Cousteau, Jacques. "Attack and Defense." In *Jacques Cousteau: The Ocean World.* New York: Harry N. Abrams, 1985.

Crawford, R.; Campbell, D. G.; and Ross, J. "Carbon monoxide poisoning in the home: recognition and treatment." *British Medical Journal* 301 (October 27, 1990): 977–979.

Delaney, Lisa. "Dictionary of Healing Techniques and Remedies," part 31. *Prevention* 43 (December 1991): 26–30.

Derelanko, Michael J., and Hollinger, Mannfred A., eds. *CRC Handbook of Toxicology.* London: CRC Press, 1995.

Der Marderosian, A. H., and Roia, F. C. *Toxic Plants.* New York: Columbia University Press, 1979.

De Wolf, G. P. *1987 Taylor's Guide to Houseplants.* New York: Houghton Mifflin, 1987.

Dozier, Thomas A. *Dangerous Sea Creatures.* New York: Time-Life Films, 1977.

Duffy, David Cameron. "Land of Milk and Poison: A Mysterious Death Overtook Many of America's Pioneers." *Natural History* 99 (July 1990): 4–7.

Duke, James A. *CRC Handbook of Medicinal Herbs.* Boca Raton, Fla.: CRC Press, 1985.

Du Pont, Herbert L.; Chappell, C. L.; et al. "The infectivity of Cryptosporidium parvum in healthy volunteers." *New England Journal of Medicine* 332 (March 30, 1995): 855–860.

Edlow, Jonathan. "Gut Reactions: Preventing Food Poisoning." *American Health* 11 (June 1992): 66–70.

Eisenga, B. H., et al. "Identification of unknown mushrooms: the good, the bad, and the ugly." *Journal of Toxicology—Clinical Toxicology* 36, no. 6 (1998): 635–636.

Ellenhorn, Matthew, ed. *Ellenhorn's Medical Toxicology: Diagnosis and Treatment of Human Poisoning.* 2nd ed. Philadelphia: Lippincott, Williams & Wilkins, 1996.

Ellis, M. D. *Dangerous Plants, Snakes, Arthropods and Marine Life.* Hamilton, Ill.: Drug Intelligence Publications, 1978.

Erickson, Deborah. "Demonic Toxin Found in Shellfish." *Scientific American* 266 (May 1992): 129–130.

Everett, Thomas H. *The New York Botanical Garden Illustrated Encyclopedia of Horticulture.* New York: Garland Publishing, 1981.

Fackelmann, Kathy A. "Device Sounds Out Salmonella-Infected Eggs." *Science News* 141 (March 7, 1992): 150.

Farley, Dixie. "Dangers of lead still linger." *FDA Consumer* (January/February 1998): 16–22.

Fatovich, D. M. "Aconite: A Lethal Chinese Herb." *Annals of Emergency Medicine* 21, no. 3 (March 1992): 309–311.

FDA Consumer. "New Drug to Treat Lead Poisoning." *FDA Consumer* 25 (June 1991): 2.

———. "Safe handling of fruits and vegetables." *FDA Consumer* (March 1997): 19–20.

———. "Plans to reduce health risk from unpasteurized juice." *FDA Consumer* 31, no. 7 (November/December 1997): 2.

———. "A test to detect potentially dangerous *E. coli* bacteria." *FDA Consumer* 31, no. 7 (November/December 1997): 37.

———. "Two Agencies Look at Lead in Wine." *FDA Consumer* 25 (November 1991): 2–3.

Fischer, Arlene. "Would Your Kitchen Pass a Health Inspection?" *Family Circle* 105 (August 11, 1992): 144–148.

Fleisher, G. R. "Gastric Decontamination in the Poisoned Patient." *Pediatric Emergency Care* 7, no. 6 (December 1991): 378–381.

Fogden, Michael. "A Tiff Over Turf (Strawberry Poison Dart Frogs)," *Natural History* 100 (June 1991): 76–77.

Foley, Denise. "Case of the 'Anemic' Diagnosis." *Prevention* 43 (September 1991), p. 106–112.

Food and Drug Administration. "Succimer (DMSA) Approved for Severe Lead Poisoning," *Journal of the American Medical Association* 265 (April 10, 1991): 1,802.

Fox, Nichols. "Danger for Dinner: Why our food is making us sick." *Atlanta Journal-Constitution* (September 21, 1997): B1, B2.

———. *Spoiled: The Dangerous Truth About a Food Chain Gone Wild.* New York: Basic Books, 1997.

Franklin, Deborah. "The Case of the Paralyzed Travelers." *Health* 5 (December/January 1992): 28–30.

———. "Germ crazy." *Health* (May/June 1998): 95–101.

———. "Lead: Still Poison After All These Years," *Health* 5 (September/October 1991): 38–50.

Freethy, Ron. *From Agar to Zenry: A Book of Plant Uses, Names and Folklore.* Dover, N.H.: Tanager Books, 1985.

Fritz, Cheryl. "Household Hazards; Protecting Your Pets from Poisons." *Better Homes and Gardens* 70 (August 1992): 116.

Gadd, L. *Deadly Beautiful: The World's Most Poisonous Animals and Plants.* New York: Macmillan, 1980.

Garrettson, L. K. "Ipecac Home Use." *Journal of Toxicology, Clinical Toxicology* 29, no. 4 (1991): 515–519.

Gibson, Janice T. "Beware of Poisonous Plants." *Parents' Magazine* 66 (October 1991): 160.

Gill, Paul. "Fatal Fumes: Preventing Carbon Monoxide Poisoning," *Outdoor Life* 189 (June 1992): 94–96.

Gillyatt, Peta. "Testing the waters." *Harvard Health Letter* 18 (June 1993): 1–2.

Graf, A. B. *Tropica: A Color Encyclopedia of Exotic Plants.* East Rutherford, N.J.: Roehrs, 1985.

Griffith, H. Winter. *Complete Guide to Prescription and Non-Prescription Drugs.* New York: Putnam, 1992.

Griggs, Barbara. *Green Pharmacy: A History of Herbal Medicine.* New York: Viking Press, 1981.

Gutman, W. E. "A Poison in Every Cauldron; Chemical and Biological Weapons," *Omni* 13 (February 1991): 42–51.

Haddad, Lester M., and Shannon, Michael W., eds. *Clinical Management of Poisoning and Drug Overdose.* Philadelphia: W B Saunders Co, 1998.

Hall, Richard L. "Foodborne Illness: Implications for the Future." *Emerging Infectious Diseases, CDC.* Available http://www.cdc.gov/ncidod/EID/vol3no4/hall.htm, 1998.

Hardin, J., and Arena, J. M. *Human Poisoning from Native and Cultivated Plants.* Durham, N.C.: Duke University Press, 1974.

Harris, Ben Charles. *The Compleat Herbal.* Barre, Mass.: Barre Publishers, 1972.

Harvard Health Letter. "Therapeutic Poison: Botulinum toxin used to treat blepharospasm and strabismus." *Harvard Health Letter* 16 (February 1991): 7–8.

HealthFacts. "Susceptibility to Food Poisoning: Certain Foods, Certain People." *HealthFacts* 17 (May 1992): 4.

Heiser, Charles B., Jr. *Nightshades.* San Francisco: W. H. Freeman, 1969.

Hennessy, T. W.; Hedberg, C. W.; et al. "A national outbreak of Salmonella enteritidis infections from ice cream." *New England Journal of Medicine* 334 (1996): 1,281–1,286.

Hevesi, Dennis. "After New Testing, Parents Worry About Levels of Lead at School." *New York Times,* June 18, 1992, p. L83.

Hicks, Doris. *A Consumer Guide to Safe Seafood Handling.* Newark, Del.: University of Delaware, Sea Grant College Program, 1996.

Hingley, Audrey. "Focus on food safety." *FDA Consumer* (September/October 1997): 8–11.

———. "Rallying the troops to fight food-borne illness." *FDA Consumer* (November/December 1997): 7–16.

Hodgson, Ernest, and Levi, Patricia. *A Textbook of Modern Toxicology.* Stamford, Conn.: Appleton & Lange, 1997.

Hoffman, R. S., et al. "Association Between Life-Threatening Cocaine Toxicity and Plasma Cholinesterase." *Annals of Emergency Medicine* 21, no. 3 (March 1992): 247–253.

Hoffman, Robert S., and Barsan, William G. "Emergency Treatment of Acute Drug Ingestions." *Journal of the American Medical Association* 266 (November 27, 1991): 2,831–2,832.

Holloway, Marguerite. "A Great Poison: Dioxin Helps Elucidate the Function of Genes." *Scientific American* 263 (November 1990): 16–17.

Hoppu, Kalle; Tikanoja, Tero; Tapanainen, Paivi; et al. "Accidental Astemizole Overdose in Young Children." *Lancet* 338 (August 31, 1991): 538–540.

Horowitz, Janice; Lafferty, Elaine; and Thompson, Dick. "The New Scoop on Vitamins." *Time* (April 6, 1992): 59.

Huebner, Albert L. "Get the Lead Out." *American Baby* 54 (August 1992): 32–37.

Huff, J., and LaDou, J. "Aspartame bioassay findings portend human cancer hazards." *International Journal of Occupational and Environmental Health* 13, no. 4 (October–December 2007): 446–448.

Hunter, Beatrice Trum. "Dietary Lead: Problems and Solutions." *Consumers' Research Magazine* 75 (May 1992): 18–22.

———. "Paralytic Shellfish Poisoning: A Growing Problem." *Consumers' Research Magazine* 75 (February 1992): 8–9.

———. "Short-Term Illness, Long-term Health Disorders." *Consumers' Research Magazine* 73 (September 1990): 8–9.

Hunter, Linda Mason. *The Healthy Home: An Attic-to-Basement Guide to Toxin-Free Living.* New York: Pocket Books, 1990.

Hutchens, Alma. *Indian Herbalogy of North America.* Boston: Shambhala, 1991.

In Health. "Talcum Takes a Powder." *In Health* 5 (September/October 1991): 11.

Institute of Medicine. *Emerging Infections, Microbial Threats to Health in the United States.* Washington, D.C.: National Academy Press, 1992.

JAMA. "Request for Assistance in Preventing Lead Poisoning in Construction Workers." *Journal of the American Medical Association* 267 (April 15, 1992): 2,012.

Jaroff, Leon. "Is Your Fish Really Foul?" *Time* 139 (June 29, 1992): 70–71.

Johnson, Howard M.; Russell, Jeffry K.; and Pontzer, Carol H. "Superantigens in Human Disease." *Scientific American* 265 (April 1992): 92–99.

Jones, R. L., and Allen, R. "Summary of potable well monitoring conducted for aldicarb and its metabolites in the United States in 2005." *Environ Toxicol Chem* 26, no. 7 (July 2007): 1,355–1,360.

Kaplan, Eugene. *A Field Guide to Coral Reefs.* Boston: Houghton Mifflin, 1982.

Kapperud, G.; Jenum, P. A.; et al. "Risk factors for *Toxoplasma gondii* infection in pregnancy." *American Journal of Epidemiology* 144 (1996): 405–412.

Keegan, H., and MacFarlane, L., eds. *Venomous and Poisonous Animals and Noxious Plants of the Pacific Region.* Oxford: Pergamon Press, 1963.

Kelce, W. R., et al. "Persistent DDT metabolite P,P'-DDE is a potent androgen receptor antagonist." *Nature* 375 (June 1995): 581–585.

Kerstitch, Alex. "Primates of the Sea." *Discover* (February 1992): 34–37.

Kerstitch, Alex, and Kluger, Jeffrey. "Pretty Poison: Dart Poison Frog." *Discover* 12 (July 1991): 68–71.

Kessel, Irene; O'Connor, John T.; and Graef, John W. *Getting the Lead Out: The Complete Resource on How to Prevent and Cope with Lead Poisoning.* New York: Plenum Press, 1997.

Khare, M., et al. "Poisoning in Children." *Journal of Postgraduate Medicine* 36, no. 4 (October 1990): 203–206.

Kinghorn, A. D., ed. *Toxic Plants.* New York: Columbia University Press, 1979.

Klein-Schwartz, W., et al. "Effect of milk on ipecac-induced emesis." *Journal of Toxicology, Clinical Toxicology* 29, no. 4 (1991): 505–511.

———. "Poisoning in the Elderly." *Drugs and Aging* 1 (January 1991): 67–89.

Kohn, Howard. "Dial P-O-I-S-O-N-S." *Reader's Digest* 140 (March 1992): 119.

———. "The Poison People." *In Health* 5 (November 1991): 66–80.

Korn, Peter. "The Persisting Poison: Agent Orange in Vietnam." *Nation* 252 (April 8, 1991): 440–445.

Kowalchik, Claire, and Hylton, William H., eds. *Rodale's Illustrated Encyclopedia of Herbs.* Emmaus, Penn.: Rodale Press, 1987.

Kozma, J. J. *Killer Plants: A Poisonous Plant Guide.* Jacksonville, Ill.: Milestone Publishing, 1969.

Kurtzweil, Paula. "Can Your Kitchen Pass the Food Safety Test?" *FDA Consumer* (November 1996): n.a.

———. "Safer Seafood." *FDA Consumer* (November/December 1997): 10–14.

Ladies' Home Journal. "How Clean Is It?" *Ladies' Home Journal* (February 1998): 124–177.

Lampe, K. F., and McCann, M. C. *AMA Handbook of Poisonous and Injurious Plants.* Chicago: American Medical Association, 1985.

Lederberg, J.; Shope, R. E.; and Oaks, S. C. *Emerging Infections: Microbial Threats to Health in the United States.* Washington, D.C.: National Academy Press, 1992.

Lee, W. J., et al. "Pesticide use and colorectal cancer risk in the Agricultural Health Study." *International Journal of Cancer* 121, no. 2 (July 15, 2007): 339–346.

Lefferts, Lisa Y., and Schmidt, Stephen. "Molds: The Fungus Among Us." *Nutrition Action Healthletter* 18 (November 1991): 1–3.

———. "Name Your (Food) Poison." *Nutrition Action Healthletter* 18 (July/August 1991): 1–4.

Levy, C. K., and Primack, R. B. *A Field Guide to Poisonous Plants and Mushrooms of North America.* Brattleboro, Vt.: Stephen Greene Press, 1984.

Lewis, Rick. "The rise of antibiotic-resistant infections." *FDA Consumer* (September 1995): 11–15.

Lewis, W. H., and Elvin-Lewis, M. *Medical Botany: Plants Affecting Man's Health.* New York: John Wiley, 1977.

Lichtenstein, Grace. "They're Poisoning Our Children." *Woman's Day* (November 27, 1990): 56–58.

Lovejoy, Frederick H., Jr. "Corrosive Injury of the Esophagus in Children: Failure of Corticosteroid Treatment Re-emphasizes Prevention." *New England Journal of Medicine* 323 (September 6, 1990): 668–670.

Lund, Barbara M. "Foodborne Disease due to Bacillus and Clostridium Species." *Lancet* 336 (October 20, 1990): 982–986.

McKnight, Kent, and McKnight, Vera. *Peterson Field Guides to Mushroom.* Boston: Houghton Mifflin, 1987.

McLeod, Michael. "Death on the Doorstep." *Reader's Digest* 139 (August 1991): 135–140.

Magnuson, B. A., et al. "Aspartame: a safety evaluation based on current use levels, regulations, and toxicological and epidemiological studies." *Critical Review of Toxicology* 37, no. 8 (2007): 629–727.

Mahon, B. E.; Ponka, A.; et al. "An international outbreak of Salmonella infections caused by alfalfa sprouts grown from contaminated seed." *Journal of Infectious Diseases* 175 (1997): 876–882.

Malloy, Julia. "Straight Answers About Produce and Pesticides." *Better Homes and Gardens* (August 1992): 37–38.

Martinez, H. R., et al. "Clinical diagnosis in Karwinskia humboldtiana polyneuropathy." *Journal of the Neurological Sciences* 154, no. 1 (January 21, 1998): 49–54.

Massaro, Edward J. *Handbook of Human Toxicology.* London: CRC Press, 1997.

Mayo Clinic. "Seafood Safety: Fish Is Low in Fat, but What About Pollutants?" *Mayo Clinic Health Letter* 9 (November 1991): 6–7.

Michaels, Evelyne. "Holiday Food Safety." *Chatelaine* 64 (December 1991): 34.

Millard, Peter S.; Gensheimer, Kathleen F.; et al. "An outbreak of cryptosporidiosis from fresh-pressed cider." *Journal of the American Medical Association* 272 (November 23, 1994): 1,592–1,597.

Mills, Simon. *The Dictionary of Modern Herbalism: A Comprehensive Guide to Practice Herbal Therapy.* New York: Thorsons Publishers, 1985.

Mitchell, J., and Rook, A. *Botanical Dermatology: Plants and Plant Products Injurious to the Skin.* Vancouver: Greengrass, 1979.

MMWR. "Hepatitis A associated with consumption of frozen strawberries—Michigan." *Morbidity and Mortality Weekly Report (MMWR)* 46 (1997): 288, 295.

Moll, Lucy. "Getting the Lead Out of Dinner." *Vegetarian Times* (March 1992): 30.

Morris, C. C. "Pediatric iron poisoning in the United States." *Southern Medical Journal* 93, no. 4 (April 2000): 352–358.

Morrow, Jason D., and Jackson, L. "Was the Tuna a Red Herring? Scombroid Fish Poisoning Caused by Improper Storage." *Patient Care* 26 (May 15, 1992): 245–247.

Morrow, Jason D.; Margolies, Gary R.; Rowland, Jerry; et al. "Evidence That Histamine Is the Causative Toxin of Scombroid-Fish Poisoning." *New England Journal of Medicine* 324 (March 14, 1991): 716–720.

Mullins, M. E. "Identification of unknown mushrooms: if it ain't broke, don't fix it." *Journal of Toxicology—Clinical Toxicology* 36, no. 6 (1998): 637–638.

Murphy, Cullen. "Something in the Water." *Atlantic Monthly* (September 1997): 26–28.

Murray, Mary. "Are You Serving Poison?" *Reader's Digest* 137 (December 1990): 129–133.

Nakanishi, Y., et al. "Monosodium glutamate (MSG): a villain and promoter of liver inflammation and dysplasia." *Journal of Autoimmunity* 30, no. 1–2 (February–March 2008): 42–50.

New, Amy Hoffman. "Home (Sniff!) Home: Household Allergies Are Nothing to Sneeze At." *Better Homes and Gardens* (April 1992): 446.

NY Times. "Iron Pills Lead the List in Killing of the Young." *New York Times,* June 9, 1992, p. N88.

Olson, Kent R., et al. *Poisoning and Drug Overdose.* Norwalk, Conn.: Appleton and Lange, 1990.

Olson, Kent R. *Poisoning & Drug Overdose.* Stamford, Conn.: Appleton & Lange, 1998.

Pantridge, Margaret. "Fish." *Boston Magazine* 84 (April 1992): 62–69.

Pappas, Nancy. "Controlling Poison Ivy." *Country Journal* 17 (July/August 1990): 15–16.

Parker, H. W., and Grandison, A. G. C. *Snakes—A Natural History.* Ithaca, N.Y.: Cornell University Press, 1977.

Pennisi, Elizabeth. "Pharming Frogs: Chemist finds precious alkaloids in poisonous amphibians" *Science News* 142, no. 3 (July 18, 1992): 40–42.

People. "Japan's Fugu Is a Delicacy: But Is It Poisson or Poison?" *People Weekly* 33 (January 22, 1990): 95.

Perl, Trish M.; Bedard, Lucie; Kosatsky, Tom; et al. "An Outbreak of Toxic Encephalopathy Caused by Eating Mussels Contaminated with Domoic Acid." *New England Journal of Medicine* 322 (June 21, 1990): 1,775–1,780.

Phelps, Tony. *Poisonous Snakes.* Poole, England: Blandford Press, 1981.

Potterton, David, ed. *Culpeper's Color Herbal.* New York: Sterling Publishing, 1983.

Purdy, Candy. "House Plants: What You Don't Know Can Hurt You." *Current Health* 18 (December 1992): 24–25.

Rangel, J. M., et al., "Epidemiology of *Escherichia coli* O157:H7 outbreaks, United States, 1982–2002." *Emerging Infectious Diseases* [serial on the Internet]. Available online. URL: http://www.cdc.gov/ncidod/EID/vol11no04/04-0739.htm. Accessed April 2005.

Reitbrock, N., and Woodcock, B. G. "Two hundred years of foxglove therapy: *Digitalis purpurea.*" *Trends of Pharmacology Science* 6 (1985): 277–284.

Repetto, R., and Sanjay, B. *Pesticides and the Immune System: The Public Health Risks.* Washington, D.C.: World Resources Institute, 1996.

Ricaurte, G. A., and McCann, U. D. "Experimental studies on 3,4-methylenedioxymethamphetamine (MDMA, "ecstasy") and its potential to damage brain serotonin neurons." *Neurotoxicity Research* 3, no. 1 (2001): 85–99.

Ricciuti, E. R. *The Devil's Garden: Fact and Folklore of Poisonous Plants.* New York: Walker Publishing, 1978.

Rios, C., et al. "Efficiency of Prussian Blue Against Thallium Poisoning." *Proceedings of the Western Pharmacology Society* 19, no. 34: 61–63.

Robinson, Arnold G. "Painful Mistakes: An Emergency-Room Doctor Tells How to Avoid the Common Blunders That Keep Him So Busy." *Men's Health* 6 (April 1991): 32–33.

Rock, C. L. "Mutivitamin-multimineral supplements: who uses them?" *American Journal of Clinical Nutrition* 85, no. 1: 277S–279S.

Rosenthal, Elizabeth. "Poison Berries." *Discover* 11 (February 1990): 80–83.

Russell, F. E. *Snake Venom Poisoning.* Philadelphia: J.B. Lippincott, 1980.

Sacks, Jeffrey J. "Points of Potential IQ Lost From Lead." *Journal of the American Medical Association* 264 (November 7, 1990): 1,044–1,046.

Satchell, Michael. "A Vicious Circle of Poison: New Questions About American Exports of Powerful Pesticides." *U.S. News & World Report,* June 10, 1991, pp. 31–32.

Schmidt, Karen F. "Puzzling Over a Poison: On Closer Inspection, the Ubiquitous Pollutant Dioxin Appears More Dangerous Than Ever." *U.S. News & World Report,* April 6, 1992, pp. 60–61.

Schulte, Brigid. "Hamburger Disease Called a Growing Risk." *Philadelphia Inquirer,* May 21, 1995, pp. A1, A16.

Science News. "Parasitic Strategy for Poison Control: How Plasmodium falciparum Protects Itself from Toxins." *Science News* 139 (February 9, 1991): 92.

———. "Pesticide May Cause Allergy." *Science News* (February 15, 1992): 141.

———. "Wine: Getting the Lead Out." *Science News* 140 (September 21, 1991): 189.

Segal, Marian. "Botulism in the Entire United States." *FDA Consumer* 26 (January/February 1992): 27.

Shannon, Michael, and Graef, John. "Hazard of lead in infant formula." *New England Journal of Medicine* 326 (January 9, 1992): 137.

Shepard, Thomas. *Catalog of Teratogenic Agents.* Baltimore: Johns Hopkins University Press, 1998.

Sherman, S. E., et al. "Comparing the tolerability and effectiveness of two treatment regimens in a smoking clinic." *Military Medicine* 173, no. 6 (June 2008): 550–554.

Shiffman, S., et al. "Real world efficacy of prescription and over-the-counter nicotine replacement therapy." *Addiction* 97 (2001): 505–516.

de Silva, H. J.; Wijewickrema, R.; and Senanayake. "Does Pralidoxime Affect Outcome of Management in Acute Organophosphorus Poisoning?" *Lancet* 339 (May 9, 1992): 1,136–1,138.

Snyder, Solomon H., and Bredt, David S. "Biological Roles of Nitric Oxide." *Scientific American* (May 1992): 68–77.

Soffritti, M., et al. "Life-span exposure to low doses of aspartame beginning during prenatal life increases cancer effects in rats." *Environmental Health Perspectives* 115, no. 9 (September 2007): 1,293–1,297.

Spencer, Peter L. "Poison Oak, Ivy." *Consumers' Research Magazine* 73 (March 1990): 2.

Spongberg, Stephen A. "Deck the Halls: Poisonous Plants." *Harvard Health Letter* 17 (December 1991): 4.

Stapleton, Richard M. *Lead Is a Silent Hazard.* New York: Walker and Co, 1995.

Stephens, H. A. *Poisonous Plants of the Central United States.* Lawrence, Kans.: University of Kansas, 1980.

Stevens, S. D., and Klarner, A. *Deadly Doses.* Cincinnati, Ohio: Writer's Digest Books, 1990.

Stone, A. L., Storr, C. L., and Anthony, J. C. "Evidence for a hallucinogen dependence syndrome developing soon after onset of hallucinogen use during adolescence." *International Journal of Methods in Psychiatric Research* 15 (2006): 116–130.

Stone, R. "Name Your Poison: Toxicologists Meet." *Science* 255, no. 5050 (March 13, 1992): 1,356–1,357.

Street, Robin. "Safety First for Summertime Foods." *Better Homes and Gardens* 69 (August 1991): 40–41.

Stroder, Mark. "No bugs on our watch." *Costco Connection* (May 1998): 26.

Swain, T., ed. *Plants in Development of Modern Medicine.* Cambridge: Harvard University Press, 1972.

Swann, Lauren. "When Food Bites Back: Sage Advice on How to Savor Food Safety." *Weight Watchers Magazine* 24 (July 1991): 16–17.

Tait, Elaine. "What You Don't Know About Food Poisoning Can Hurt You," *Philadelphia Inquirer (Sunday),* January 8, 1995, p. H1.

Tappero, J. W.; Schuchat A.; et al. "Reduction in the incidence of human listeriosis in the United States." *Journal of the American Medical Association* 273 (1995): 1,118–1,122.

Tauxe, Robert V. "Emerging Foodborne Diseases: An Evolving Public Health Challenge." *Emerging Infectious Diseases.* Available http://www.cdc.gov/ncidod/EID/vol3no4/tauxe.htm, 1998.

Taylor, D. M., et al. "Treatment of human contamination with plutonium and americium: would orally administered ca- or zn-DTPA be effective?" *Radiation Protection Dosimetry* 127 (June 7, 2007).

Teitelbaum, S. L., et al. "Reported residential pesticide use and breast cancer risk on Long Island, New York." *American Journal of Epidemiology* 165, no. 6 (March 15, 2007): 643–651.

Telzak, Edward E.; Budnick, Lawrence D.; Zweig Greenberg, Michele S.; et al. "A Nosocomial Outbreak of *Salmonella Enteritidis* Infection due to the Consumption of Raw Eggs." *New England Journal of Medicine* 323 (August 9, 1990): 394–397.

Tenenbein, M. "Unit-dose packaging of iron supplements and reduction of iron poisoning in young children." *Archives of Pediatric and Adolescent Medicine* 159, no. 6 (June 2005): 557–560.

Tenenbein, Milton; Kowalski, Stephen; Sienko, Anna; et al. "Pulmonary Toxic Effects of Continuous Desferrioxamine Administration in Acute Iron Poisoning." *Lancet* 339 (March 21, 1992): 699–671.

Time. "Scrambled: After 2,000 Food-Poisoning Cases, Fear of Salmonella Is No Yolk." *Time* 137 (May 13, 1991): 50.

Tranter, Howard S. "Foodborne Staphylococcal Illness." *Lancet* 336 (October 27, 1990): 1,044–1,046.

Trestrail, J. H. *Mushrooms and Mushroom Poisoning.* Grand Rapids, Mich.: Blodgett Regional Poison Center, 1989.

Tufts Diet & Nutrition Letter. "Before You Head for the Raw Bar." *Tufts University Diet & Nutrition Letter* 9 (November 1991): 1.

Turkington, Carol A. *Protect Yourself from Contaminated Food and Drink.* Paramus, N.J.: Prentice Hall, 1999.

Turkington, Carol, and Ashby, Bonnie. *The Encyclopedia of Infectious Diseases.* New York: Facts On File, 1998.

UCBerkeley. "Should You Drink from Crystal?" *University of California, Berkeley Wellness Letter* 7 (June 1991): 7.

University of Minnesota. "Fast-acting Cyanide Antidote Discovered." *ScienceDaily,* January 1, 2008. Available online. URL: http://www.sciencedaily.com/releases/2007/12/071227183912.htm. Accessed June 26, 2008.

USA Today. "Hidden Danger in the Home." *USA Today,* February 1991, p. 12.

USA Weekend. "Lead Poisoning." *USA Weekend,* January 3, 1992, p. 8.

USDA Food Safety Research Information Office. Available online. URL: http://fsrio.nal.usda.gov/document_fsheet.php?product_id=48.

Van Etten, C. *Toxic Constituents of Plant Foodstuffs.* New York: Academic Press, 1969.

Warner, M., et al. "Serum dioxin concentrations and breast cancer risk in the Seveso Women's Health Study." *Environmental Health Perspectives* 110, no. 7 (July 2002).

Warrell, D. A. "Treatment of bites by adders and exotic venomous snakes." *BMJ* 331 (November 26, 2005): 1,244–1,247.

Warrick, Sheridan. "The Milk Cow, the Rat Poison and the President: How Dicumerol and Warfarin Were Developed as an Anticoagulant." *In Health* 4 (July/August 1990): 14.

Wasco, James. "Was It Something You Ate?" *Woman's Day* (July 21, 1992): 10.

Wasley, A., et al. "Incidence of hepatitis A in the United States in the era of vaccination." *Journal of the American Medical Association* 294, no. 2 (July 13, 2005): 194–201.

Waters, Tom. "The Fine Art of Making Poison." *Discover* (August 1992): 29–32.

Watson, W. A., et al. "Toxic exposure surveillance system." *Morbidity and Mortality Weekly Report* 53 (Suppl.) (September 24, 2004): 262.

WFPHA (World Federation of Public Health Associations). "Persistent Organic Pollutants and Human Health." Washington 2000.

Williams, W. K. *A Handbook for Physicians and Mushroom Hunters.* New York: Van Nostrand Reinhold, 1987.

Wojcik, D. P., et al. "Mercury toxicity presenting as chronic fatigue, memory impairment and depression: diagnosis, treatment, susceptibility, and outcomes in a New Zealand general practice setting (1994–2006)." *Neuro Endocrinology Letter* 4 (August 27, 2006): 415–423.

Woodward, L. *Poisonous Plants: A Color Field Guide.* New York: Hippocrene Books, 1995.

Xu, Y. K., et al. "Alkaloids from *Gelsemium elegans*." *Journal of Natural Products* 69, no. 9 (September 2006): 347–350.

Yamada, E. G., et al. "Mushroom poisoning due to amatoxin." *Western Journal of Medicine* 169, no. 6 (December 1998): 3,804.

Yeih, D-F., et al. "Successful treatment of aconitine induced life threatening ventricular tachyarrhythmia with amiodarone." *Heart* 84, no. 8 (October 2000).

Zamula, Evelyn. "Contact Dermatitis: Solutions to Rash Mysteries." *FDA Consumer* 24 (May 1990): 28–32.

Zyla, Gail. "Vitamin Vigilance: Preventing Vitamin Poisoning." *Reader's Digest (Canada)* 140 (April 1992): 115–116.

INDEX

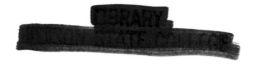